# Dawn and Evolution of Cardiac Procedures

Marco Picichè
Editor

# Dawn and Evolution of Cardiac Procedures

## Research Avenues in Cardiac Surgery and Interventional Cardiology

Foreword by Alain Carpentier

Springer

*Editor*
Marco Picichè
Cardiac Surgery Unit
San Filippo Neri Hospital
Rome
Italy

ISBN 978-88-470-2399-4 ISBN 978-88-470-2400-7 (eBook)
DOI 10.1007/978-88-470-2400-7
Springer Milan Heidelberg New York Dordrecht London

Library of Congress Control Number: 2012943630



Printed on acid-free paper

Springer is part of Springer Science+Business Media (www.springer.com)

*To my father, a man of the utmost integrity*
*and a devoted parent*
*To my little Elsa; Mirta and Bernardo*
*To my mentors of surgery*

# Foreword

One century ago, no surgeon would have dared touch a living human heart, which represented the last frontier in the development of surgery. End-stage heart disease was regarded as the normal termination of life. A few surgeons and cardiologists, however, did not accept this fatality and began dreaming about sophisticated procedures to take up this challenge. Development of novel cardiac surgery procedures required imagination and faith and, indeed, took decades of strenuous work in research laboratories by unknown pioneers. Nothing is more instructive than the history of these developments and that of the men and women who served them and brought them to be. A sterling example is the behaviour of John Gibbon facing the tragic last hours of life of a woman suffering from a massive pulmonary emboli. He felt guilty of not having the means to save her life. During the very night he stood at her bedside, he conceived the heart–lung machine and drew the energy and perseverance required to develop it. It took 20 years to do it and today millions of patients have benefited from this invention. At the opposite end of the complex chain of innovation, stands the charismatic figure of the first interventional cardiologist, Andreas Gruentzig who conceived and developed the transcutaneous balloon dilatation technique for arterial stenosis, which also benefited millions of patients.

Between its two extremities, the chain comprises many research scientists, surgeons and cardiologists who should be strongly commended for having turned cardiac surgery and interventional cardiology into the disciplines we practise today. A 50-year old saga during which millions of patients have been saved from diseases that hitherto had been invariably fatal: tuberculosis, bacterial endocarditis, myocardial ischemia and rheumatic valvulopathies. Fifty years of tireless, daring work and tenacity from the pioneers who made our specialty what it has become today. From bench to bedside, these pioneers explored new procedures in a time when the price of a few victories was paid for by an appalling number of defeats. They often faced bitter criticism and scepticism from their peers or the public, but had the courage and the faith to persist, to go forward, to persevere.

The editor Marco Picichè and the authors of this fascinating story should be congratulated for having brought these pioneers and their contributions into the limelight. The readers, and particularly the younger ones, will find not only a precious source of information and inspiration in this book, but also the forces they need to contribute to the opening of new avenues of research which will hopefully lead to yet further progress in the field.

Since we know that time, wind and rain tend to erase human tracks in the sands of life, this beautiful book will serve in addition as a vibrant homage to pioneers in cardiac surgery and interventional cardiology. A true masterpiece!

Alain Carpentier

# Preface

Like the history of peoples, wars, geopolitical conflicts, and all great social movements and developments, the history of cardiac surgery must be constantly questioned and reviewed as new documents come to light or new interpretations suggest themselves for old documents. Just as courageous and determined individuals have faced down the forces of nature over the centuries to make history with great explorations of land and sea or amazing discoveries of flight, so too has the indomitable human spirit shaped the history of cardiac surgery.

The origins of cardiac surgery are dramatic. It took root in suffering and has developed and evolved through an incalculable number of deaths. It is the product of the effort and abnegation of visionaries who were often criticized and at times dismissed as mad, as well as the despair of patients willing to subject themselves to new and untried procedures in the hope of cheating death.

While often disregarded, the history of scientific inquiry has much to teach us. It can establish important links between past and present, providing a better understanding of current practice and charting a more realistic and imaginative path to the future. Old ideas and experiments, released from the technological constraints of their time, can also be very useful in current research with its modern tools and enhanced knowledge. Ingenious theories that have fallen by the wayside can be brought back and explored again. What is more, when we learn and know about history, we pay tribute to those whose forward-thinking ideas formed the embryo of our daily practice.

This book's potential usefulness to research was its main inspiration. From the outset I conceived the book not as a mere history text but as a history text for researchers. Each author of each chapter was asked to gather original writings from libraries and the Internet and look at them anew, to offer current and future cardiovascular researchers a detailed overview of previous investigative efforts and an understanding of the thinking and mentality of our predecessors.

With interventional cardiology and cardiac surgery on a course of convergence likely to culminate in hybrid management of coronary revascularization and transcatheter aortic valve replacement, this book also includes the history of percutaneous cardiac procedures. Increasingly, therapeutic heart procedures are considered as a whole, with some observers maintaining that these disciplines will some day join together in a single residency program. One of this text's objectives is to offer future residents a complete overview of the field and thus deepen their personal understanding of the issues at play. Pages on mini-invasive and sutureless valve surgery have also been included, to further assist the reader in transitioning from past to present and future.

From the Internet and high-speed transportation to genetics and robotic surgery, we are living in an era of frenetic scientific progress. Although no one can predict the future frontiers of medicine, it is worthwhile remembering what Theodore Billroth had to say: "A surgeon who tries to suture a heart wound deserves to lose the esteem of his colleagues" (1883). And the words of Stephan Paget: "Surgery of the heart has probably reached the limits set by Nature to all surgery. No method, no new discovery, can overcome the natural difficulties that attend a wound of the heart" (1897). After millions of open heart operations since 1953—the date of the first successful cardiopulmonary bypass operation—such statements give pause.

To help speed the dawn of progress for the heart's "two sister disciplines," I have brought together an international team of cardiac surgeons, interventional cardiologists, anesthesiologists, biomedical engineers, and perfusionists, for a grand total of 60 authors from 22 centers and six countries: Canada, Australia, France, Switzerland, Belgium, and Italy. Allow me to express my gratitude to each of them for their enthusiastic support of the project and the very high quality of their writings.

As it is my pleasure to personally know almost all of them, I have attempted to fit each chapter to the profile and interests of each author, so as to offer the reader the best in quality and knowledge. I feel particularly honored as some have been surgery mentors of mine, making their contributions particularly meaningful to me.

Besides the above-mentioned objectives, I also wish to salute the many investigators who, despite the value and innovativeness of their work, are still unjustly ignored by a great part of the scientific community. It is my hope that this book will finally earn their names their rightful place in the annals of the history of science.

Marco Picichè

# Introductory Remarks

It is fascinating and inspiring to look at the past and consider the incredible efforts of the scientific community to create innovative solutions for the benefit of patients with heart diseases. The extraordinary progress in cardiology and cardiac surgery has had a great impact on the natural history of these diseases, with constant improvement in survival and quality of life over recent decades.

At this point in time, however, more radical changes in clinical practice are expected owing to the pronounced variation in the epidemiology of heart disease in different patient populations and the widespread availability of new technologies.

There is no question that in the future, all patients with heart disease will be treated in a multidisciplinary integrated environment by different specialists with access to a wide variety of therapeutic options. The care will be personalized according to individual needs, taking into account the specificity of the disease, the clinical condition, the general risk profile, and the personal wishes of the patient. Such a scenario is consistent with the concept of patient-centered care. Patient-centered care is defined as "care that is respectful of and responsive to individual patient needs, preferences, and values." A multidisciplinary integrated environment which includes specialists with different responsibilities and skills who work together as a "disease-focused" team is mandatory for tailored patient management.

Let us consider, for example, a relatively common disease affecting the heart: ischemic cardiomyopathy. Many diverse pathophysiological conditions are recognized as being responsible for left ventricular dysfunction, contributing to the picture of heart failure. Patients differ considerably depending on their pathophysiology. Ischemia, stunning, hibernation, LV remodeling with or without dyskinetic areas, mitral regurgitation, LV dyssynchrony, various types of arrhythmia, etc. can be identified in the individual patient and specifically addressed by appropriate treatment. In extreme cases, even heart transplantation or ventricular assist devices can be considered. It is clear that, due to the complexity of the disease and the variety of possible procedures, different cooperating and interacting specialists are necessary for diagnosis, decision-making, and therapy. These include imaging experts for viability studies; anesthesiologists, cardiac surgeons, interventional cardiologists, and electrophysiologists for most possible interventions; and clinical cardiologists for medical therapy.

Advances in technology have had a marked impact on the spectrum of therapeutic modalities available for many heart diseases. For instance, the treatment options for patients with structural heart diseases (congenital heart defects, valve dysfunctions, and other anomalies) have increased enormously with the advent of percutaneous approaches and hybrid procedures. The various cardiac specialists have to cooperate and contribute according to their specific knowledge, skill, experience, and expertise. As part of this process, the boundaries between disciplines are expected to become less well-defined. The possibility of treating structural heart diseases with less invasive methods using ad hoc devices is particularly attractive, and conventional cardiac surgery will become limited to special circumstances for which superiority in outcome can be definitely documented.

Awareness of the differences among patients with the same disease has been increasingly acquired in the era of post-genomic medicine, and the great advantage of having a wide spectrum of available solutions has been recognized. As a consequence, new technologies are continuously being proposed by industry with the intention of fulfilling the requirements of physicians for their patients.

Until recently, the only therapy for a symptomatic patient with severe aortic stenosis was aortic valve replacement with conventional surgery. Nowadays, many alternative solutions are available for management of this lethal disease, and even inoperable or very high risk patients can be offered treatment to increase survival and improve quality of life. Transcatheter aortic valve implantation (TAVI) is possible with a variety of devices, using different approaches according to the individual situation. Thus, the valve can be inserted through the femoral artery, the apex of the left ventricle, the axillary artery, or the ascending aorta. In special circumstances a sutureless aortic prosthesis can be implanted with a minimally invasive approach or an apicoaortic conduit can be inserted through a left thoracotomy in a beating heart. Similarly, patients with mitral regurgitation can be treated conventionally or with a minimally invasive approach or even percutaneously with new devices addressing the leaflets and the annulus.

The opportunities offered by this new scenario of patient care, and its consequences, are obvious. First, the benefit for the patient is quite evident. Tailored pathways of care and less traumatic solutions can be conveniently applied with versatility to face the most demanding situations, even in patients with a high-risk profile. Secondly, standardized approaches are becoming less common. Attention to individual differences in conjunction with rapidly evolving technology often results in original, creative, innovative, and almost "artistic" ways of treating patients, with new achievements being recorded almost every day. Thirdly, learning opportunities are being greatly enhanced by new clinical experiences and by the daily interaction with other specialists with different backgrounds, knowledge, and expertise. Fourthly, opportunities for invention and innovation in the treatment of heart diseases are once again wide and real, continuing the glorious tradition of the past.

A glance at the ongoing and anticipated changes in clinical practice might help in placing the past in the correct perspective.

Ottavio Alfieri

# Acknowledgments

I wish to thank Fabio De Gobbi and Alessandro Meggio of Arsmedicaitalia for their invaluable technical assistance in drawing the cover image. Since I wanted the cover to represent both cardiac surgery and interventional cardiology from different periods of their technical evolution, saphenous vein grafts (1960s–1970s), stents inside the vein grafts (1980s–1990s), and a prosthesis similar to the last aortic valve prostheses ever used were included. In truth, the latter is a hybrid of a transcatheter and a sutureless prosthesis, which represents current and future technology, but is not intended to be a reproduction of any specific design available on the market. After countless sketches, the artists rendered the subject just as I imagined it, in a drawing that pays great respect to every detail.

I wish to thank Grant Hamilton, Robert Cory, Corinne Tourtois, John Long, and biomedical engineer Maurizio Allegri for their valuable support.

Thanks also to Elena Roncastri of the Vicenza's San Bortolo Hospital medical library, Jocelyne Bellemare, and Hélène Girard of the Québec Heart and Lung Institute medical library, Laval University, for their assistance in unearthing old and forgotten manuscripts. I would also like to express my gratitude to the medical libraries that offered similar support in Montpellier, Bern, Saint Etienne, Toulouse, Caen, Melbourne, Brussels, Brescia, Pisa, Milan, and Rome.

Finally, I express my deepest gratitude to Juliette Ruth Kleemann, Donatella Rizza, Roberto Garbero, Mr. Sundari and Catherine Mazars, of Springer Verlag, for accompanying me on such a challenging but exciting editorial adventure.

Marco Picichè

# About the Editor

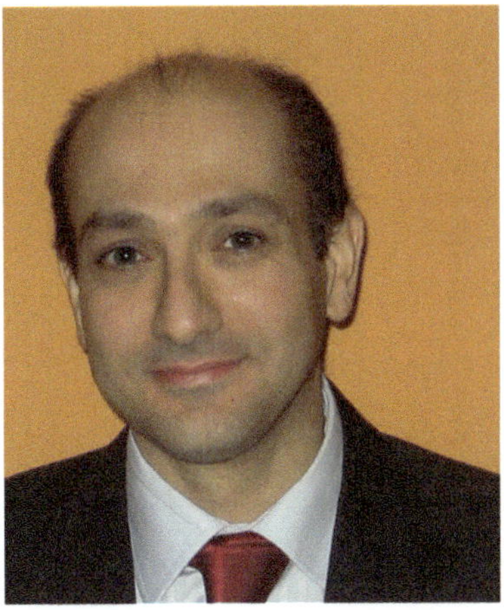

Marco Picichè (MD, Ph.D.) graduated with a degree in medicine from the University of Florence in 1995 (where he attended the Air Force military medical academy) and completed his cardiac surgery residency at the Tor Vergata University of Rome in 2000, both summa cum laude.

He has worked as an assistant at Saint Luc Hospital, Catholic University of Louvain, Brussels (1999–2001), as a clinic head/hospital assistant at the universities of Clermont-Ferrand (2003–2004) and Montpellier (2004–2007), and he attended a research and clinical fellowship at the Québec Heart & Lung Institute, Laval University, Canada (2007–2009).

He held regular teaching appointments at the university of Montpellier school of medicine, obtained certification by the French Board in cardiac surgery (Paris, 2007), earned his research master in surgical science (Paris, 2007), and received a university diploma in vascular surgery (Paris, 2007).

In March 2007 he presented research on the history of cardiac surgery in Narbonne, France, and he had the privilege of being asked to give the presentation to the French Society of Thoracic and Cardiovascular Surgery, which is published on the Society's website at http://www.sfctcv.net/pages/college.php ("Dossiers").

In May 2009 he had the honor of opening the 44th Congress of the European Society for Surgical Research with a lecture on "The history of surgical research."

In Canada he authored a research project on "Noncoronary collateral circulation," which was submitted to the annual research competition at Québec Heart & Lung Institute, Laval University, and received the competition's highest grant.

Since 1998 he has written many publications and has worked as a guest reviewer for several international leading journals. He is a member of the International Committee of the French Journal of Thoracic and Cardiovascular Surgery.

In September 2011 he received a doctor of philosophy (Ph.D.) in therapeutic innovations from Paris-Sud University.

In Italy he has worked as a cardiac surgeon at San Bortolo Hospital in Vicenza (2001–2002; 2009–2012). Currently he is a cardiac surgeon at San Filippo Neri Hospital in Rome.

# Contents

# Part I

# Research on Cardiac Surgery and Right Cardiac Catheterization Before the Advent of Cardiopulmonary Bypass

# The Discovery of Blood Circulation

1

Yves Glock

*Vita brevis, ars longa, occasio praeceps, experimentum periculosum, iudicium difficile.*

Hippocrates

**Abstract**

Throughout history and in various cultures the beating heart was always considered anatomically, metaphorically, and symbolically to be a major organ. As early as the prehistoric period (Magdalenian era to 15,000 years BC) the heart seems to have been represented on the painted rocks in the Pindal cave (Spain): a splash of red in the centre of a painted elephant can be interpreted as a primitive cardiac symbol. In the terracotta tablets from the King's Assurbanipal library in Assyria (700–453 BC) the spurt of blood is described as the liver. This organ was used during animal sacrifices to read oracles. The term "circulation of blood" can be found early in the ancient Chinese medical literature. However, the mechanism was attributed to the opposite forces of the Yin and Yang. Egyptians (Eber's papyrus, 1550 BC) believed that air inhaled through the nose went to the heart and lungs to be distributed throughout the body. However, they did describe the concept of a pulse. Alcemeon of Crotona (500 BC) described the difference between arteries and veins.

Throughout history and in various cultures the beating heart was always considered anatomically, metaphorically and symbolically to be a major organ. As early as the prehistoric period (Magdalenian era—15,000 years BC) the heart seems to have been represented on the painted rocks in the Pindal cave (Spain): a splash of red in the centre of a painted elephant can be interpreted as a primitive cardiac symbol. In the terracotta tablets from the King's Assurbanipal library in Assyria (700–453 BC) the spurt of blood is described as the liver. This organ was used during animal

Y. Glock (✉)
Department of Cardio-vascular Surgery, Rangueil University Hospital,
1, Avenue J. Poulhes, TSA 50032, Toulouse, Cedex 09 31059, France
e-mail: glock.y@chu-toulouse.fr

M. Pichè (ed.), *Dawn and Evolution of Cardiac Procedures*,
DOI: 10.1007/978-88-470-2400-7_1, © Springer-Verlag Italia 2013

sacrifices to read oracles. The term "circulation of blood" can be found early in the ancient Chinese medical literature. However, the mechanism was attributed to the opposite forces of the Yin and Yang. Egyptians (Eber's papyrus, 1550 BC) believed that air inhaled through the nose went to the heart and lungs to be distributed throughout the body. However, they did describe the concept of a pulse.

Alcemeon of Crotona (500 BC) described the difference between arteries and veins [1–10].

## 1.1 The Hippocratic Era

Born in 460 BC and considered the father of medicine, Hippocrates the Great was the Master of a school that built between the fifth and the fourth centuries BC the basis of an era extending into the 2nd century AC. Their anatomical considerations describing the two ventricles of the cardiac muscle and the sigmoid leaflets were pertinent, but their physiological interpretation was fanciful: considering that the left ventricle in a dead animal appears empty of blood they believed that the left atrium expired the air to blow it into the left ventricle. They also misunderstood the valve's function, considering it to be regurgitant and never closed. Plato (426–347 BC) confirmed these beliefs: for him the role of the "pneuma" entering into the lungs was to cool the blood. Widely referenced in William Harvey's book, "de motu cordis", the Greek philosopher and biologist Aristotle (384–322 BC), while performing animal dissections, realised the relationship between the beats of the arteries and the motion of the heart and felt the perception of death as a cardiac arrest. He also described the modification of the blood consistency on contact with air, to guess the coagulation phenomenon. Anatomically, he attributed three ventricular chambers to the heart and described the main artery exiting from the heart, which he named "aorta". Herophile (340–300 BC) was the first to dissect human cadavers and counting the pulse rate with reference to a clepsydra. Erasistrate from Ceos (320–250 BC) believed that the blood's origin comes from the liver. He considered two circulatory systems: the air into the arteries and the blood into the veins. In event of overload, he considered that a communication between arteries and veins was possible, describing special communications that he named the "synastomoses". In his treaty of medicine, Celse (1st century AC) described arterial bleeding in wounds and ascertained the presence of blood in the arteries. Arete from Cappadocia (120–200 AC) confirmed the relationship between syncope and the heart's function [1–10].

## 1.2 The Galenic Era

Galen was born (130–201 AC) in Pergamum on the Aegean coast in Asia Minor. He was famed as an anatomist, philosopher and physician. His medical authority remained uncontested during the 15th century. He had dissected many animals as well as a few human corpses.

The cardio-vascular system was well described in his book: "de usu partibus".

He describes anatomically the aorta arising from the left ventricle with a tricuspid aortic valve, the "venous artery" (pulmonary vein) penetrating the lungs and two membranous epiphyses (mitral valve). For Galen, the atria were not part of the heart, but only "vascular diverticles" playing a role to full the ventricle. He described the cardiac vascularisation with its coronal disposition. Physiologically, he observed the two types of blood: the bright red carried by the arteries and the dark red carried by the veins.

He explained that the forward arterial flow was due to pulsations in the walls of the arteries: for him, the arterial wall had its own "pulsific" virtue. Galen observed that the arterial ligature stopped the distal pulsation, but he explained the phenomenon by the stopping of this arterial intrinsic propriety. He confounded cause and effect. He also believed that the liver produced the dark blood in the veins and that the heart was seen to produce the bright red arterial blood. The two types of blood were distributed into the visceral tissues and totally consumed.

Like Erasistrate, Galen also attempted to explain the communication between the two circulation systems using the "synastomoses" and invented the theory that the interventricular septum was perforated by invisible pores allowing the passage of blood from the left to the right ventricle. He remained ignorant of the pulmonary circulation. This concept remained uncontested for many centuries despite the anatomical objective observations. In his book entitled "The Book of al-Mansouri", the Persian physician Abu Bakr Mohammad Zakaria Razi, known as Rhazes (865–925 AC), followed the Galenic tradition describing the interventricular pores. He specified the anatomy of the coronary arteries in crown disposition, arising from the aorta and distributing their branches to the cardiac muscle, the "ears" aspect of the atrial appendage. He affirmed the closure of the aortic tri-membranous valve from the outside inwards to allow the free exit from the heart of the blood and "pneuma", and the filling of the right ventricle, with dark red blood coming from the liver across a trimembranous valve opening forwards and closing backwards. Haly Abbas (Ali Ibn Abbas Majusi) was an Iranian physician from the 10th century who also shared the views of Galen regarding blood circulation. He wrote two famous books: "The Perfection of the Art of Medicine" and the "Royal Book" known in Latin as "Liber regius".

This author described the digestive system with the extraction from the small intestine by the veins of the nutritional essences to transport them to the liver by the portal vein and distribute them throughout the body via the vena cava. He pointed out the soft uni-layer of the vein and the two layers of the arteries, and the several layers of strong muscle fibres of the cardiac wall whose function was to dilate and contract. Ibn An Nafis (Ala ad-Din Abu al-Hassan Ali Ibn Abi-Hazm akl Qarshi, 1210–1285) was a philosopher, theologist and physician born near Damascus in a small village called Quarsh. He was 80 years old when he died in Damascus after spending most of his life in Egypt.

He wrote an encyclopaedia of medicine and other books such as the "Avicenn's Canon of Medicine". In this book, contradicting Galen's belief, he made an essential discovery: "...there is no communication between the two ventricles...The opinion of some people who pretend that this part is porous is thus archifalse. The passage of the blood into the left ventricle is made across the lungs. After that this blood os warmed and goes up from the right ventricle". He described the constitution of the lungs, bronchi and interaction between air and blood and the role of the coronary vessels in perfusing the cardiac muscle.

Andrea Alpago de Belluno, who was physician in the consulate of Venetia in Damascus, translated one of Ibn Nafis' books in 1527. It is possible that Servet, Vesale, Colombo and Harvey read this text, but not one of them referred to it. This discovery was forgotten for centuries. Up to the early 20th century, Michael Servet was considered to have discovered pulmonary circulation. In Hebraic medicine, two authors published in the field of cardiology with a poor contribution to the approach of the blood circulation. Assaph de Tiberiade (6th century AC) described different types of pulses and palpitations. In the "Aphorisms", Maimonides (1135–1204) confesses this belief of Galen's and Hippocrates's assertions.

In the Occidental Middle Age the creation of many universities was the bedrock of the future "Renaissance" of medicine: University of Salerno in the 9th century, Bologna (1123), Paris (1215) and Montpellier (1220) [1, 2, 5, 8].

## 1.3 The Renaissance

During the 16th century the concept of the "real" circulation of blood was born. It was established on the basis of better anatomical knowledge, to which many authors contributed. Berengario da Capri (1470–1530), in his book *Isagogae* described the arterial anatomy using injections of water in the vessels to dissect them. Leonardo da Vinci (1452–1519) studied as a painter the anatomy in dissecting cadavers: he well designed the heart, valves, vessels, but his work was more artistic than scientific because of the absence of names given to the structures. Pupil of the Parisian masters, Jean Gonthier d'Andernach and Jacques Dubois (surname Sylvius), Andrea Van Wessel (1514–1564) was one of the greatest anatomists of this period. Arriving in France he changed his name in Andrea Vesalius. As professor of anatomy in Padua, he realized a major anatomical work in collaboration for the designs of the dissected pieces with a pupil of Veronese, the painter Stefano Calcar. This work was entitled "De corporis humani fabrica", and the first edition was published in Basel in 1543. In the books number III and VI (out of eight volumes) he dealt with the cardio-pulmonary and vessel anatomy. Even though the anatomical descriptions are fine, the author remained faithful to Galen. In his view, in effect, the veins distribute blood to the organs and the arteries distribute the "pneuma", the vital spirit. However, he proclaimed the absence of microscopic trans-septal communications.

Michael Servetus (1511–1553), an anatomist and theologian, was initially credited with the discovery of pulmonary circulation. Unfortunately, by denying the Holy Trinity in his book, the "Christanismi restitutio (The restoration of Christianity)" published in Vienna (Austria), he was condemned by both Protestants and Catholics to be burned. He died on Friday, 27 October 1553, in Champel near Geneva on the orders of John Calvin. His book was at his side. All the editions were destroyed and only three copies of this first edition remained.

In the fifth book he described the pulmonary circulation, specifying that the "subtle blood arising from the right ventricle is shacked up into the lung to be transformed into red blood".

In agreement with Galen's assertions, he did not contest the patency of the inter-ventricular septum, specifying the possibilities of partial transudation of blood across it. It is probably that Servetus knew about Ibn An Nafi's Work and this paternity regarding the discovery of pulmonary circulation was contested in 1933 by Max Meyerhof and in 1948 by Binet and Herpin. Realdo Colombo's book "De re anatomica" in which he denied inter-ventricular communication and affirmed the existence of the pulmonary circulation was published in Venetia in 1559, after his death. The authors of the end of the 16th century, mainly Ambroise Pare, attributed this important discovery to him. He demonstrated that the contraction was the active movement of the heart. He slowed down the hearts of vivisected dogs and cold-blooded animals like snakes and fish to study their action.

He studied the heart valves and affirmed their competence in not allowing the blood to leak back through them.. Consecutively, he concluded that the blood had to flow from the right side of the heart to the left side across the lung via the pulmonary artery and return by the pulmonary veins. He cut the pulmonary vein in a vivisected dog and proved that it always contained blood and no air.

In the second edition of the "Questionum peripatheticarum" (libri II), in 1595, Andrea Cesalpino d'Arezzo, as Servetus, described the transpulmonary passage of the blood, but accepted the idea of the partial passage of the blood across the ventricular septum. This author was the first to use the term "circulation".

## 1.4 The Seventeenth Century

William Harvey [11–13] was born on 1 April, 1578, in Folkestone, (Kent) England. From 1599 to 1602 he studied at the Padua University as a pupil of Hieronymus Fabricius Acquapendente (1537–1619), the famous anatomist and embryologist who established that the one-way semi-lunar valves of the veins allowed the blood to flow towards the heart only.

Meeting the professor of mathematics, Galileo Galilee (1564–1642) in Padua, he understood the importance of the measures in scientific studies. Harvey's experiments were made with physiological observations in animals and dissections. In 1628, he published in Latin his book entitled: "De motu cordis et sanguinis in animalibus".

This book is clearly and simply written in the form of an academic disputation: anatomical evidence, hypothesis to explain these observations, and exposition of three levels of proof: demonstration, logical argument and arguments "consequential and a posteriori".

In the prologue, Harvey demonstrated the fragility of the previous knowledge of the function of the heart and vessels and in the first chapter he explained the reasons leading to this study. In the Chap. 2 entitled "The heart's motion in vivisection", studying the hearts of cool-blooded animals, he observed the pumping action of the heart and infirmed definitively the ancient role that was attributed to the heart, which was as a sucking muscle.

The third chapter is dedicated to the "Movement of the arteries in vivisection". Showing that a section of the artery was actively bleeding in diastole, he demonstrated that its expansion was due to the heart's work and not to an intrinsic property of the arterial wall.

In Chaps. 4 and 5, he described the two steps of the filling of the heart: the atrial systole followed by the ventricular systole ejecting the blood into the arteries. He compared the cardiac activity to a hydraulic water pump used in England. He also demonstrated the absence of inter-ventricular communication. In Chaps. 6 and 7 Harvey studied the small circulation. In the foetal circulation he noted that the blood flows across Botal's hole, the lungs remaining non-functional.

Observing the occlusion of this hole after birth, he concluded the necessity of the passage of the blood via the lungs. Chapter 8 dealt with the systemic circulation: the return of the blood from the lungs to the left cavities and aorta, the concept of a "circuit" is detailed (*De circolari motu sanguinis*).

In Chap. 9, Harvey built his theory upon the measure of heart flow. He performed a quantitative approach to the quantity of blood ejected by the ventricle. Calculating the quantity of blood passing across the heart during the course of half an hour (about 5 kg), and in one day (245 kg) he ascertained that the theory of the body consuming blood was a false one. In effect, more blood passed through the heart in half an hour than was contained in the whole body. Consecutively, he deduced the circulatory phenomenon in a closed circuit. He also observed the variations of the circulation in relation to age, external factors like exertion, sleep, rest and digestion. In Chaps. 10–13, Harvey studied venous return. He based this demonstration on experiments on ligature and compression exerted on arm veins and the vena cava.

Comparing the effects of the ligature and soft compression of veins and arteries, Harvey affirmed that the blood's flow goes from arteries to veins. A few years before the discovery of the capillaries by Malpighi, Harvey foresaw their presence and admitted that between the two vessels existed either anastomosis or intratissular porosities that allowed passage of the blood from arteries to veins. He also stated the competence of the vein's valves and compared them with the three sigmoid cusps of the aortic valve whose role is to avoid a reflux.

Continuing the fine analysis of the circulatory phenomenon, in Chaps. 15–17, Harvey underlined the different pressures between the pulmonary and the systemic network. "The impulse from the left ventricle into the aorta is stronger than that produced by the right ventricle in the pulmonary artery (arteriosus vein) explaining the different structures of the walls of the aorta and the pulmonary artery and left and right ventricle."

In Chap. 14, "Conclusio demonstrationis de sanguinis circuitu", he concluded: "...the blood in the animal body moves continuously around in a circle and ... the function of the heart is to accomplish this pumping. This is the only reason for the motion and beat of the heart."

A few years later, in 1661, the Italian anatomist Marcello Malpighi (1628–1698) achieved the schema of the circulation describing the capillary circulation: microscopically, he observed the passage of the blood from the arterioles to the venules into the tissues. This discovery allowed the complete understanding of the blood circulation to the tissues and settled Harvey's circulatory theory against his detractors like Primerose and Reid in England, Parisanus in Italy, Hofmann in Germany and Riolan and Pantin in France.

Finally, Richard Lower (1631–1691), in 1669, demonstrated the haematosis phenomenon, underlining the fact that particles of air are in contact in the lung with the dark venous blood and change it into bright red arterial blood [1, 2, 4, 6–8, 10].

## 1.5 Conclusions

Although the discovery of blood circulation received a great deal of interest in England, it was greeted with some scepticism on the mainland Europe.

Both Harvey and Malpighi were the targets of aggressive criticism because of their contestation of Galen's lessons from the conservators. Malpighi went to exile in Sicilia and Harvey was qualified as "circulator", which in Latin means "charlatan". It was mainly in the faculty of Paris that the resistance to these new ideas was strong.

In 1648 and 1649 Riolan, from the Faculty of Medicine of Paris, attacked him in two publications. However, King Louis XIV, supported the development of the new theories: in March 1673, in opposition to the Parliament Council, he decreed the opening of an anatomy lecture in the King's garden the main topic being: "the human anatomy under the blood circulation and the latest discoveries". Pierre Dionis, a 33-year-old French anatomist and physician was charged with diffusing the new theory.

The French retrograde Faculty of Medicine (Riolan and Guy Patin) was losing this ideological fight and the existence of blood circulation was definitively admitted.

Two French writers supported Harvey's theory: Moliere, the playwright, one of the greatest masters of comedy, wrote the "Le malade imaginaire" (the "Imaginary patient") to laugh at the anti-circulation supporters. Boileau in 1675 published his "Arrêt burlesque", mocking the ridiculous order given by the Paris Faculty of Medicine to forbid non-aristotelian teaching!

## References

1. Duffin J (2001) History of medicine. University of Toronto Press Incorporated, Canada, p 46
2. Haeger K (2000) History of surgery. Harold Starke, Eye, pp 119–122
3. Azizi M, Nayernouri T, Azizi F (2008) A brief history of the discovery of the circulation of blood in the human body. Arch Iran Med 11(3):345–350
4. Pagel W (2005) Harvey. In: Encyclopedia Americana, vol 13. Scholastic Library, Dambury, pp 838–840

5. Haddad SI, Khairallah AA (1936) The forgotten chapters in the history of circulation of the blood. Ann Surg 104:1–5
6. Friedland G (2009) Discovery of the function of the heart and circulation blood. Cardiovasc J Afr 20(3):160
7. Whitterridge G (1978) William Harvey on the circulation of the blood and on generation. Am J Med 65:888–890
8. Rullière R (1978) La cardiologie jusqu'à la fin du 18e siècle. In: Histoirede la médecine, de la pharmacie, de l'art dentaire etde l'art vétérinaire, vol VIII. Albin Michel/Laffont/Tchou, Paris 1978. pp 302–309
9. Binet L, Herpin A (1948) Sur la découverte de la circulation pulmonaire. Bull Acad Nat Med 26:542
10. Aufray C, Noble D (2009) Origins of systems biology in William Harvey's masterpiece on the movement of the heart and the blood. Int J Mol Sci 10:1658–1669
11. Harvey W (1958) Exercitation anatomica de motu cordis et sanguinis in animalibus, 4th edn. Charles Thomas, Springfield
12. Harvey W (1649) Exercitationes duae anatomicae de circulatione sanguinis. Arnold Leer, Rotterdam
13. Chauvois L (1957) William Harvey. Sedes, Paris

# The History of Surgical Research

# 2

Marco Picichè

*Imagination is more important than knowledge.*
Albert Einstein

**Abstract**

There are different options available for classifying the history of surgical research by social and cultural eras. A simple classification divides surgical research history into two periods: the first spans the centuries from Antiquity to the Early Modern and the second from the Early Modern to the present. The first "operations" were trepanations. In the ancient world, research activity that can be considered "surgical" rather than just "anatomical" may be attributed to Galen of Pergamon. Throughout the Middle Ages the Church impeded surgical research by opposing any manipulation of a dead body. During the Renaissance research flourished. To date, only nine research surgeons have been awarded the Nobel Prize in Physiology or Medicine. Many eminent research surgeons, despite lives spent pursuing experimentation and making contributions to medicine, have not been honored with such recognition.

There are different options available for classifying the history of surgical research by social and cultural eras. What follows is a simple classification divided into two periods: the first spans the centuries from Antiquity to the Early Modern and the second from the Early Modern to the present.

M. Picichè (✉)
Cardiac Surgery Unit, San Filippo Neri Hospital, Via Martinotti 20, 00135 Rome, Italy
e-mail: m.piciche@sanfilipponeri.roma.it; marcopiciche.history@libero.it

M. Picichè (ed.), *Dawn and Evolution of Cardiac Procedures*,
DOI: 10.1007/978-88-470-2400-7_2, 

## 2.1 Surgical Research from Antiquity to Early Modern

The word "surgery" derives from the ancient Greek *cheirourgia*, meaning "to work with the hands." It is a fusion of the terms *cheir* (hand) and *ergon* (work). It evolved into the Medieval Latin *chirurgia*, that evolved into Old French *cirurgerie,* which, over the centuries became anglicized to *surgery* [1, 2]. From what we know, the first "operations" were trepanations. Most evidence dates trepanation to 3000 BC, but other sources date the practice as far back as 10,000 years [3]. It was a surprisingly common practice among the Incas. The hole perimeters in the trepanned skulls of many Incas were rounded off by the ingrowth of new bony tissue, indicating that patients frequently survived the procedure. Trepanation was also a common practice in ancient Greece. Hippocrates (450–355 BC), in his tome *On the Injuries of the Head*, wrote extensively about how and when to perform trepanation [4]. The first real efforts at research were anatomical in nature. Herophilus of Calcedon (280 BC) and Erasistratus of Chios (304–250 BC) were among the first to pursue anatomical research [5]. They carried out hundreds of dissections on animals and human cadavers, and Erasistratus even performed vivisections on criminals. In Egypt in Alexandria, the Pharaohs Ptolemy I Soter and Ptolemy II Philadelphus encouraged anatomical research [5]. Research activity that can be considered "surgical" rather than just "anatomical" may be attributed to Galen of Pergamon (129–200 AD), a prominent physician and philosopher, and well known as the gladiators' surgeon. His theories dominated Western medical science for over a millennium. He merits consideration as a true research surgeon because in Rome he dissected animals with the goal of understanding anatomy, relating it to physiological function, and finding surgical solutions to pathologies. However, Rome imposed legal limitations on the dissection of human bodies, hampering his research. So Galen was obliged to dissect animals rather than human cadavers and extrapolate his findings to man. This methodology inevitably led to errors. In spite of the limitations, Galen performed some audacious operations and it seems he was the first to carry out cataract surgery [5]. Throughout the Middle Ages the Church impeded surgical research by opposing any manipulation of a dead body. Some popes, such as Innocent III, Gregorius IX, Sixtus VI, and Bonifatius VIII, excommunicated anybody who dissected cadavers. Only on rare occasions did the Church tolerate dissections, e.g., in the suspicious circumstances surrounding the deaths of high priests, popes, or nobility. Despite these limitations Mondino de Liuzzi (1270–1326) in Italy was the first to publicly use cadaver dissections as a teaching tool. The dissections were performed in the amphitheater of Bologna University with a horizontal rather than a vertical cadaver [5]. Church restrictions on surgery led to the development of barber–surgeon corporations. At that time, monks were the traditional practitioners of medicine, but were forbidden to spill blood and hence were unable to practice surgery. Barbers replaced the monks as surgeons and in addition to cutting hair, amputated limbs, administered leeches, carried out blood-letting, and extracted teeth. Barber schools were established, but their medical culture was limited. They embodied a medieval paradox, i.e., "physici" (hence the modern term "physician"), who understood anatomy and pharmacology, did not perform surgery, while barber–surgeons, who had a poor grasp of anatomy and pharmacology, did [5]. Henri de Mondeville, an eminent surgeon from Montpellier and Paris, and author of a five-volume textbook on surgery, addressed this paradox head on. Mondeville defended the fusion of artisan surgery and intellectual medicine, and defined the ideal surgeon as *cyrurgicus* and *medicus*, i.e., representing the union of medical culture, science, and manual work. He also sought to circumvent church-based obstacles to surgery by elevating the image of surgeons, despite their work with blood. Frenchman Guy de Chauliac took another step in that direction [5]. His surgical activities emerged from the combination of a strong medical and philosophical background with an anatomical and surgical approach. More progress was made by Flemish-born Andreas Vesalius and Frenchman Ambroise Paré, the latter a leader in the use of surgical techniques and battlefield medicine during the Renaissance. At one time he cared for two soldiers who lay side by side with similar wounds. He treated one wound by the standard method (cauterization with boiling oil) and the second wound with debridement, cleansing, and application of a clean dressing. He spent a restless night pondering the outcome and the next morning discovered that the second patient had no symptoms, while the first suffered from fever and tachycardia [5]. This was among the first medical applications of comparative methodology and helped lay the groundwork for *controlled experiments*.

During the Renaissance the Italian Fabrizi d'Acquapendente dissected animals in order to investigate the progressive development of the fetus [5]. In Padua he discovered membranous folds in the lumina of veins, which he called valves. William Harvey, a father of cardiovascular physiology and one of d'Acquapendente's disciples at the University of Padua, also studied under Galileo Galilei, professor of mathematics at the same university. Harvey applied the Galilean mathematical method to his research on blood circulation, which led to the publication of *Motu Cordis*, a landmark text in Renaissance medicine [6]. Fabrizi d'Acquapendente was one of many researchers who participated in the 16th century enlightenment. Matteo Realdo Colombo, Gabriele Falloppio, Bartolomeo Eustachi, and Gaspare Aselli in Italy; Jean Pecquet and Jean Riolan (the Younger) in France; Thomas Bartholin in Denmark; and Pieter Pauw in Holland all contributed to the flourishing of innovative theories and notions about anatomy, physiology, and surgery in the 16th and 17th centuries [5, 6].

## 2.2 Surgical Research from Early Modern to the Present

The first figure of note in the Contemporary Era was John Hunter [7]. Born near Glasgow in 1728, Hunter was interested in comparative anatomy and in the natural history of disease. He was a true research surgeon whose inquiries often led to experiments and to operations. Many students attended his London school to study his research methods. To him we owe the understanding that smaller vessels may, through necessity, take on the work of larger vessels. He is famous for an operation performed on a coachman in 1785—later called the Hunterian operation.

Joseph Lister (1827–1912) was the father of surgical antisepsis [7]. Before Lister's discoveries, nearly every wound became infected and suppurated. Following Pasteur's lead he chose phenol (carbolic acid) rather than dry heat to ensure adequate sterilization during surgery. Lister developed his theories on surgical antisepsis by examining infected surgical wounds, performing experiments, and applying the results clinically. At first, the scientific community rejected his ideas and at the third meeting of the American Surgical Association he encountered strong opposition.

The 19th century witnessed the birth of the first surgical and research training program in Europe thanks to Bernard von Langebeck, professor of surgery at the University of Berlin [7]. He was also founder of the first journal dedicated entirely to surgery (*Archiv für klinische Chirurgie*) and taught some renowned research surgeons such as Theodor Billroth, Frederick Trendelembourg, and Theodor Kocher. In North America the first surgical and research training programs were developed at the newly established Johns Hopkins Medical School (1886) by William Halsted [7]. As for John Hunter, he experimentally tested all his surgically related theoretical concepts, which led to the emergence of new types of operations: radical mastectomy, radical hernia cures, goiter operations, etc. At Johns Hopkins, staff members received broad support to pursue surgical research. As new research centers cropped up in the 19th and 20th centuries, ideas about surgery evolved rapidly. In a famous painting by Thomas Eakins, *The Gross Clinic*, one sees people huddled around the surgical team. This was the custom in the 19th century—surgeons operated while observed by students and admirers. At the start of the 20th century there was a shift in the way surgeons worked. They began operating alone or with few assistants. Eugene Doyen, a French surgeon at the beginning of the 19th century, performed surgery with almost no one around—in the modern way. But he still worked with no hat, mask, or sterile gloves—in the old way [8]. Overall, these work habits signaled a transition period in which surgery edged closer to the use of modern techniques.

### 2.2.1 The Nobel Prizes

To date, only nine research surgeons have been awarded the Nobel Prize in Physiology or Medicine. Alexander Fleming, who received the Nobel Prize in 1945 for the discovery of penicillin, had been trained as a surgeon but never practiced surgery and was primarily regarded as a bacteriologist [9].

The first Nobel laureate surgeon was Emil Theodor Kocher from Switzerland [10]. He intensively studied hypothyroidism-related myxedema, which he called "cachexia stumipriva". He solely performed more than 2,000 thyroidectomies, and a further 7,000 were performed in his clinic. The 1909 Nobel Prize was awarded to him for his work on the physiology, pathology, and surgery of the thyroid.

Allvar Gullstrand, from Denmark, began his career in 1890 at the Royal Caroline Institute with a dissertation on the origins of astigmatism. He applied his knowledge of mathematics and physics to ophthalmology. He performed the first operation for symblepharon and received the Nobel Prize in 1911 for his work on dioptrics and accommodation [10].

Alexis Carrel was a French surgeon who moved first to Canada and then to the United States [11]. He developed the vascular anastomosis technique and in 1910 performed an experimental descending thoracic aorta to left coronary artery bypass using a cold temperature-preserved bovine carotid artery [12]. He was interested in organ storage and preservation and artificial organ perfusion. He was able to perfuse the thyroid gland of a cat for 18 days, after which he achieved perfusion of the heart and other organs for several days [8, 11]. He was awarded the Nobel Prize in Physiology or Medicine in 1912 [13]. Charles Lindbergh, the famous aviator (and neither a Nobel laureate nor a physician), worked with Carrel to discover a treatment for a family member suffering from mitral stenosis for which the corrective procedure required stopping the heart. They aspired to create a machine capable of carrying on heart function while the surgeon accessed the mitral valve. Together, they built a new organ perfusion apparatus capable of doing the job [11].

Robert Barany, from Austria, studied the vestibular canals, vertigo, and nystagmus. During the First World War, he was captured by the Russian army and while interned received news that he had been awarded the Nobel Prize. Upon returning to Vienna, despite the acclaim, he was accused of plagiarism by his colleagues. He was fully exonerated of these defamatory charges, but, tired of the injustice he endured, eventually left Austria and moved to Sweden, where he accepted the rather modest appointment of assistant professor at the University of Uppsala [10].

Frederick Banting was a Canadian surgeon who studied the endocrine function of the pancreas by removing its exocrine function [10]. He approached John James Rickard Macleod, chief of a research laboratory in Toronto, with his research proposal, but was repeatedly rebuffed. But Banting persisted and eventually Macleod relented. He allowed the young surgeon to use his Toronto laboratory in his absence. Charles Best, a medical student, was assigned to work with Banting. They observed that an extract of the atrophic pancreas could reverse diabetic coma in dogs [14]. In 1922 a crude preparation was used to treat a young boy with diabetic ketoacidosis. Banting was awarded the Nobel Prize in 1923 for his discovery of insulin. The Nobel Prize was also conferred upon Macleod, despite his initial resistance to Banting's proposals. The exclusion of Best wounded Banting's sense of fairness. By sharing half the award with Best he ignited a controversy on the "anatomy" of scientific collaboration [10, 15].

Walter Hesse, from Switzerland, studied the biological control of emotions. He observed that electrical stimulation of the hypothalamus elicited a rage response in experimental animals. His research led him to attribute specific physiological functions to specific areas of the brain [16]. In 1949 he received the Nobel Prize for his work on the diencephalon (interbrain) as coordinator of internal organ activities [10].

The German physician Werner Theodor Otto Forssmann was a surgery resident who sought a method by which drugs could be introduced directly into the heart. He performed a cardiac catheterization on himself through the basilic vein! Rather than being lauded he was fired by his department chief, who told him he was a clown and that the department was not a circus. In spite of this reaction, Forssmann continued his experiments elsewhere and stopped only when he had no veins left to access. A historical X-ray of Forssmann's thorax shows the catheter through the arm vein reaching the superior vena cava, the innominate vein, and finally the right atrium [17]. Sometimes life has its compensations—for the very reason Forssmann was humiliated he was awarded the Nobel Prize in 1956. He shared the prize with Andre Cournaud, a French researcher who worked in the USA, and the American, Dickinson Richards [8, 10].

The Canadian Charles Huggins observed that in the canine model, normal prostatic secretion is regulated by androgens and estrogens. He noted that orchiectomy reduced serum levels of acid phosphatase, a marker of metastatic prostatic cancer [18]. He received the Nobel Prize in 1966 for the discovery of hormonal therapy as a treatment for prostate cancer [10].

Finally, in the United States in 1954 Joseph Murray performed the first human kidney transplant in identical twins [19]. He was actually a plastic surgeon with wide experience in skin grafting. He performed many animal experiments in which he induced host tolerance for transplanted organs and he concluded that transplantation is feasible when the host immune response can be suppressed [20]. Murray shared the 1990 award with E. Donnall Thomas for discoveries in the field of organ and cell transplantation [21].

It is worth noting that many eminent research surgeons, despite pursuing lives of experimentation and contributions to medicine, were not honored with the Nobel Prize. There is still hope that those alive will in time receive due recognition. Among those deserving the highest praise are John Heymann Gibbon, for the first clinically functional heart–lung machine [22]; Norman Shumway, for heart transplantation techniques [23]; Thomas Starzl, for liver transplantation [24]; and Alain Carpentier, still active in research and a pioneer in valve reconstructive surgery, valve-prosthesis-preservation methods, radial-artery-arterial revascularization, and current investigations into a new intraventricular assist device [25–27].

Not all who helped revolutionize surgical outcomes were surgeons. Three worth recalling are Jonathan Rhoads, Stanley Dudrick, and Harry Vars [28]. They collaborated in the area of parenteral nutrition to dramatically improve postoperative outcome for millions of chronic intensive care patients.

The history of surgical research is too complex to be covered in these few pages, and many deserving research surgeons had to be excluded from this record. In forthcoming chapters the work of surgeons who specialized in cardiac research will be elaborated.

## References

1. Answers.com. American heritage dictionary. www.answers.com/topic/surgery. Accessed 3 July 2011
2. My etymology. http://www.myetymology.com/english/surgery.html. Accessed 3 July 2011
3. Arnott R, Finger S, Smith CUM (eds) (2003) Trepanation. History, discovery, theory. Swets & Zeitlenger, Abingdon

4. Hippocrates. On injuries of the head. (Trans: Francis Adams) 2007 eBooks@Adelaide http://ebooks.adelaide.edu.au/h/hippocrates/head/
5. Cosmacini G (2003) La vita nelle mani. Storia della chirurgia. Laterza, Rome
6. Argenteri A, Felici R (2005) L'avventura della circolazione. In: Spartera C (ed) Chirurgia delle arterie. Masson, Milan, pp 1–12
7. Chitwood WR, Sabiston DC Jr (1998) Selected historical perspectives on the evolution of surgical science. In: Troidl H, McKneally MF, Mulder DS, Wechsler AS, McPeek B, Spitzer WO (eds) Surgical research: basic principles and clinical practice. Springer, Berlin, pp 23–38
8. Picichè M. Histoire de la Chirurgie Cardiaque. Site de la Société Française de Chirurgie Thoracique et Cardiovasculaire. http://www.sfctcv.net/pages/college.php (Item College; Item Dossier) Accessed 3 July, 2011
9. Ligon BL (2004) Penicillin: its discovery and early development. Semin Pediatr Infect Dis 15(1):52–57
10. Yee J, Mulder DS (1998) Surgeons who have won the Nobel Prize. In: Troidl H, McKneally MF, Mulder DS, Wechsler AS, McPeek B, Spitzer WO (eds) Surgical research: basic principles and clinical practice. Springer, Berlin, pp 39–47
11. Comroe JH (1979) Who was Alexis who? Cardiovasc Dis 6(3):251–270
12. Carrel A (1910) On the experimental surgery of the thoracic aorta and heart. Am J Surg 52:83–95
13. Carrel A (1967) Nobel lectures in physiology or medicine. Elsevier, Amsterdam, pp 437–466
14. Banting FG, Best CH (1922) Internal secretion of pancreas. J Lab Clin Med 7:251–326
15. Harris H (1946) Banting's miracle: the story of the discovery of insulin. Lippincott, Philadelphia
16. Hess WR (1967) Causality, consciousness, and cerebral organization. Science 158:1279–1283
17. Forssman WO (1974) Experiments on myself: memoirs of a surgeon in Germany. St. Martin's, New York
18. Huggins CB, Hodges CV (1941) Studies on prostate cancer. I. The effect of castration, estrogen, and androgen injection on serum phosphatases in metastatic carcinoma of the prostate. Cancer Res 1:293–297
19. Murray JE, Merrill JP, Harrison JH, Guild WR (1956) Successful homotransplantations of the human kidney between identical twins. JAMA 160:270–282
20. Murray JE, Merrill JP, Harrison JH, Wilson RE (1963) Prolonged survival of human kidney homografts by immunosuppressive drug therapy. N Engl J Med 268:1315–1323
21. Jurkiewicz MJ (1990) Nobel laureate: Joseph E. Murray, clinical surgeon, scientist, teacher. Surgery 125:1423–1424
22. Gibbon JH (1954) Application of a mechanical heart and lung apparatus to cardiac surgery. Minn Med 37:171–185
23. Lower RR, Stofer RC, Hurley EJ, Dong E Jr, Cohn RB, Shumway NE (1962) Successful homotransplantations of the canine heart after anoxic preservation for seven hours. Am J Surg 104:302–306
24. Starzl TE (1992) The puzzle people: memoirs of a transplant surgeon. University of Pittsburgh Press, Pittsburgh
25. Carpentier A (1983) Cardiac valve surgery–"the French correction". J Thorac Cardiovasc Surg 86(3):323–337
26. Carpentier A, Guermonprez GL, Deloche A, Frechette C, DuBost C (1973) The aorta-to-coronary radial artery bypass graft. A technique avoiding pathological changes in grafts. Ann Thorac Surg 16(2):111–121
27. Carpentier A, Lemaigre G, Robert L, Ladislas R, Carpentier S, Dubost C, Gerbode C, Gerbode F (1969) Biological factors affecting long-term results of valvular heterografts. J Thorac Cardiovasc Surg 58(4):467–480
28. Thompson JC (2000) Gifts from surgical research. Contributions to patients and to surgeons (2). Am Coll Surg 190(5):509–521

# The Ignored Birth of Cardiac Surgery: The History of the Surgical Treatment of Heart Wounds and Pericardial Effusions

3

Vladimir Saplacan, Fabio Cuttone and Massimo Massetti

*The road to the heart is only 2–3 cm in length in a direct line, but it has taken surgery nearly 2,400 years to travel it.*
William Randolph Smith

**Abstract**
This chapter retraces the history of cardiac injuries and pericardial effusions from its very beginning in Antiquity until the first years of the 20th century. From Homer and Galen to Romero, Cappelen and other pioneers, the ignored birth of cardiac surgery is presented as described by the historical documents.

## 3.1 Introduction

The history of cardiac injuries was classified by Beck in a reference article published in 1926 into three periods: mysticism, experimentation and observation, and cardiac repair [1].

The first mention of a cardiac wound appears in Homer's Iliad. Of the 147 wounds described in Guido Majno's work [2] we find that of Alkathoos: "The hero Idomeneus smote him in the midst of the breast with the spear…and he fell with a crash, and the lance fixed in his heart that, still beating, shook the butt end of the spear." [3]. The poor prognosis for a haemorrhage, with only the use of rest and chants being encouraged as treatments [2], is also mentioned by Hippocrates [4] and Aristotle: "The heart alone of all the viscera cannot withstand serious injury" [5].

V. Saplacan (✉) · F. Cuttone · M. Massetti
Cardiac Surgery Department, University Hospital of Caen,
Avenue De La Cote de Nacre, Caen, Basse Normandie 14033, France
e-mail: vladimirsaplacan@yahoo.com

F. Cuttone
e-mail: fabiocutto@tiscali.it

M. Massetti
e-mail: massetti-m@chu-caen.fr

M. Picichè (ed.), *Dawn and Evolution of Cardiac Procedures*,
DOI: 10.1007/978-88-470-2400-7_3, 

"Medical treatises written in a language other than Greek have no prestige" wrote Pliny [6]: this historical context meant that the treatise in Latin by Cornelius Celsus "De Medicina" fell into obscurity until the Renaissance. In it we find the picture of a haemorrhagic shock following cardiac injuries: "When the heart is wounded much blood is lost, the pulse weakens, pallor becomes extreme, a cold and foul sweat arises from the stricken body, the extremities become cold and speedy death follows" [7]. Celsus describes the characteristics of a surgeon: "nearer youth, with strong and steady hand which never trembles and ready to use the left hand as well as the right; with vision sharp and clear and spirit undaunted" [2], stressing the importance of his anatomical knowledge: "when a man's viscera are exposed in a wound, he who is ignorant...may be unable to recognize which part is intact...then he cannot relieve the damaged part" [2].

Galen, gladiators' surgeon in Pergamon around 160 AD, was powerless in the face of cardiac wounds in the amphitheatres despite his knowledge of arterial haemostasis: "When a perforation penetrated in one of the cardiac ventricles, they died on the spot, mainly by blood loss, and even faster if the left ventricle was injured. When the penetrating object did not pass through the cardiac cavity but stopped at the cardiac muscle, some of the wounded gladiators lived through the very day on which they were wounded as well as the following night; they eventually died later because of an inflammation (of the heart)" [8].

Ambroise Paré, surgeon to four kings of France would write almost 1,500 years later: "The Heart is the chief mansion of the Soule, the organ of the vital faculty, the beginning of life, the fountain of the vital spirits, and so consequently the continual nourisher of the vital heat, the first living and last dying" [9]. He studied the semiology of cardiac wounds: "By these signs you may know that the heart is wounded: if a great quantity of blood gush out, if a trembling possess all the members of the body, if the pulse be little and faint, if the color become pale...then death's at hand" [9]. During the Italian campaign (1537) he described the famous case of the gentleman from Turin: "I saw a gentleman who fighting a duel with another, received a wound under his left breast which pierced into the substance of his heart....I found a wound in the substance of the heart, so large as would contained one's finger" [9].

The first physicians to call into question the absolute mortality of cardiac wounds appear to have been Hollerius (1498–1562) and Cabriolanus (1604) [10], who were ignored completely, as shown by statements made by Herman Boerhaave (1668–1738): "All wounds of the heart deep enough to penetrate into either of its ventricles are mortal" [11]. Any treatment is prohibited, the surgeon being encouraged to cure every organ in the chest except the heart [4].

It was in Paris that the first suggestions about evacuating a pericardial collection appeared. Riolan in 1649 and Senac, Louis XV's physician, in 1749, imagined the trephination of the sternum [12, 13]. Morgagni described the danger of tamponade in 1769 [14] and Bichat in 1814 reported the first pericardial drainage performed by Desault at the end of the 18th century, contested by Trousseau, who validated only a left pleural drainage [15].

The Catalonian surgeon Francisco Romero begins his memoir (Fig. 3.1) on the treatment of thoracic effusions presented before the Society of the Medical School of Paris in 1815 with the words: "Novum posteritati sanitatis condidi signum, anno 1801" ("I have established a new medical landmark for posterity, in the year 1801"). His patient, Antonio de Mira, who had an operation for a pericardial collection in 1801, was the first successful case of cardiac surgery ever recorded [16]. According to his memoir, Romero performed two successful open pericardial and five open pleural drainages. According to a paper by Aris [17], he voluntarily did not mention a third case of pericardial drainage because the patient had died. Hence, his experience represents not only the beginning of cardiac surgery history, but also the first case of a hidden fatality!

In his memoirs, Dominique-Jean Larrey, chief surgeon of Napoleon's armies, describes several cases of cardiac wounds, the surgical technique of opening the pericardium, crossing the diaphragm at the point that would later take his name, and also the first drainage for post-traumatic tamponade. Bernard St Ogne, a soldier of the Imperial Guard, was brought to Larrey 45 days after stabbing himself in the chest on 18th March 1810: "… I incised the skin and the cellular tissue in the intercostal space between the fifth and the sixth ribs… I cut the intercostal muscle …when I reached the costal pleura, I moderated the action of the bistoury in order that I may not go beyond this last partition in case the heart was very close. I inserted a button bistoury into the cavity and enlarged the opening with a proper incision … I pushed my finger far down into the chest and actually felt the apex of the heart."

The patient died 3 weeks after the operation from suppurated pericarditis found at the autopsy. A grenadier of the Imperial Guard, Chapron, pierced by a sword was, according to Larrey, the first documented case of survival after opening of the pericardium [18].

At the same time, a famous English surgeon, George Guthrie (1785–1856), a "British Larrey", also questioned the lethality of cardiac wounds: "Wounds of the heart are for the most part immediately fatal. Many persons have however been known to live for hours, nay days and even weeks. That the heart when wounded is capable of recovery in a few rare instances is indisputable" [19].

Dupuytren states in his "On the lesions of the vascular system disease": "It is well ascertained … that injuries involving the substance of the heart are not incurable, however deeply the instrument may have penetrated or whatever cavity may have been implicated in the lesion", "indeed this conclusion is generally admitted by educated surgeons". The recommended treatment is: "bloodletting, rest, a single dressing of the wound, sometimes enlargement of the wound and exhibition of acidulated drinks". He also presents cases of "famous" cardiac injury patients, like the Duke of Berry, killed on 13th February 1830, by a lesion of the right atrium [20]. In the *Treatise on weapons of war wounds*, published in 1834, he evokes a principle later used in surgery: cardiac suture is easier on an unloaded heart (in our time using the cardiopulmonary bypass, in his time by venisection)—"If we had to retrieve an instrument involved in the substance of the heart it would be necessary before to reduce the quantity of blood" [21].

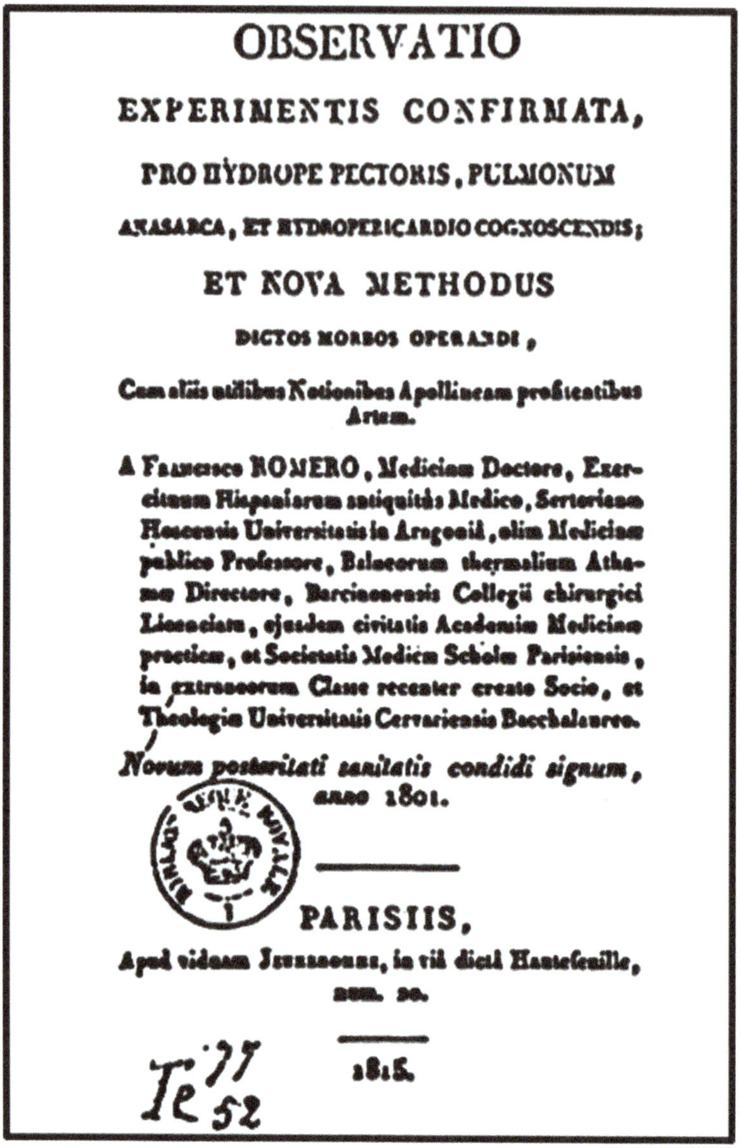

OBSERVATIO

EXPERIMENTIS CONFIRMATA,

PRO HYDROPE PECTORIS, PULMONUM

ANASARCA, ET HYDROPERICARDIO COGNOSCENDIS;

ET NOVA METHODUS

DICTOS MORBOS OPERANDI,

Cum aliis utilibus Nationibus Apollineam profitentibus Artem.

A Francisco ROMERO, Medicinae Doctore, Exercituum Hispaniarum antiquitùs Medico, Sertorianae Hoscensis Universitatis in Aragoniâ, olim Medicinae publico Professore, Balneorum thermalium Athaenae Directore, Barcinonensis Collegii chirurgici Licenciato, ejusdem civitatis Academiae Medicinae practicae, et Societatis Medicae Scholae Parisiensis, in extraneorum Classe recenter creato Socio, et Theologiae Universitatis Cervariensis Bacchalaureo.

*Novum posteritati sanitatis condidi signum,* anno 1801.

PARISIIS,

Apud viduam Jeunehomme, in viâ dictâ Hautefeuille, num. 20.

1815.

**Fig. 3.1** Front page of Francisco Romero's memoir, proof of the birth of cardiac surgery

The first needle pericardiocentesis into the third left space was performed by the Viennese Franz Schuh in 1840 [22] followed in 1841 by Karawagen, who, during an outbreak of scurvy in Kronstadt, drained a pericardial effusion by aspiration in the fifth left space [23].

Several case reports began to appear in the literature on cardiac injuries. Purple in 1850 published a monograph in New York, referring to 50 patients in the USA, UK and Europe [24]. In 1868 Fischer analysed 50 survivors out of 452 patients [25].

At the time, the medical community discouraged any attempts to repair a cardiac injury. Billroth, the famous Viennese surgeon said in 1875: "Paracentesis of the pericardium is an operation which in my opinion approaches very closely to that kind of intervention which some surgeons would term a prostitution of the surgical act and other madness" [26].

In 1882, in Danzig, Block proved, on an animal model, the possibility of recovery after a cardiac injury was repaired [27], but the medical community did not allow itself to be influenced. Billroth pronounced in 1883: "the surgeon who should attempt to suture a wound of the heart would lose the respect of his colleagues", supported by Riedinger: "the suggestion to suture a wound of the heart, although made in all seriousness, scarcely deserves notice" [28].

Despite these difficulties, Del Vecchio, in Naples, proved once again, on a canine model, the possibility of the repair of cardiac wounds [29].

The 1890s marked a turning point in the history of cardiac surgery: two pericardial sutures were performed in the USA by Dalton (1891) and Williams (1893, reported in 1897) and several repairs of cardiac stab wounds made in Europe—by Cappelen in 1894 (Christiana—the former name of Oslo), Farina (Rome) and Rehn (Frankfurt) in 1896 and by Parrozzani (Rome) in 1897 [30].

The unfavourable environment for the birth of cardiac surgery is well described by Stephen Paget, one of the most influential surgeons of the era, who begins the chapter on heart wounds in his treatise *Surgery of the chest*, published in 1896, as follows: "Surgery of the heart has probably reached the limits set by nature to all surgery. No new method and no new discovery can overcome the natural difficulties that attend a wound of the heart. It is true that heart sutures have been vaguely proposed as a possible procedure, and has been done on animals. But I cannot find that it has ever been attempted in practice" [31].

Dalton's patient, 22-year-old Eugene L., having been stabbed in the chest, "entered the City Hospital, September 6, 1891... I might have let it alone, and trusted to Providence, luck, or adhesions to shut it off from the injured pleural cavity, and prevent its possible infection by that route... I had no precedent to guide me, no authority to uphold me in attempting to sew up this wound over a heart that was beating at the rate of 140 per minute. With a long needle-holder, armed with a sharply curved needle and catgut, I was able, with very great difficulty, to close the pericardial wound by continuous suture" [32].

Despite the hostility of the medical world, a first attempt to suture a heart wound in humans was made by Axel Hermansen Cappelen, a 37-year-old surgeon at the National Hospital in Christiana (Oslo). On 4 September 1895, a 24-year-old man who received a stab wound to the left thorax was addressed with: "an imperceptible pulse and distant, faint heart sounds. Bleeding from the wound had ceased. Camphor stimulated the heart so that the pulse could be felt and consciousness returned. At operation chloroform anesthesia was used". Cappelen opened the chest in the fourth left space: "The left pleural cavity contained

1,400 cc. of blood. The lung was not injured… A wound in the left ventricle of 2 cm long was sutured with chromic catgut and a bleeding coronary artery was ligated. The rhythm of the heart was regular throughout the operation." Despite the technical success, the patient died on the third postoperative day of sepsis [33, 34].

In March 1896, at Ospedale della Consolazione in Rome, Guido Farina made a second attempt to suture a left ventricular wound, but the patient died 5 days later of bronchopneumonia. "The patient… received a blow from a very fine and sharp dagger, in the fifth intercostal space in the parasternal line… It wounded the pericardium and penetrated into the right ventricle. The wound in the myocardium was about 7 mm long… I sutured the wound with three silk sutures, and between these three particular points I placed two others of less importance…" The heart was healed at the autopsy. "I begged our judicial authorities to let me have the heart for further study of the process of healing, but met with an energetic refusal. It was precisely because of my irritation at this fact that I have not published any communication on this interesting case." Farina "had the courage to apply to a heart that had been stabbed the simplest and greatest canon of surgery concerning accidental haemorrhage, namely, arrest bleeding…" [35].

Ludwig Rehn reported the first success at the 26th Congress of the German Surgical Society in 1897. In Frankfurt on 9th September 1896 he had repaired a wound of 1.5 cm from the right ventricle of a 22-year-old florist [36]. "There remained one question: what was injured—the heart or its great vessels, an intercostal artery, or the internal mammary…? The tract of the wound lay in the direction of the heart. I decided to attempt to arrest the bleeding" [37]. "It was very disquieting to see the patient pause in diastole with each pass of the needle. The heart gave a laboured beat and then resumed with forceful contractions as we breathed a sigh of relief" [37, 38]. The outcome was favourable, despite a post-operative empyema. Rehn writes: "The feasibility of cardiorrhaphy no longer remains in doubt… I trust that this case will not remain a curiosity, but rather, that the field of cardiac surgery will be further investigated. Let me speak once more my conviction that by means of the cardiorrhaphy, many lives can be saved that were previously counted as lost" [37].

After the success of Rehn, Parrozzani in Rome reported the repair of a wound in the left ventricular apex so large that "the little finger could be passed into the ventricular cavity… from which the blood spurted in small jets at every beat of the organ" [36]. The case was reported by Brock in The Lancet in 1896, who ironically added: "Happily it is only in Italy that surgeons have many opportunities of practicing cardiac surgery, opportunities that they owe to the terrible frequency to which the dagger is resorted to in this country in the quarrels of the lower orders" [39].

A famous date in the history of cardiac wounds remains 10 September 1898, when Luigi Lucheni in Geneva stabbed Elizabeth of Wittelsbach, empress of Austria and Queen of Hungary, known as Sissi, in the left breast. She died soon afterwards in tamponade, as the autopsy proved: "The lesions described have been produced by a long instrument of triangular shape with more or less blunted edges. This instrument entered the thoracic wall with violence, breaking a rib and completely perforating the left ventricle… Death was undoubtedly caused by a progressive and slow blood leak, sufficient to compress the heart and to suspend its functions. The finding of a voluminous blood clot occupying the pericardium is the absolute proof of it" [40].

Beck, in his article on cardiac wounds, considered the lesion treatable, "... but at this late date, recent as it may seem, the pulsating heart of the human being had been exposed to view only a few times and the veil of mystery (to the surgeon) was just being lifted" [2].

Fontan, a Navy surgeon in Toulon in 1902 reported two cases of the suturing of cardiac wounds, the first dating back to 1 January 1900: "One must take advantage of the moment when the wound presents itself most favourably to the hand of the operator and be careful not to do penetrating bites with the needle, for avoiding haemorrhage and also clot formation on the suture material" [41].

Hill entered history as the first American surgeon to successfully suture a wound of the heart with his famous intervention of 4 September 1902 on a 13-year-old boy who underwent surgery on the kitchen table by the light of two kerosene lamps [42].

Mortality from these repairs remained high, 59 % in the series of 17 patients (review of the literature), published by Hill in 1900 [43] and 60 % in the series by Rehn of 124 patients (1907) [44]. Peck demystified the high lethality of auricular wounds in 1909: "Nearly all writers on heart wounds considered wounds of the auricles more dangerous than those of the ventricles, but of the 11 reported cases 7 had recovered—a mortality of 36.3 %, while general mortality of sutured heart wounds is about 64 %" [45].

Pool in 1912 presented a new vision of therapy on heart wounds: "The rationality of immediate surgical treatment for wounds of the heart has been thoroughly established by 15 years of relatively good and constantly improving results. Even in suspected wounds of the heart, when the diagnosis is probable but not positive, exploratory operation is an approved procedure". As Peck before him, he emphasised the importance of asepsis of the surgical field [46]. He raised the possibility of internal cardiac massage, useful in arrhythmias frequent enough after haemostasis manoeuvres like the "Sauerbruch grip" (compression of the base of the heart) [47].

On 27 October 1913, the Russian surgeon Djanelidze carried out the first successful repair of a wound on the ascending aorta [48].

The outbreak of the First and especially the Second World War provided the premise for surgery involving the removal of intra-cardiac foreign bodies. Dr Dwight Harken performed research in this field and developed his surgical technique by operating on dogs. In three groups of animals undergoing operations, the first group had a 100 % death rate, the second 50 % and the third 14 %. He was then director of the Fifteenth Thoracic Centre based at Cirencester in England, and in the 10 months after D-Day, 134 operations were performed to remove retained shell particles in and around the heart, among which 56 were intrapericardial and 13 intracavitary. Remarkably, he reported that there were no deaths among these patients [49].

In conclusion, it took 50 years for surgeons to prove that both Paget and Billroth were wrong about operating on the heart, largely because of the pioneering efforts of war surgeons working under desperate circumstances.

## References

1. Beck CS (1926) Wounds of the heart. Arch Surg 13:205–227
2. Majno G (1991) The healing hand—Man and wound in the ancient world. Harvard University Press, Harvard
3. Homer (1922) The iliad (trans: Lang et al) Macmillan and Co, New York, vol 8, 259 as quoted by Beck CS (1926) Wounds of the heart. Arch Surg 13:205–227
4. Asensio JA, Petrone P, Pereira B et al (2009) Penetrating cardiac injuries: a historic perspective and fascinating trip through time. J Am Coll Surg 3:462–473
5. Aristotle (384–322 BC) The partibus animalium. Lib III, Chap 4. Opera edidit academia regia borrusca, vol 3, p 328. As quoted by Beck CS (1926) Wounds of the heart. Arch Surg 13:205–227
6. Pliny (The elder) (1991) Natural history. In: Majno G (ed) The healing hand—man and wound in the ancient world. Harvard University Press, Harvard, p 353
7. Celsus (1st century A. D.): Medicinae Libri Octo, Lib. V, cap. 26, L Targae, Lugduni Batavorum, by S. and J. Luchtmans, 1791, p 307 As quoted by Beck CS (1926) Wounds of the heart. Arch Surg 13:205–227
8. Galen M (1976) De locis affectis (trans: siegel RE), New York. As quoted by Blatchford JW III, Anderson R (1985) The evolution of the management of penetrating wounds of the heart. Ann Surg 5:615–623
9. Pare A (1634) The workes of that famous chirurgion ambrose parey (trans: Johnson T). T Cotes, London. As quoted by Beck CS (1926) Wounds of the heart. Arch Surg 13:205–227
10. Cabriolanus B (1614) Alphabet anatomic. P Rigaud, Lyon. As quoted by Asensio JA, Petrone P, Pereira B et al (2009) Penetrating cardiac injuries: a historic perspective and fascinating trip through time. J Am Coll Surg 3:462–473
11. Boerhaave De vulnere in genere, Aphorismi de Coognoscendis et Curandis Morbis, Aphorism 170, 43. As quoted by Beck CS (1926) Wounds of the heart. Arch Surg 13:205–227
12. Riolan J (1649) Encheiridium Anatomicum et Pathologicum Lugduni Batavorum, Ex Officina Adriani Wyngaerden. As quoted by Hurt Raymond (1996) History of Cardiothoracic Surgery from Early Times, The Parthenon Publishing Group, Casterton Hall, Carnforth Lancs, LA6 2LA, UK, p 411
13. Senac JB (1749) Traité de la Structure du Coeur, de son Action et de ses Maladies. As quoted by Hurt Raymond (1996) History of cardiothoracic surgery from early times. The Parthenon Publishing Group, Casterton Hall, Carnforth Lancs, LA6 2LA, UK, p 411
14. Morgagni GB (1769) The seats and causes of diseases (trans: Alexander B). Millar and Cadell, London. As quoted by Hurt, Raymond (1996) History of cardiothoracic surgery from early times. The Parthenon Publishing Group, Casterton Hall, Carnforth Lancs, LA6 2LA, UK, p 411
15. Bichat MFX (1814) The Surgical works, or statement of the doctrine and practice of dessault (trans: Smith ED). Dobson, Philadelphia. As quoted by Hurt Raymond (1996) History of cardiothoracic surgery from early times. The Parthenon Publishing Group, Casterton Hall, Carnforth Lancs, LA6 2LA, UK, p 411
16. Van Thielen J, Van Hee R (2008) Pericardiotomy: the first cardiac operation. Acta Chir Belg 108:133–138
17. Aris A (1997) Francisco Romero, the first heart surgeon. Ann Thorac Surg 64:870–871
18. Larrey DJ (1829) Clinique Chirurgicale, exercée particulièrement dans les camps et les hopitaux militaires, depuis 1792 jusqu'en 1829. Gabon Libraire-Editeur, Paris

19. Guthrie GJ (1848) On wounds and injuries of the chest. Henry Renshaw, London
20. Dupuytren G (1854) Lesions of the vascular system, diseases of the rectum and other surgical complaints. The Syndeham Society, London
21. Dupuytren G (1834) Traité Theorique et Pratique des Blessures par Armes de Guerre. J-B Baillière, Paris
22. Kilpatrick ZM, Chapman CB (1965) On pericardiocentesis. Am J Cardiol 16:722–728
23. Karawagen (1841) On scorbutic pericarditis and pleuritis and the cure by paracentesis. Br Foreign Med Rev 12:250. As quoted by Hurt Raymond (1996) History of cardiothoracic surgery from early times, The Parthenon Publishing Group, Casterton Hall, Carnforth Lancs, LA6 2LA, UK, p 413
24. Purple SS (1855) Statistical observations on wounds of the heart and on their relations to forensic medicine with a table of forty-two recorded cases. NY Med 14:411. As quoted by Asensio JA, Petrone P, Pereira B et al (2009) Penetrating cardiac injuries: a historic perspective and fascinating trip through time. J Am Coll Surg 3:462–473
25. Fischer G (1868) Die Wunden des Herzeus und des Herzbeutels. Arch Klin Chir 9:571. As quoted by Asensio JA, Petrone P, Pereira B et al (2009) Penetrating cardiac injuries: a historic perspective and fascinating trip through time. J Am Coll Surg 3:462–473
26. Billroth T. Quoted by Jeger E (1913) Die Chirurgie der Blutgefasse und des Herzens. Berlin, 295. As quoted by Beck CS (1926) Wounds of the heart. Arch Surg 13:205–227
27. Block MH (1882) Verhandlunge der Deutschen Gessellshof fur Chirurgie. Elfren Congress, Berlin, part I:108. As quoted by Beck CS (1926) Wounds of the heart. Arch Surg 13:205–227
28. Riedinger F (1888) Verletzungen und Chirurgische Krankheiten des Thorax und Seines Inhaltes. F Enke, Stuttgart. As quoted by Beck CS (1926) Wounds of the heart. Arch Surg 13:205–227
29. Del Vecchio S (1895) Sutura del cuore. Riforma Med 11, 38. As quoted by Beck CS (1926) Wounds of the heart. Arch Surg 13:205–227
30. Hurt Raymond (1996) History of Cardiothoracic Surgery from Early Times, The Parthenon Publishing Group, Casterton Hall, Carnforth Lancs, LA6 2LA, UK
31. Paget S (1896) Surgery of the chest. Wright, Bristol
32. Dalton HC (1895) Report of a case of Stab-wound of the Pericardium, terminating in recovery after resection of a rib and suture of the pericardium. Ann Surg 21:147–152
33. Cappelen AH (1896) Vulnus Cordis. Sutur af Hjertet. Norsk Mag Laegevidensk 11:285–288. As quoted by Beck CS (1926) Wounds of the heart. Arch Surg 13:205–227
34. Søreide K, Krüger AJ (2006) Penetrating cardiac injuries—A century from Cappelen to current care. Scand J Trauma Resusc Emerg Med 14:142–146
35. Bland-Sutton J (1910) Treatment of the injuries of the heart. Br Med J 1:1273–1276
36. Erlsberg CA (1899) An experimental investigation of the treatment of wounds of the heart by means of suture of the heart muscle. J Exp Med, IV, 5–6:33–75
37. Blatchford JW III, Anderson R (1985) The evolution of the management of penetrating wounds of the heart. Ann Surg 202:615–623
38. Rehn L (1897) Ueber Penetrerende Herzwunden und Herznaht. Arch Klin Chir 55:315. As quoted by Beck CS (1926) Wounds of the heart. Arch Surg 13:205–227
39. Brock GS (1897) Penetrating wound of the pericardium and left ventricle; suture; recovery. Lancet, 2:260. As quoted by Hurt Raymond (1996) History of cardiothoracic surgery from early times, the parthenon publishing group, Casterton Hall, Carnforth Lancs, LA6 2LA, UK, p 402
40. Meyer P, Keller P-F, Spodick DH (2008) Empress Sissi and cardiac tamponade: a historical perspective. Am J Cardiol 102:1278–1280
41. Le Dentu M (1902) Sur un travail du Dr J. Fontan intitulé: Contribution à la Chirurgie du Coeur. Bull Acad Nat Med, XL7:381–389
42. Hill LL (1902) A report of a case of successful suturing of the heart, and table of 37 other cases of suturing by different operators with various terminations and conclusions drawn. Med Record 62:846–848. As quoted by Asensio JA, Petrone P, Pereira B et al (2009) Penetrating cardiac injuries: a historic perspective and fascinating trip through time. J Am Coll Surg 3:462–473

43. Hill LL (1900) Wounds of the heart with a report of 17 cases of heart suture. Med Record 58:921–924. As quoted by Asensio JA, Petrone P, Pereira B et al (2009) Penetrating cardiac injuries: a historic perspective and fascinating trip through time. J Am Coll Surg 3:462–473
44. Rehn L (1907) Zur Chirurgie des Herzens und des Herzbeutels. Arch Klin Chir 83:723–778. As quoted by Blatchford JW III, Anderson R (1985) The evolution of the management of penetrating wounds of the heart. Ann Surg 5:615–623
45. Peck CH (1909) The operative treatment of heart wounds. Ann Surg 50:100–134
46. Pool EH (1912) Treatment of heart wounds. Ann Surg 55:485–512
47. Sauerbruch F (1907) Uber die Verwendbarkeit der pneumatischen Kammer fur die Herzschirurgie. Central Chir 34:44. As quoted by Asensio JA, Petrone P, Pereira B et al (2009) Penetrating cardiac injuries: A historic perspective and fascinating trip through time. J Am Coll Surg 3:462–473
48. Alexi-Meskishvili V, Konstantinov IE, Yustin Y (2000) Djanelidze and the first successful repair of an injured ascending aorta. Tex Heart Inst J 27:113–116
49. Harken DE (1946) Foreign bodies in, and in relation to the thoracic blood vessels and heart; techniques for approaching and removing foreign bodies from the chambers of the heart. Surg Gynecol Obstet 83:117–125

# The History of Pulmonary Embolectomy Before the Advent of CPB

# 4

Marco Vola and Jean-Francois Fuzellier

*In this way the false conception has developed that the majority of emboli are instantly fatal.*

Friedrich Trendelenburg

**Abstract**

The history of the surgical approach to pulmonary embolism before the advent of CPB was exclusively limited to acute forms and very much associated with the person of Friederich Trendelenburg. He observed that the time between the onset of the embolism and ensuing death allowed time for acute surgical treatment. He developed in animal studies (1907) a surgical procedure for pulmonary embolectomy, later known as the Trendelenburg operation. Only after his death, his pupil, Martin Kirschner successfully removed clots from the arterial pulmonary artery of a 38-year-old woman. Sporadic reports of the procedure were issued until the advent of cardiopulmonary bypass, which increased the opportunities for disseminating the practice of surgical embolectomy. Chronic constrictive pericarditis had been anatomically described by Galen (AD 160), but the surgical usefulness of liberating the ventricles was suggested by Weill in 1895. A surgical technique of pericardial decortication was presented by Delorme in 1898, and was performed by Rehn in 1913 on a human being. Current surgical decortications follow the same principles, but are practiced after an accurate topographic evaluation of the pericardium.

The gravity of pulmonary embolism as a life-threatening condition and the need to find surgical solutions was presented by Friedrich Trendelenburg, Director of the University Surgical Clinic at Leipzig, on 21 April 1908 at the 37th Annual Congress

M. Vola (✉) · J.-F. Fuzellier
Service de Chirurgie Cardiovasculaire, Centre Hospitalier Universitaire,
Avenue Albert Raymond, 42270 St-Priest en Jarez, France
e-mail: marco.vola@univ-st-etienne.fr

J.-F. Fuzellier
e-mail: j.francois.fuzellier@chu-st-etienne.fr

M. Picichè (ed.), *Dawn and Evolution of Cardiac Procedures*,
DOI: 10.1007/978-88-470-2400-7_4, © Springer-Verlag Italia 2013

of the German Surgical Association. The history of the surgical approach to pulmonary embolism before the advent of CPB was exclusively limited to acute forms and very much associated with Friederich Trendelenburg. This giant among innovators is generally linked in the mind of most physicians to the famous Trendelenburg operating position. In reality, Trendelenburg's contributions were multidisciplinary. He administered the first endotracheal anesthesia (inventing a cannula to close the trachea and prevent blood entering after a tracheotomy), focused on advancing the field of genitourinary surgery, and developed a surgical approach to pulmonary embolism [1]. The curiosity surrounding this eccentric surgeon probably had its origins in his proclivity for observation—a trait transmitted to him by his mother and his father Adolf, a professor of philosophy. Young Friedrich was able to attend anatomy courses in Glasgow taught by Professor Allen Thompson. He graduated with a degree in medicine in Berlin, and subsequently had seminal exchanges with major figures in the German surgical world, who at that time dominated the international scientific community. He was a disciple of Ludwig Traube and an assistant to Bernhard Langenbeck in Berlin, where he demonstrated a recognized "facility of innovation and a particular enjoyment of plastic surgery" [2].

In Trendelenburg's report he noted that in 7 out of 9 cases of massive pulmonary embolism, the time between the onset of the embolism and ensuing death was between 10 and 60 min. He observed that in the most favorable outcomes the interval could be extended to 15 min to allow time for acute surgical treatment, but unfortunately medical efforts at the time were only concerned with the patient's medical stabilization. The concept of a surgical procedure for pulmonary embolectomy, later known as the Trendelenburg operation, was first developed in animal studies. In the first series on animals, Trendelenburg incised the conus arteriosus of the right ventricle and introduced a cannula into the pulmonary artery to aspirate the venous emboli. These preliminary results were presented in Dresden in 1907. In the next series of animal studies, he showed that direct incision of the pulmonary artery was the best option for accessing and extracting emboli. Extraction was performed with a polyp forceps after proximal occlusion of the vessel. He also discussed the critical topic of the maximum clamping time of the pulmonary artery, i.e., 45 s to 2 min before death in rabbits, 45 s to 1 min in sheep. Trendelenburg described the technique in detail and attempted it in humans. Surgical access was well described. A skin incision was made laterally for 10 cm in the left hemithorax from the end of the second rib close to the sternal margin. A second vertical incision met the first along the sternum to produce a final T incision. The two resulting skin flaps with the underlying pectoralis major muscle were then returned and fixed laterally. The second rib was divided, the costal cartilage was ablated while sparing the internal mammary artery, and the pleura opened. The pericardium was opened vertically, anterior to the phrenic nerve, which was visualized. The pulmonary artery was then localized in the pericardium, and the author refers to insertion of a rubber tube through the transverse sinus to encircle the aorta and the pulmonary artery together. Previously, he had used a wet band to occlude by traction the great vessels, but this resulted in rupture of the posterior wall of the vessels. The surface of the pulmonary artery had to be cleaned to facilitate rapid incision and emboli extraction. Constriction and compression of the great vessels was then applied, clamping them proximally. A short 0.75-cm incision was reported on the anterior–lateral side of the pulmonary artery to permit emboli extraction for a maximum of 45 s. Then, Trendelenburg described lateral clamping of the open pulmonary artery in order to reestablish circulation. The aspiration maneuver could be repeated to extract a maximum amount of material. Trendelenburg emphasized that the most difficult part of the procedure was the closure with running suture of the pulmonary artery performed with fine silk outside the side-occluding clamp.

The first human patient operated on by Trendelenburg, using the above-mentioned wet band occlusion technique, died of a hemorrhage. He reported another relevant limitation to the technique related to opening the left pleural cavity with obvious impacts on the ventilation of a non-intubated patient. Trendelenburg reported that only one patient survived the procedure, but died 48 h after the operation. Nonetheless, he reaffirmed the possibility for success based on the positive results from animal studies. He insisted that the procedure be performed by a skilled team and only after accurate and rapid symptom identification.

Friederich Trendelenburg died in 1924. That same year his pupil, Martin Kirschner, successfully removed clots from the arterial pulmonary artery of a 38-year-old woman. Except for sporadic reports on Trendelenburg's techniques in intervening years, these techniques did not resurface in full view until Denton A. Cooley and colleagues published in 1961 their successful application during pulmonary embolectomies using cardiopulmonary bypass [3]. The advent of cardiopulmonary bypass increased the opportunities for disseminating the practice of surgical embolectomy. The necessity for emergency interventions of this type decreased with the advent of thrombolytic therapy.

## 4.1 The History of Chronic Constrictive Pericarditis Before the Advent of CPB

Constrictive pericarditis was identified and described anatomically in 160 AD by Galen, but its physiopathological significance in the genesis of cardiac failure was not understood. In the 18th century Lancisi performed an autopsy in which he related the condition of abdominal and jugular swelling to the thickened pericardium constricting of a small heart [4]. Pick in 1896 identified constriction of the pericardium in three patients whose clinical course had been attributed to hepatic cirrhosis [5]. As Holmann pointed out in 1951, "it is amongst patients who are regarded as having heart failure, but in whom the ordinary causes are lacking, i.e., hypertension, coronary sclerosis, valvular disease, hyperthyroidism, or who are thought to have cirrhosis of the liver, in whom constrictive pericarditis will be found" [6]. Weill suggested the possibility of surgical treatment for constrictive pericarditis. He emphasized that diagnostic uncertainty was the main impediment to the use of surgery in treating pericardial decortications, and stated that "one should try to approach this by releasing part of the heart, the apex for example and the surface. It will be up to surgery to free the heart from this jacket that strangles it" [7].

In 1898, Delorme, after his detailed observations on cadavers, spoke of the possibility of eliminating adhesions between the lung and the pericardium with scissors and fingers. He defined the concept of decortication of the heart. He was supported in his ideas by his previous experiences with the decortication of the lung. He recommended actual ablation of pericardial tissue, and when that was not possible, sections of the pericardium and anterior adherences. He presented his procedure at several meetings in France [8], but the medical community considered his operation to be more tricky than the mere ablation of costal precordial cartilage proposed by Brauer [9].

The first operation reported using Delorme's technique was performed by Rehn in 1913 [10]. In the following decade, Rehn and others in Europe and the USA increasingly used Delorme's technique. These surgeons acquired experience in physiopathology in order to pre-operatively prepare for cardiac decortication. The advent of fluoroscopic examination enabled evaluation of ventricular movements and particularly the portion of the ventricle and right atrium constricted by the pericardium.

We need to acknowledge Claude S. Beck's seminal work, which led to a better understanding of the physiopathology of constrictive pericarditis. This eclectic surgeon contributed many scientific innovations, including in the field of the operating room management of cardiac arrest [11]. On the subject of pericardial constrictive syndrome, he pointed out, after some animal experimentation, that in order to cause constrictive syndrome, the pericardium must be thick and inextensible, and that ablation of this membrane can be effective in restoring physiological function [12].

## References

1. Trendelenburg F (1908) Über die Operative Behandlung der Embolie der Lungenarterie. Arch Klin Chir 86:686–700
2. Bernstein AM, Koo HP, Bloom DA (1999) Beyond the Trendelenburg position: Friedrich Trendelenburg's life and surgical contributions. Surgery 126(1):78–82
3. Cooley DA, Beall AC Jr, Alexander JK (1961) Acute massive pulmonary embolism. Successful surgical treatment using temporary cardiopulmonary bypass. JAMA 5(177):283–286
4. Lancisi GM (1728) De Motu Cordis et Aneurysmatibus. Salvioni, Rome, pp 38–39
5. Pick F (1896) Über chronische unter dem Bilde dem Lebercirrhose verlaufende Perikarditis (perikardische Pseudolebecirrhose) nebst Bermerkungen über die Zuckergussleber (Curschmann). Z Klin Med 29:385
6. Holman E (1951) The surgical treatment of constrictive pericarditis: clinical and experimental observations. Ann R Coll Surg Engl 9(5):309–317
7. Weill E (1895) Traité clinique des maladies du coeur chez les enfants. Doin, Paris, p 128
8. Delorme E (1898) Sur un traitement chirurgical de la Symphyse cardo-pericardique. Bull Mem Soc Chir Paris 24:918
9. Brauer L (1903) Die Kardiolyse und ihre Indikationen. Arch Klin Chir 71:258
10. Rehn L (1913) Die Chirurgie des Herzens und des Herzbeutels. Berliner Klin Wchnschr, 50:241–246
11. Meyer JA (1988) Claude Beck and cardiac resuscitation. Ann Thorac Surg 45(1):103–105
12. Beck CS (1929) The effect of surgical solution of chlorinated soda (Dakin's solution) in the pericardial cavity. Arch Surg 18(4):1659–1671

13. Meyer JA (1990) Friedrich Trendelenburg and the surgical approach to massive pulmonary embolism. Arch Surg 125(9):1202–1205
14. Griswold RA (1993) The Trendelenburg operation for pulmonary embolism. Ann Surg 98(1):33–42

# Right Cardiac Catheterization Before the Advent of Cardiopulmonary Bypass

5

Achille Gaspardone and Giulio G. Stefanini

*Pulchra sunt quae videntur, pulchriora quae sciuntur, longe pulcherrima quae ignorantur.*

Niels Stensen [Steno]

**Abstract**

Right cardiac catheterization is an important tool in current cardiology practice for diagnostic and therapeutic purposes and one of the most frequently performed procedures yearly worldwide. Right cardiac catheterization has the accuracy of intracardiac pressure, blood volume, cardiac output measurements, and permits right chamber visualization throughout angiography. The development of this invasive technique has been an ongoing journey starting in the 18th century with the cannulation of an equine artery for the measurement of systemic arterial pressure performed by Stephen Hale (1677–1761), on to the catheterization of both ventricles in a horse by Claude Bernard in 1844, right heart catheterization in dogs and human cadaver by Arrigo Montanari in 1928, and finally, the self-catheterization by Werner Forssmann in 1929 leading to the development of more sophisticated procedures by Cournand and Richards in 1944. After more than 50 years from its inception, right heart catheterization continues to be the gold standard in diagnosing patients with elevated right heart pressure and in the management of complex patients, although the use of the pulmonary artery catheter is a monitoring procedure and not a treatment. When viewed in this context, the pulmonary artery catheter provides the clinician with the advantage of continuous hemodynamic monitoring that could assist the trained health care professional in the application of therapeutic treatments.

A. Gaspardone (✉) · G. G. Stefanini
Division of Cardiology, Department of Medicine, Ospedale S. Eugenio,
Piazzale dell'umanesimo 10, 00144 Rome, Italy
e-mail: a_gaspardone@yahoo.com

M. Picichè (ed.), *Dawn and Evolution of Cardiac Procedures*,
DOI: 10.1007/978-88-470-2400-7_5, 

Right cardiac catheterization represents an important tool in current cardiology practice for diagnostic and therapeutic purposes, with over 20 million procedures performed yearly in the USA [1–8]. Right cardiac catheterization ensures the accuracy of intracardiac pressure, blood volume, cardiac output measurements and permits right chamber visualization throughout angiography [7, 9–12].

## 5.1 The Precursors

The development of this invasive technique has been an ongoing journey starting in the 18th century with the cannulation of an equine artery for the measurement of systemic arterial pressure by Stephen Hales (1677–1761), on to the catheterization of both ventricles in a horse by Claude Bernard in 1844, right heart catheterization in dogs and human cadavers by Arrigo Montanari in 1928, and finally, the self-catheterization by Werner Forssmann in 1929, which led to the development of more sophisticated procedures by Cournand and Richards in 1944 [7, 9–13]. The early history and the development of right cardiac catheterization provides the reader with a greater appreciation of current clinical applications and the limitations of this important procedure.

It was 1711 when the Reverend Stephen Hales (Fig. 5.1), in England, first measured blood pressure and cardiac output in a horse, with the use of brass pipes [14–17]. Some years later, Auguste Chauveau and Étienne-Jules Marey made graphic records of the auricular and ventricular pressure using a double cardiac catheter technique, once again in a horse [14–18]. Two hypotheses followed these experiences, namely the pulmonary combustion and the tissue combustion hypotheses [19, 20]. In the late 18th century Antoine-Laurent de Lavoisier proposed the former hypothesis, based on his theory that heat is produced when respiratory gas exchange occurs in the lungs [4, 19, 20]. The latter hypothesis was proposed by the chemist Gustav Magnus in 1837, who suggested that tissues serve as the site of heat production [4]. The well-known physiologist Claude Bernard (Fig. 5.2), who stressed the importance of the physiological understanding of disease from the very beginning of his career, attempted to verify these two hypotheses by directly correlating the physics of the circulation through the use of thermodynamic principles [4, 19]. Bernard hypothesized that the pulmonary combustion model would result in blood being warmer in the left side of the heart after passing through the pulmonary system; in order to test this he performed the first cardiac catheterization in 1844 [4, 6, 21]. This catheterization procedure involved exposing a horse's jugular vein and carotid artery to insert a glass tube into the right and left ventricles by a retrograde approach. The renowned physiologist finally inserted a mercury thermometer into the left and right sides of the heart to obtain the respective temperatures, verifying the validity of the tissue combustion hypothesis [4, 18, 21]. These experiments showed that right cardiac catheterization could be used for monitoring potential cardiac events and in the second half of the 19th century Bernard and two other French physiologists,

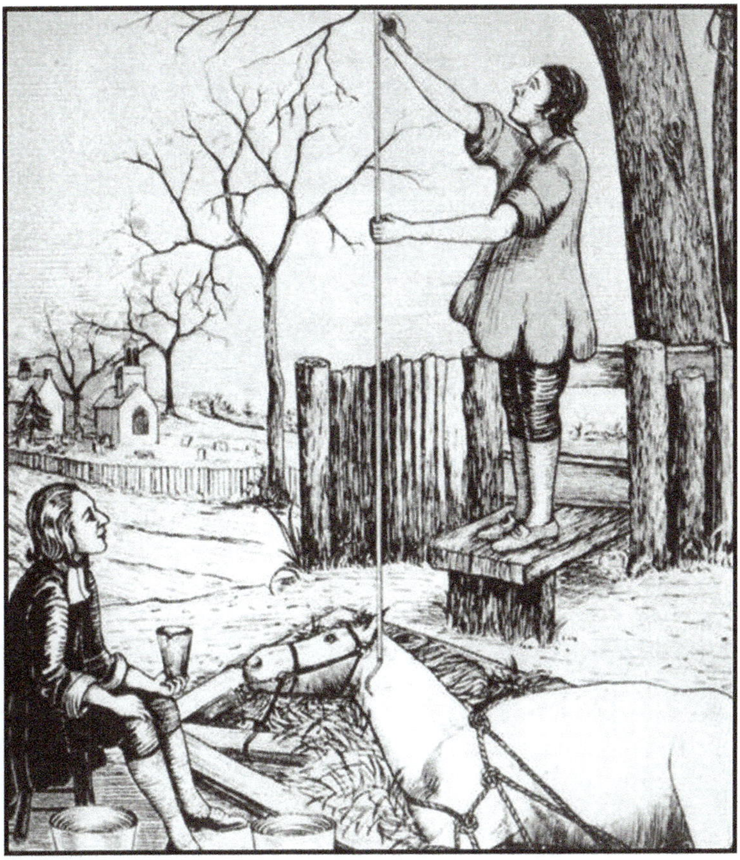

**Fig. 5.1** Stephen Hales measuring blood pressure in a mare

Jean-Baptiste Chauveau and Étienne Marey, continued to use cardiac catheterization in the horse to measure intracardiac pressure (Fig. 5.3) [4].

At the beginning of the 20th century Fritz Bleichroder and Ernst Unger performed cardiac catheterization in dogs, and finally Fritz Bleichroder was the first reported human subject to undergo three invasive catheter-based procedures performed by Ernst Unger through the basilic vein and into the axillary, and on separate occasions through the femoral vein and into the inferior vena cava [4]. During one of these maneuvers, Bleichroder experienced severe chest pain, leading the researchers to believe that they may have performed the first human heart catheterization; however, they failed to document the catheter position by either X-ray or pressure recording. In 1928, Arrigo Montanari performed in Florence several accurate autopsy studies confirming the possibility of precisely localizing a catheter in the right ventricle through a brachial vein [13].

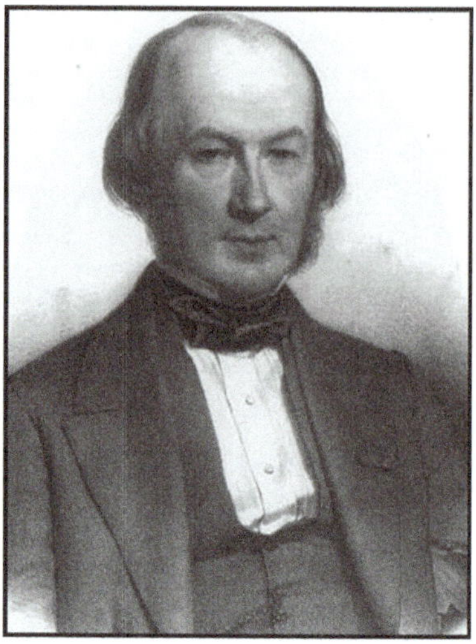

**Fig. 5.2** Claude Bernard (1813–1878)

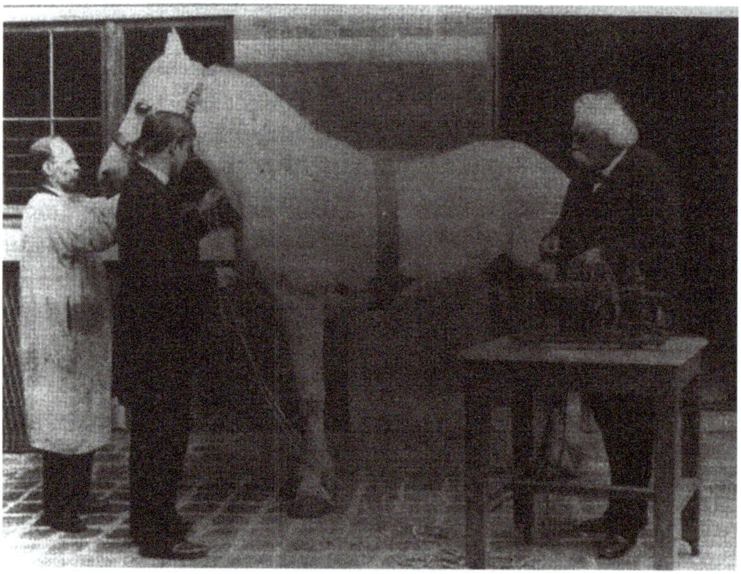

**Fig. 5.3** First cardiac catheterization in a horse by Chauveau and Marey

## 5.2 In Vivo Human Right Cardiac Catheterization

In 1929, a 25-year-old German physician named Werner Forssmann—unaware of Bleichroder and Unger's experiments—reported the first "in vivo" recorded human cardiac catheterization [22, 23]. Forssmann, well aware of Bernard's safe cardiac catheterization experiments in animals, believed that cardiac catheterization could have represented a solid tool for the investigation of circulatory and metabolic mechanisms, as well as a possible vehicle for the administration of cardiac medications [18, 22, 24]. The young Dr Forssmann inserted into himself a ureteral catheter, pushed it into the right auricle and documented this self-catheterization with an X-ray without suffering pain or complications (Fig. 5.4) [23]. He then repeated the procedure in a septic patient, believing in the benefit of injecting suprarenin and strophanthin (i.e., adrenalin and a digitalis preparation respectively) directly into the central circulation. Disregarding the innovative approach, this procedure was strongly criticized by the scientific community and the media of that time, and Dr Forssmann had his clinical license suspended [14, 22, 24]. This drawback notwithstanding, the use of right cardiac catheterization in humans finally became a popular method in the 1930s, when Dr Klein in Prague used this technique to sample mixed venous blood and to quantify cardiac output in 30 patients [25]. However, it was not until 1941 that three medical doctors—André Cournand, Hilmert Ranges, and Dickinson Richards—further developed right cardiac catheterization techniques in order to perform hemodynamic measurements [7, 9, 26]. André Cournand and Dickinson Richards, experts in pulmonary physiology and cardiovascular medicine respectively, teamed up at Bellevue Hospital in New York to redesign the catheter used by Forssmann in his studies [26–31]. In 1945, they reported a series of more than 260 right cardiac catheterizations [9], showing the safety of this technique. The right catheterization approach was then used for the collection of mixed venous blood and the measurement of cardiac output through the direct Fick principle [32–35]. The concept behind the Fick principle is that blood flow to an organ in the body can be calculated using any dissolved indicator in the blood, given that the indicator's uptake by the organ over time is constant, and the initial concentration of the indicator as well as the concentration of the indicator leaving the organ are known. The cardiac output can then be calculated by dividing the indicator's uptake by the concentration difference measured in arterial blood and mixed venous blood samples. In Fick's original description oxygen was used as the indicator; however, until the introduction of right cardiac catheterization this method was rarely used because of the difficulty in obtaining a mixed venous blood sample unless direct cardiac puncture was performed. Thus, the application of right cardiac catheterization allowed the measurement of cardiac output through the direct Fick principle to become a standard medical procedure [9, 24].

In 1946, Cournand and Richards published a further study reporting a comparison of right atrial pressure and right ventricle pressure in healthy subjects and in patients with chronic pulmonary disease or cardiac disease [36]. Integrating his

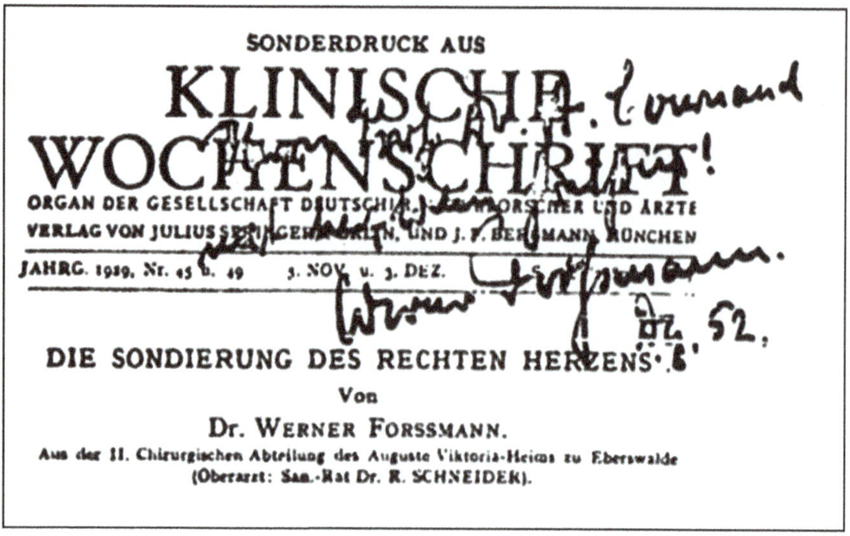

SONDERDRUCK AUS

KLINISCHE WOCHENSCHRIFT

ORGAN DER GESELLSCHAFT DEUTSCHER NATURFORSCHER UND ÄRZTE
VERLAG VON JULIUS SPRINGER, BERLIN, UND J. F. BERGMANN, MÜNCHEN

JAHRG. 1929, Nr. 45 u. 49 5. NOV. u. 3. DEZ.

DIE SONDIERUNG DES RECHTEN HERZENS.

Von

Dr. WERNER FORSSMANN.

Aus der II. Chirurgischen Abteilung des Auguste Viktoria-Heims zu Eberswalde
(Oberarzt: San.-Rat Dr. R. SCHNEIDER).

**Fig. 5.4** Cover page of the initial paper by Werner Forssmann describing self-catheterization

personal experience with the evidence available at that time, Cournand described the dynamics of the pulmonary circulation concluding that:

1. The pulmonary flow equals the system flow; however, momentary differences are present owing to rhythmic changes related to breathing.
2. The pulmonary vascular bed is a low-pressure system resulting from the great distensibility of the main pulmonary artery and distal branches, and from the very large capacity and deformability of arteriolar, pre-capillary, and the capillary beds.
3. The distribution of blood in the pulmonary circulation is controlled by local mechanical mechanisms rather than by the central nervous system [37, 38].

In 1953, Richards and his co-workers reported the simultaneous measurement of cardiac output by right heart catheterization (i.e., the direct Fick method) and by the ballistocardiograph method among hospitalized patients and healthy controls. They showed that measurement of cardiac output using the ballistocardiographic method produced unreliable results, concluding that the ballistocardiographic measurements were no longer to be used to assess cardiac output [39].

Overall, Cournand and Richards developed the right cardiac catheterization as a versatile tool for hemodynamic measurements as well as for blood gases measurements and respiratory gas exchange [39–42], providing several important breakthroughs as it relates to cardio-pulmonary physiopathology and significantly improving the diagnostic abilities of physicians. In recognition of these achievements, in 1956 the Nobel Prize in Physiology and Medicine was awarded to doctors André Cournand, Dickinson Richards, and Werner Forssmann (Figs. 5.5, 5.6) [43].

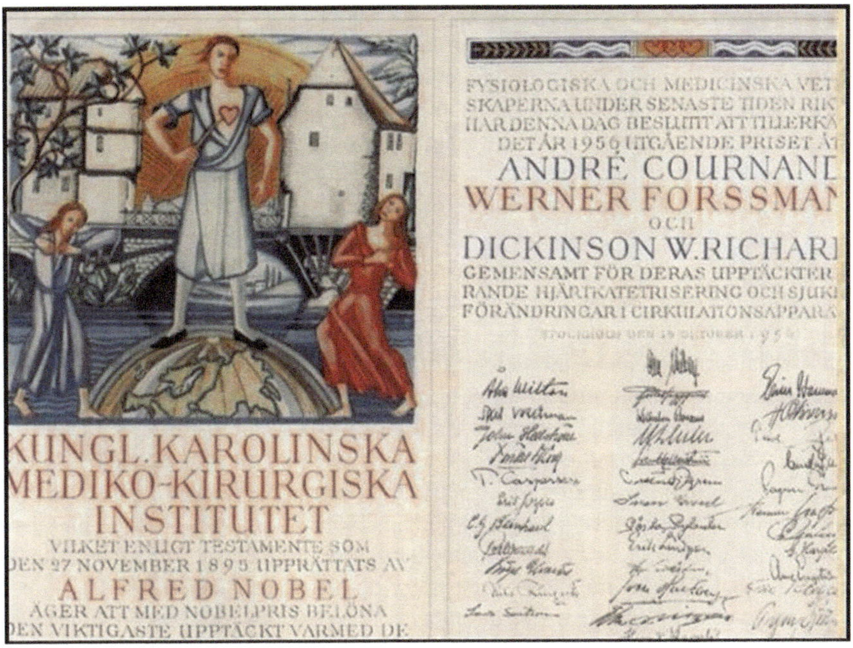


Fig. 5.5 The Nobel prize in medicine or physiology: October 1956

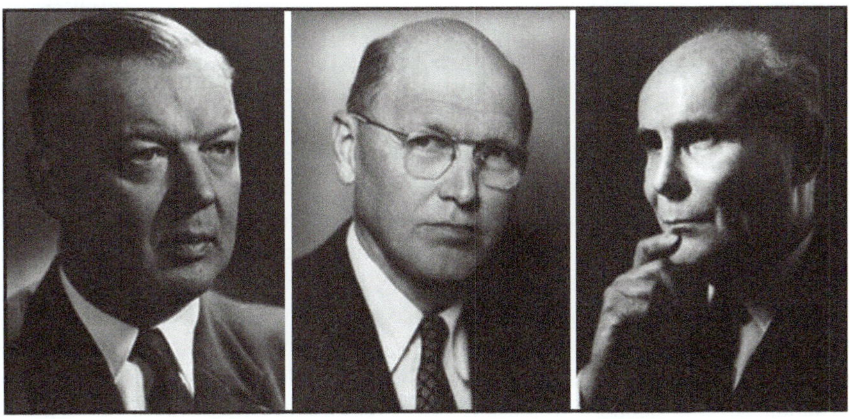

Fig. 5.6 The three awardees of the Nobel prize in 1956: Werner Forssmann, Dickinson W. Richards, and André F. Cournand

Although Cournand believed that blood withdrawn from the right atrium was mixed venous blood, in 1944 Holt and Knoefel suggested that true mixing did not occur in the right atrium [11]. Moreover, Warren found significant differences in oxygen saturation between the right atrium and the right ventricle [12]. In 1947, Dexter confirmed these findings and remarked that in order to obtain true mixed venous blood, sampling from the pulmonary artery is required [44]. During the same year, Dexter and co-workers applied the use of right cardiac catheterization to the study of complex congenital heart diseases, reporting the following findings:

1. In patent ductus arteriosus, blood from the pulmonary artery is more highly oxygenated than blood from the right ventricle.
2. In ventricular septal defects, blood from the right ventricle is more highly oxygenated than blood from the right atrium.
3 In tetralogy of Fallot, pulmonary stenosis can be identified by a higher systolic pressure in the right ventricle compared with the pulmonary artery, and in some patients the catheter can be introduced through the ventricular septal defect and into the aorta.
4. In atrial septal defects, the defect itself may be recognized by passage of the catheter into the left atrium, or by the evidence of arterial oxygenated blood in the right atrium among patients with a left to right shunt [45].

The assessment of pulmonary flow dynamics was further advanced in 1948, when Hellems and Dexter first described and measured pulmonary capillary wedge pressure in animal models and then in humans [46, 47]. Hellems, Dexter, and their co-workers were able to advance under fluoroscopic guidance a cardiac catheter into a small branch of the pulmonary artery obstructing the arterial vessel lumen (i.e., the wedge position) in an attempt to measure downstream pressure. The authors were correctly convinced that the pressure transmitted to the obstructing catheter was from the pulmonary capillary bed of the lung. They reported that the average mean occlusion pressure was 10 mmHg, ranging from 7 to 15 mmHg; the average systolic pulmonary artery pressure was 24 mmHg, ranging from 19 to 30 mmHg; and the average diastolic pulmonary artery pressure was 10 mmHg, ranging from 6 to 17 mmHg. In addition, by performing blood samples for the catheter the authors also observed the absence of significant pre-capillary admixture of bronchial arterial with pulmonary arterial blood (venous saturated blood) [48]. In a further investigation of healthy patients, the same authors calculated that the average work of the right ventricle at rest was 0.89 kg/m/min/BSA $m^2$ [49]. In 1953, Lategola and Rahn published an interesting report on their 2-year experience with a pulmonary artery catheter with a balloon fixed to the tip [50]. They showed that this catheter followed the blood flow into the pulmonary artery without the need for fluoroscopic guidance. Notably, the authors successfully verified the ease of catheter placement by asking medical students and other non-experienced staff members to place the catheter into the pulmonary artery only by watching pressure changes on the manometer.

## References

1. Greenberg SB, Murphy GS, Vender JS (2009) Current use of the pulmonary artery catheter. Curr Opin Crit Care 15:249–253
2. Kahwash R, Leier CV, Miller L (2009) Role of the pulmonary artery catheter in diagnosis and management of heart failure. Heart Fail Clin 5:241–248

3. Fife WP, Lee BS (1965) Construction and use of self-guiding, right heart and pulmonary artery catheter. J Appl Physiol 20:148–149
4. Cournand A (1975) Cardiac catheterization; development of the technique, its contributions to experimental medicine, and its initial applications in man. Acta Med Scand Suppl 579:3–32
5. Goldhaber SZ (1993) Angioplasty or coronary bypass graft? Lancet 341:599–600
6. Baim DS (2005) Cardiac catheterization-history and current practice standards. Grossman's cardiac catheterization, angiography, and intervention. Lippincott Williams and Wilkins, Philadelphia
7. Cournand AF, Lauson H, Bloomfield R et al (1944) Recording of right heart pressures in man. Proc Soc Exp Biol Med 55:34–36
8. Richardson MS, Reddy VD (1994) Floating around. Use of the pulmonary artery (Swan-Ganz) catheter in critical care. Chest 105:643
9. Cournand A, Riley RL, Breed ES et al (1945) Measurement of cardiac output in man using the technique of catheterization of the right auricle or ventricle. J Clin Invest 24:106–116
10. Valentine PA, Fluck DC, Mounsey JP et al (1966) Blood-gas changes after acute myocardial infarction. Lancet 2:837–841
11. Holt JP, Knoefel PK (1944) Oxygen content of blood in right auricle and right ventricle. Fed Proc 3:19
12. Warren JV, Stead EA Jr, Brannon ES (1946) The cardiac output in man: a study of some of the errors in the method of right heart catheterization. Am J Physiol 145:458–464
13. Baroni W (1972) Arrigo montanari e il sondaggio cardiovasale. In: Proceedings of the 23rd Congress of the History of Medicine, London, 2–9 Sept 1972
14. Berry D (2009) Pioneers in cardiology. Werner Forssmann—sowing the seeds for selective cardiac catheterization procedures in the twentieth century. Eur Heart J 30:1296–1297
15. Lewis O (1994) Stephen Hales and the measurement of blood pressure. J Hum Hypertens 8:865–871
16. Felts JH (1977) Stephen Hales and the measurement of blood pressure. N C Med J 38:602–603
17. Hoff HE, Geddes LA, McCrady JD (1965) The contributions of the horse to knowledge of the heart and circulation. 1. Stephen Hales and the measurement of blood pressure. Conn Med 29:795–800
18. Bourassa MG (2005) The history of cardiac catheterization. Can J Cardiol 21:1011–1014
19. Acierno LJ (1994) Radiologic methods. Taylor and Francis, London
20. Welch GR (1991) Thermodynamics and living systems: problems and paradigms. J Nutr 121:1902–1906
21. Cournand A (1980) Historical details of Claude Bernard's invention of a technique for measuring the temperature and the pressure of the blood within the cavities of the heart. Trans N Y Acad Sci 39:1–14
22. Forssmann-Falck R (1997) Werner Forssmann: a pioneer of cardiology. Am J Cardiol 79:651–660
23. Forssmann W (1929) Die Sondierung der rechten Herzens. Klin Wchnschr 8:2085
24. Mueller RL, Sanborn TA (1995) The history of interventional cardiology: cardiac catheterization, angioplasty, and related interventions. Am Heart J 129:146–172
25. Klein O (1930) Zur Bestimmung des zirkulatorischen Minutenvolumens beim Menschen nach dem Fickschen Prinzip mittels Herzsondierung. Munchen Med Wchnschr 77:1311–1312
26. Cournand A, Ranges HA (1941) Catheterization of the right auricle in man. Proc Soc Exp Biol Med 46:462
27. Cournand A, Bryan NA, Richards DW (1935) Cardiac output in relation to unilateral pneumothorax in man. J Clin Invest 14:181–189
28. Lassen HC, Cournand A, Richards DW (1937) Distribution of respiratory gases in a closed breathing circuit. I. In normal subjects. J Clin Invest 16:1–7
29. Cournand A, Lassen HC, Richards DW (1937) Distribution of respiratory gases in a closed breathing circuit. II. Pulmonary fibrosis and emphysema. J Clin Invest 16:9–14

30. Richards DW, Cournand A, Rappaport I (1935) Relation of the regulatory mechanism of respiration to clinical dyspnea. Proc Natl Acad Sci U S A 21:498–501
31. Richards DW, Cournand A, Bryan NA (1935) Applicability of rebreathing method for determining mixed venous CO2 in cases of chronic pulmonary disease. J Clin Invest 14:173–180
32. Berseus S, Lagerlof H, Werko L (1950) A comparison between the direct Fick and the Grollman methods for determination of the cardiac output in man. Acta Med Scand Suppl 239:258
33. Hamilton WF, Riley RL, Attyah A et al (1948) Comparison of the Fick and dye injection methods of measuring the cardiac output in man. Am J Physiol 153:309–321
34. Cournand A, Ranges HA, Riley RL (1942) Comparison of results of the normal ballistocardiogram and a direct Fick method in measuring the cardiac output in man. J Clin Invest 21:287–294
35. Richards DW (1945) Cardiac output by the catheterization technique, in various clinical conditions. Fed Proc 4:215–220
36. Bloomfield RA, Lauson HD, Cournand A et al (1946) Recording of right heart pressures in normal subjects and in patients with chronic pulmonary disease and various types of cardio-circulatory disease. J Clin Invest 25:639–664
37. Cournand A (1947) Recent observations on the dynamics of the pulmonary circulation. Bull N Y Acad Med 23:27–50
38. Cournand A (1950) Some aspects of the pulmonary circulation in normal man and in chronic cardiopulmonary diseases. Circulation 2:641–657
39. 'Cathcart RT, Field WW, Richards DW Jr (1953) Comparison of cardiac output determined by the ballistocardiograph (Nickerson apparatus) and by the direct Fick method. J Clin Invest 32:5–14
40. Harvey RM, Enson Y, Cournand A et al (1965) Cardiac output in cor pulmonale. Arch Kreislaufforsch 46:7–16
41. Cournand A, Motley HL, Werko L et al (1948) Physiological studies of the effects of intermittent positive pressure breathing on cardiac output in man. Am J Physiol 152:162–174
42. Fritts HW Jr, Harris P, Chidsey CA III et al (1957) Validation of a method for measuring the output of the right ventricle in man by inscription of dye-dilution curves from the pulmonary artery. J Appl Physiol 11:362–364
43. Raju TN (1999) The Nobel chronicles. 1956: Werner Forssmann (1904–1979); Andre Frederic Cournand (1895–1988); and Dickinson Woodruff Richards, Jr (1895–1973). Lancet 353:1891
44. Dexter L, Haynes FW, Burwell CS et al (1947) Studies of congenital heart disease. II. The pressure and oxygen content of blood in the right auricle, right ventricle, and pulmonary artery in control patients, with observations on the oxygen saturation and source of pulmonary "capillary" blood. J Clin Invest 26:554–560
45. Dexter L, Haynes FW, Burwell CS et al (1947) Studies of congenital heart disease. III. Venous catheterization as a diagnostic aid in patent ductus arteriosus, tetralogy of Fallot, ventricular septal defect, and auricular septal defect. J Clin Invest 26:561–576
46. Hellems HK, Haynes FW, Dexter L (1949) Pulmonary capillary pressure in man. J Appl Physiol 2:24–29
47. Hellems HK, Haynes FW, Dexter L et al (1948) Pulmonary capillary pressure in animals estimated by venous and arterial catheterization. Am J Physiol 155:98–105
48. Hellems HK, Haynes FW, Dexter L (1948) Pulmonary capillary pressure in man. J Clin Invest 27:540
49. Dexter L, Dow JW, Haynes FW et al (1950) Studies of the pulmonary circulation in man at rest; normal variations and the interrelations between increate pulmonary blood flow, elevated pulmonary arterial pressure, and high pulmonary "capillary" pressures. J Clin Invest 29:602–613
50. Lategola M, Rahn H (1953) A self-guiding catheter for cardiac and pulmonary arterial catheterization and occlusion. Proc Soc Exp Biol Med 84:667–668

# The History of Mitral and Tricuspid Valve Surgery Before the Advent of Cardiopulmonary Bypass

6

Luigi Chiariello, Paolo Nardi and Giovanni Alfonso Chiariello

*Intellectuals solve problems, geniuses prevent them.*
Albert Einstein


**Abstract**

The history of mitral valve surgery runs parallel to the development of heart surgery, as at the turn of the last century rheumatic fever was an epidemic disease that led to late cardiac valve lesions, mostly to mitral stenosis. The year 1948 was historically an important step in the development of closed mitral surgery: on 10 June Bailey performed his first successful commissurotomy and on 16 June Harken performed his first valvuloplasty. Closed mitral valve surgery should be considered one of the most relevant landmarks of heart surgery especially because, focusing on the basic concepts of anatomy and physiopathology of the mitral valve, a simple and effective therapeutic procedure was developed, that briefly became one of the most diffuse cardiac operations performed. Once satisfactory results were obtained and mortality became consistently low, the fate of thousands of patients with rheumatic mitral stenosis dramatically changed. Closed mitral valvuloplasty was considered for long time to be a very effective procedure, in spite of the introduction and diffusion of open heart surgery: thus, until the 1970s most surgeons advised closed valvulotomy as the primary operation in all patients with mitral stenosis.


The history of mitral valve surgery runs parallel to the development of heart surgery, as at the turn of the last century rheumatic fever was an epidemic disease that led to late cardiac valve lesions, mostly to mitral valve stenosis [1, 2]. In fact, cardiac surgery has its origins in closed mitral valve surgery.


L. Chiariello (✉) · P. Nardi · G. A. Chiariello
Department of Cardiac Surgery, Tor Vergata University of Rome,
Fondazione Policlinico Tor Vergata, Viale Oxford 81, 00133 Rome, Italy
e-mail: lchiariello@tiscali.it



M. Picichè (ed.), *Dawn and Evolution of Cardiac Procedures*,
DOI: 10.1007/978-88-470-2400-7_6, © Springer-Verlag Italia 2013

In 1902 Sir Lauder Brunton, a Scottish physician, after preliminary experiments on human cadavers and cats, suggested that stenotic lesions of the mitral valve might be susceptible to surgical intervention [3, 4]. Sir Brunton focused on three major problems: the method of enlarging the valve orifice, the surgical approach to the heart, the appropriate surgical instruments. He stated that "elongating the natural opening" of the valve was possible just by incising the leaflets in the middle. Regarding the surgical approach, he chose the left ventricle, believing that the thick ventricular wall would be less prone to bleeding than the thinner left atrium. However, Sir Brunton was criticized by surgeons of his day because he did not provide convincing experimental evidence that could subvert the current opinion of the "inviolable heart" [2, 5, 6]. Carrel and Tuffier in 1914 published their important paper "Chirurgie des orifices du coeur", in which they concluded, based on animal experiments, that mitral stenosis under certain well-defined conditions might benefit from surgical intervention [2, 3].

## 6.1 Elliot Cutler and Sir Henry Souttar

It took another 10 years before the first clinical successes were reported by Cutler and Souttar. Elliot Cutler in 1923 performed 7 valvulotomies at the Peter Bent Brigham Hospital in Boston with a transventricular mitral valvotome. Only one patient survived and, consequently, after 6 postoperative deaths from massive mitral regurgitation, he abandoned the procedure. While describing his intervention, Cutler underlined the difficulty in locating the mitral valve: "we feel at the present time that the orientation within the heart is one of the most serious problems". Another problem was conceptual: in the blind valvulotomy, mitral stenosis could progress into regurgitation, which had been the leading cause of death in the Cutler's series [5, 7, 8].

On 6 May 1925, at the London Hospital, Sir Henry Souttar performed the first finger dilatation of the mitral valve, using a transatrial approach. He inserted his right index finger into the left atrium of Lily Hines, a 19-year-old girl who had mitral stenosis and regurgitation. The patient improved clinically and survived for 5 years, subsequently dying from cerebral embolus. However, Souttar's first successful valvuloplasty was also his last one, as he explained in his letter to Dwight Harken: "I did not repeat the operation because I could not get another case" [5, 9]. The lack of progress in mitral valve surgery was likely caused by the fact that physicians at that time believed that patient's clinical problems were related to the cardiomyopathy rather than to the narrowed valve orifice [2, 5]. Moreover, in the 1920s the number of failed cases was high enough to discourage continuation of such an experimental operation: it is therefore not surprising that two more decades elapsed before surgery on the mitral valve became a reality.

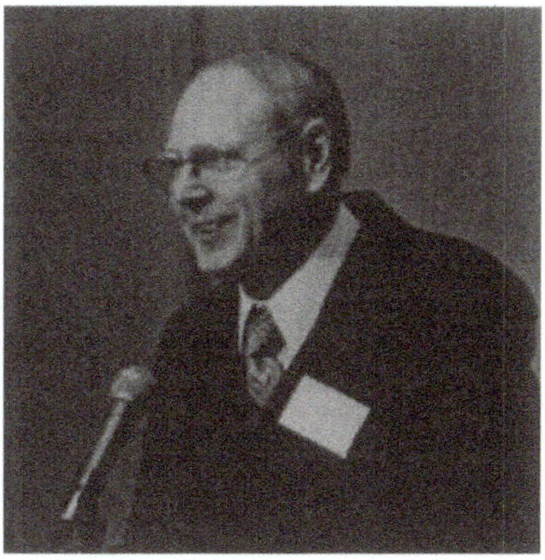

**Fig. 6.1** Charles P. Bailey (1910–1993) (With the permission of Elsevier [1], Copyright Elsevier, 1998)

## 6.2 The Golden Year

Charles Philamore Bailey (1910–1993), Dwight Harken (1910–1993), and Russell Brock (1903–1981) represented the new generation of pioneering surgeons believing in mitral valve surgery. In the 1940s, several American teams were facing the problem of mitral stenosis. Bland and Sweet (1949) proposed a venous shunt operation in which an anastomosis was made between the azygos vein and a branch of the inferior pulmonary vein, aiming to reduce the high pressure in the pulmonary circulation [6]. However, these operations, although possibly offering symptomatic relief, did not treat the valvular obstruction and the impaired function of the right side of the heart.

The year 1948 represented historically a step in the development of closed mitral valve surgery: on 10 June the first successful Bailey's commissurotomy and on 16 June Harken's first valvuloplasty were performed (Figs. 6.1, 6.2) [1, 2, 5, 8, 10–12].

It is questionable whether, under today's ethical standards, they could have gone through those failures, but once the techniques as well as the indications were established, hundreds and thousands of patients were relieved from the misery of terminal mitral stenosis.

Bailey's first surgical success was preceded by four deaths [1, 10]. His first patient died in the operating room because of bleeding from the distended left atrium before anything had been done to the mitral valve (14 November 1945, Hahnemann Medical College). In his second case (12 June 1946), the patient's clinical condition deteriorated rapidly during anesthesia and the surgeon initially decided to desist. However, encouraged by his colleagues, Bailey once again reattempted to open the mitral valve, unsuccessfully with an instrument and subsequently with his finger, this time eliminating the murmur. The patient died 48 h later and at the autopsy the valve was widely open. After these two deaths Bailey became the target of numerous derogatory comments and some colleagues termed him "the butcher".

Bailey's third attempt was performed on 22 March 1948 at the Memorial Hospital in Wilmington: the patient had a very tight valve with severe calcification, which was opened with a hooked knife. Because of the thrombotic

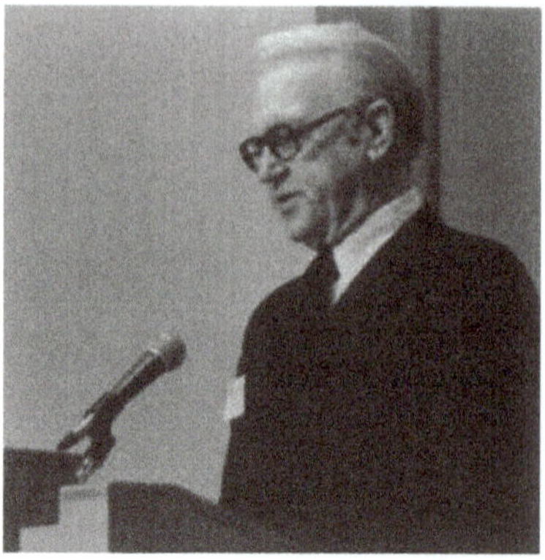

**Fig. 6.2** Dwight E. Harken (1910–1993) (With the permission of Elsevier [1], Copyright Elsevier, 1998)

complications in his second case, this time he did use heparin in the postoperative period. The patient's clinical condition significantly improved in the first 2 days, but then the patient began to bleed and required a large amount of transfusion leading on the third postoperative day to a fatal pulmonary edema.

The fourth and fifth operations were performed on the same day (10 June 1948). In the fourth case Bailey decided to operate with the patient in the face-down position (probably because of a history of bronchiectasis). The heart arrested and during cardiac massage a digital mitral dilatation was performed, but the patient died. The fifth patient was operated upon on the same day at the Episcopal Hospital in Philadelphia: the patient, Mrs. Melville Claire Ward, a young woman who had been affected by rheumatic fever since the age of 7 years, presented long-lasting symptoms of severe dyspnea and congestive heart failure. A hooked knife and the surgeon's finger were used to open the anterolateral mitral commissure; the entire operation lasted 80 min.

After the operation Mrs. Claire Ward was out of bed on the third postoperative day and went home after a week. On her 10th postoperative day she attended the Annual Meeting of the College of Chest Physicians in Chicago, to which she had travelled by train from Philadelphia. Subsequently, Bailey reported 8 % surgical mortality in a series of 811 cases of mitral commissurotomy that had been performed using various forms of knife and guillotine adapted to the curve of the index finger. Two years after the operation at the Episcopal Hospital, mitral valve surgery was being performed widely throughout the world.

Dwight Harken, the first surgeon who had performed a series of elective operations on the heart against the backdrop of the Second World War, performed his first successful operation on the mitral valve in Boston on 16 June 1948, only 6 days after Mrs. Melville's operation, although he was completely unaware of the earlier event. Previously, he had lost only one patient on 22 March 1947: the valve had been approached through the pulmonary vein. In his second, successful case, the left atrial appendage approach was preferred. In both cases he used an instrument to cut out the fused leaflets at the commissures (Harken's punch valvulotome): Harken believed that a certain amount of mitral regurgitation would inevitably result from the procedure, but this would be better tolerated than the preoperative severe mitral stenosis.

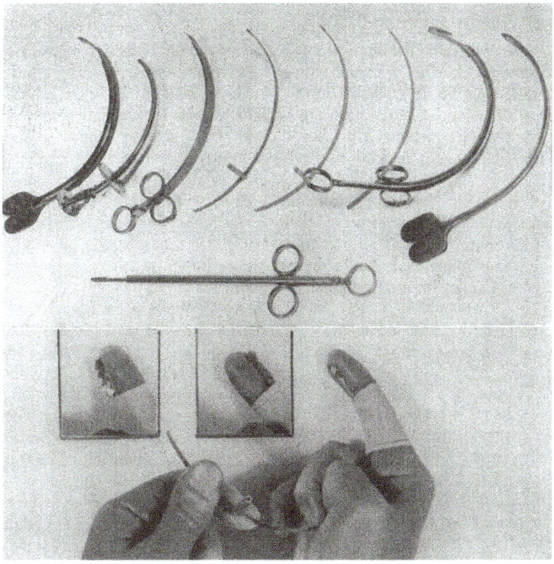

**Fig. 6.3** Several types of valvulotomes *top* developed by Bailey and Harken. Bread knife valvulotome *bottom* with finger recess for insertion into the auricle to treat anterior and posterior fusion. (With the permission of the Copyright Clearance Center. Publisher: Wolters Kluwer health, [12], Copyright, the Copyright Clearance Center, 1951)

Therefore, he proposed to name this kind of operation "mitral valvuloplasty". Moreover, the initially adopted cutting instruments were subsequently abandoned, because he found that the commissures could be better opened by lateral or medial digital pressure (finger-fracture valvuloplasty) [1, 9–12].

Bailey and Robert Glower (Bailey's partner at the Episcopal Hospital) performed mitral commissurotomy in 932 patients with a mortality rate improving from 33 % in 1949 to 5 % in 1959, and 6.2 % cumulative mortality over the decade. In 1964, Harken and his group reported similar results in 1,571 patients over a 12-year period [13]. Bailey and Harken were true pioneers of closed heart surgery: they learned to suture cardiac lesions, to control blood loss from the appendage, to defibrillate the heart and, later on, progressively learned to be selective in indications. They also developed several types of valvulotomes to treat mitral stenosis (Fig. 6.3).

In Europe Lord Russell Claude Brock (1903–1986), a surgeon already well-known for the so-called Brock operation, a closed pulmonary valvulotomy and infundibulectomy for congenital pulmonic stenosis, performed his first mitral valvulotomy on 16 September 1948, reaching the same gratifying results of the two American pioneering surgeons, although unaware of their experience [14]. He described his own cases at the 1949 meeting of the American College of Surgeons where Bailey, Glover, and O'Neill also presented their famous paper on a number of successful commissurotomies (Fig. 6.4).

Another important contribution to closed mitral surgery was made by Charles Dubost (1914–1991). The French surgeon made mitral commissurotomy a much easier and more effective operation by introducing in 1951 a new mechanically expandable dilatator inserted safely through the auricular appendage; however, nowadays, this instrument is called the Tubbs dilatator, after the name of the British surgeon, Oswald Tubbs [2]. Also, a major contribution should be attributed to Horace Smithy, who

**Fig. 6.4** The Brock technique to treat mitral stenosis. **a** The correct way to incise the stenosed valve is along the line of the lateral and medial commissures. The mobility of the valve cusps is restored without impairment of mitral regurgitation. **b** If circular portions of the valve are incised, even at the site of the commissures, regurgitation will certainly follow. **c** A thin sliver can be excised along the line of the commissures and may confer greater valvular mobility. (With the permission of British Medical Journal Publishing Group [12], copyright British Medical Journal Publishing Group Ltd, 1950)

operated on a young woman with an end-stage mitral stenosis in Charleston, South Carolina, USA, 5 months before Harken and Bailey. Smithy himself suffered from rheumatic aortic stenosis and died of progressive congestive heart failure at the age of 34 (28 October 1948), 270 days after his first mitral operation. Unfortunately, his premature death prevented him from receiving acknowledgment of his achievements [15, 16]. Bailey, in his unpublished manuscript in 1988, mentioned Smithy's cases and noted that 2 of the 5 original survivors were still alive in 1955 [1]. Another important contribution to the development of mitral surgery was made by the Russian surgeon Nikolai Terebinski (1880–1959), who in Moscow, between 1920 and 1930, had experimented with a device intended to exclude the circulatory system in animals and to perform open heart valve surgery. From 1929 to 1937 he performed a total of 298 closed heart procedures in dogs, 216 of them consisting of creating stenosis or insufficiency of the mitral and tricuspid valves. Terebinski also described the excellent exposure provided by left ventriculotomy [17, 18].

## 6.3 Mitral Regurgitation and Multiple Valvular Disease

Before the advent of cardiopulmonary bypass some valve repair techniques for mitral insufficiency had also been developed by Bailey and Harken, who faced the problem of the correction of regurgitation onset in patients primarily operated on for mitral stenosis. Bailey's approach was to try to control the regurgitation with a pericardial patch placed across the left ventricular inflow below the valve orifice [19]. Harken, instead, proposed a spindle baffle passed obliquely through the mitral valve orifice and anchored in the ventricular wall [20].

The first surgical treatment of multiple valvular disease in the closed heart era was performed by Trace and colleagues: on 2 May 1952, in a 24-year-old woman, after a closed mitral commissurotomy, the right auricular appendage was severely distended and the rhythm had changed into atrial fibrillation. Tricuspid commissurotomy was performed 2 weeks later and the patient made a good recovery. The paper describing this case was published by Trace et al. 2 years later [21].

**Table 6.1** Operative results of closed mitral valvuloplasty for rheumatic disease

| Reference | Number of patients | Operative mortality, *n* (%) |
|---|---|---|
| [14] | 9 | 2 (22.2) |
| [12] | 86 | 20 (23.3) |
| [27] | 100 | 13 (13) |
| [28] | 462 | 27 (5.8) |
| [1] | 932 | 58 (6.2) |
| [29] | 472 | 18 (3.8) |
| [30] | 1,000 | 87 (8.7) |
| [31] | 367 | 6 (1.6) |

Combined mitral and tricuspid commissurotomy was also performed by Brofman in 1953 [22]. In 1955, Likoff reported a series of 74 patients who underwent closed combined aortic and mitral valve commissurotomy [23]. Only after the introduction of extracorporeal circulation in 1953 were techniques for mitral commissural or prosthetic ring annuloplasty for the treatment of mitral regurgitation introduced by Kay et al. and subsequently by Carpentier and Duran et al. [24–26].

## 6.4 Conclusions

From the analysis of early surgical results in the 1950s, it was quite soon evident that closed mitral valve surgery, in selected cases, provided an effective long-term palliation with low morbidity and mortality rates. Surgical indications and technique were standardized. Some clinical and pathological conditions were recognized as relative or absolute contraindications: the presence of active rheumatism (because of the risk of a new attack especially in adolescent patients), major mitral regurgitation, heavily calcified annulus, thrombi inside the auricular appendage or left atrium, involvement of the aortic valve, and secondary right-sided heart failure.

Since 1948, the overall operative risk has decreased steadily (Table 6.1). Despite the spread of open heart surgery, closed mitral valvuloplasty has been considered for some decades to be an effective procedure; thus, up to the 1970s most surgeons would continue to recommend this procedure as the primary operation in patients with mitral stenosis.

## References

1. Davila JC (1998) The birth of intracardiac surgery: a semicentennial tribute (June 10, 1948–1998). Ann Thorac Surg 65:1809–1820
2. Naef AP (2004) The mid-century revolution in thoracic and cardiovascular surgery: part 5. Interact Cardiovasc Thorac Surg 3:415–422

3. Murray G, Wilkinson FR, Mackenzie R (1938) Reconstruction of the valves of the heart. Can Med Ass J 4:317–320
4. Brunton L (1902) Possibility of treating mitral stenosis by surgical methods. Lancet 1:35
5. Khan MN (1996) The relief of mitral stenosis. An historic step in cardiac surgery. Tex Heart Inst J 23:258–265
6. Barber JM, Smiley TB, Marshall R (1950) Valvulotomy for mitral stenosis. Ulster Med J 19:186–189
7. Cutler EC, Beck CS (1925) The present status of the surgical procedures in chronic valvular disease of the heart. Arch Surg 18:403–416
8. Gonzalez-Lavin L, Bailey C, Harken D (1992) The dawn of the modern era of mitral valve surgery. Ann Thorac Surg 53:916
9. Harken D (1967) Heart surgery—legend and a long look. Am J Cardiol 19:393–401
10. Dobell AR (1996) Rival trailblazers: the origin of successful closed valvular surgery. Ann Thorac Surg 61:750–754
11. Harken DE, Ellis LB, Ware PF et al (1948) The surgical treatment of mitral stenosis—valvuloplasty. N Engl J Med 239:801–809
12. Harken DE, Dexter L, Ellis LB et al (1951) The surgery of mitral stenosis: finger-fracture valvuloplasty. Ann Surg 134:722–741
13. Ellis LB, Harken DE (1964) Closed valvuloplasty for mitral stenosis: a twelve year study on 1571 patients. N Engl J Med 270:643
14. Baker C, Brock RC, Campbell M (1950) Valvulotomy for mitral stenosis. Report of six successful cases. Br Med J 3:1283–1293
15. Crawford FA (1996) The origins of successful closed valvular surgery. Ann Thorac Surg 62:628–629
16. Crawford FA (2010) Horace Smithy: pioneer heart surgeon. Ann Thorac Surg 89:2067–2071
17. Alexi-Meskishvili VV, Potapov EV, Beyer EA et al (1998) Nikolai Terebinski: a pioneer of the open valve operation. Ann Thorac Surg 66:1440–1443
18. Terebinski N (1938) Experimental stenosis of the atrioventricular valves of the heart and their repair. Khirurgia 12:36–43
19. Bailey CP, Jamison WL, Bakst AE et al (1954) The surgical correction of mitral insufficiency by the use of pericardial grafts. J Thorac Surg 28:551–603
20. Harken DE, Black H, Ellis LB et al (1954) The surgical correction of mitral insufficiency. J Thorac Surg 28:604–623
21. Trace HD, Bailey CP, Wendkos MH (1954) Tricuspid commissurotomy with a one year of follow-up. Am Heart J 47:613–618
22. Brofman BL (1953) Right auriculoventricular pressure gradients with special reference to tricuspid stenosis. J Lab Clin Med 42:789
23. Likoff W, Berkowitz D, Denton C et al (1955) A clinical evaluation of surgical treatment of combined mitral and aortic stenosis. Am Heart J 49:394–406
24. Kay JH, Zubiate P, Mendez MA et al (1978) Mitral valve repair for significant mitral insufficiency. Am Heart J 96:253–262
25. Carpentier A (1983) Cardiac valve surgery: the "French correction". J Thorac Cardiovasc Surg 86:323–337
26. Duran CG, Pomar JL, Revuelta JM et al (1980) Conservative operation for mitral insufficiency. Critical analysis supported by postoperative hemodynamic studies of 72 patients. J Thorac Cardiovasc Surg 79:326–337
27. Baker C, Brock RC, Campbell M et al (1952) Valvotomy for mitral stenosis; a further report, on 100 cases. Br Med J 17:1043–1055
28. Bailey CP, Zimmerman J, Likoff W (1960) The complete relief of mitral stenosis. Ten years of progress towards this goal. Chest 37:661–674
29. Glenn WW, Calabrese C, Goodyear AV et al (1969) Mitral valvulotomy. Open results after closed valvulotomy: a report of 500 cases. Am J Surg 117:493–501

30. Ellis LB, Singh JB, Morales DD et al (1973) Fifteen- to twenty-year study of one thousand patients undergoing closed mitral valvuloplasty. Circulation XLVIII:357–364
31. Augested KM, Martyushova K, Fedorov B et al (2000) Closed mitral commissurotomy in Archangel, Northern Russia, 1965–1993. Operative assessment of 367 patients operated on for rheumatic mitral stenosis. Scand Cardiovasc J 34:533–535

# 7 Surgery of the Aortic Valve Before the Era of Cardiopulmonary Bypass

Yves Glock

*On ne connaît pas complètement une science tant qu'on n'en sait pas l'histoire.*

Auguste Comte

**Abstract**

At the end of the 19th century, Stephen Paget and Theodore Billroth affirmed the unprofessional and unethical nature of the surgical approach to the human heart, with cardiac surgeons "losing the respect of their colleagues". 9 September 1896 is thus frequently not universally considered the birth of cardiac surgery, with the first successful repair of a right ventricular stab wound by Ludwig Rehn, a German surgeon. Lillehei and colleagues noted that "the outer wall of the living human heart represented a seemingly impenetrable anatomical barrier to the surgeon's knife". The challenge for the cardiac surgeons was to cross this barrier. The conquest of aortic valve surgery was carried out step by step: a blind approach first, followed a few years later by plasties under direct vision (allowed owing to techniques of hypothermia and bicaval clamping), leading to the avanguardist concept of aortic valve prosthesis implanted without cardiopulmonary bypass (CPB) by Hufnagel. Nowadays, trans-arterial aortic valve implantation is performed by the HEART TEAM, an association of surgeons, interventional cardiologists, echocardiographists and anaesthesiologists in a hybrid operating theatre.

At the end of the 19th century, Stephen Paget and Theodore Billroth affirmed the unprofessional and unethical nature of the surgical approach to the human heart, with cardiac surgeons "losing the respect of their colleagues" [1]. 9 September 1896, is not universally considered (see Chap. 3) the birth of cardiac surgery, with

Y. Glock (✉)
Department of Cardio-vascular Surgery, Rangueil University hospital,
1, Avenue J. Poulhes, TSA 50032, 31059 Toulouse, France
e-mail: glock.y@chu-toulouse.fr

M. Picichè (ed.), *Dawn and Evolution of Cardiac Procedures*,
DOI: 10.1007/978-88-470-2400-7_7, © Springer-Verlag Italia 2013

the first successful repair of a right ventricular stab wound by Ludwig Rehn, a German surgeon [2].

Lillehei and colleagues [3] note that "the outer wall of the living human heart represented a seemingly impenetrable anatomical barrier to the surgeon's knife". The challenge for the cardiac surgeons was to cross this barrier.

The conquest of the aortic valve surgery was carried out step by step: a blind approach first, followed a few years later by plasties under direct vision (allowed owing to techniques of hypothermia and bicaval clamping), leading to the avanguardist concept of aortic valve prosthesis implanted without cardiopulmonary bypass (CPB) by Hufnagel [3–27].

> As Brock wrote with an anticipatory view of the future of cardiac surgery:
> "Intracardiac surgery is not for the lone worker: TEAM Work is essential…the success is due principally to the loyal and unstained cooperation of various colleagues…" [4]

Nowadays, trans-arterial aortic valve implantation is performed by the HEART-TEAM, an association of surgeons, interventional cardiologists, echocardiographists and anaesthesiologists in an hybrid operating theatre.

## 7.1 Aortic Stenosis

### 7.1.1 First Indirect and Direct Aortic Valvulotomy

In 1872, an ophthalmologist named Becker [5] was the first to approach the aortic valve in the dog in a retrograde way: to demonstrate that in aortic valve insufficiency the magnified pulse seen in the eyegrounds was not due to something intrinsic in the eye, but to the regurgitation. He destroyed one of the cusps using a glass rod.

Haecker [6] studied experimental aortic stenosis using a constrictive suture above the origin of the aorta: only one of the three operated animals survived.

The first approach to correcting aortic valvulopathy, mainly post-rheumatic stenosis, was performed during blind operations.

In Paris, the French surgeon Theodore-Marin Tuffier (1857–1929) [7] can be considered a pioneer in thoracic and cardiovascular surgery in the field of clinical and experimental research. In collaboration at the New York Rockfeller Institute with Alexis Carrel (1873–1944), he published in 1914 many cases of valve surgery with caval occlusion in animals: all died of cerebral anoxia, but the heart tolerated these procedures. In 1913 he dilated the aortic valve by invagination of the aortic wall across the pathological valve: the improved patient survived for 10 years.

In 1946, Brock (London) designed an "operating cardioscope or combined valvoscope and valvulotome" and tried it on a patient in a case of aortic stenosis (27 March 1947) [4, 8].

By a short incision in the neck, the right subclavian artery was exposed to introduce the cardioscope: this instrument allows a good view of the "irregular calcified masses which distorted the diseased valve". Brock realized "that an attempt to cut this calcified valve semi-blindly with the small knife attached to the instrument was unlikely to be successful enough to justifiy the risk involved. The instrument was withdrawn".

### 7.1.2 The Unrealised Hope of Doctor Smithy

In the same year, Horace Smithy, using an experimental retrograde approach to the aortic valve, described the dangers of the aortic valvulotomy [11–14]. This native Virginian surgeon (born on 19 July 1914) studied medicine at Virginia University: after purchasing his first stethoscope, he detected a systolic aortic murmur in his own heart!

His experimental work on dogs about the possibilities of relieving rheumatic mitral and aortic stenosis was presented at the Surgical Forum of the American College of Surgeons in 1946 in Cleveland: he introduced a knife-like valvulotome (designed by Smithy and Coleman) through the ascending aorta and increased the opening of the stenosed aortic valve. In New York, at the 1947 American College of Surgeons he completed this demonstration. On 30 January 1948, he performed with success a mitral valvulotomy on a 21-year-old woman. The New York Times proclaimed: "New heart operation saves life of woman as surgeon cuts into valve he cannot see". Sending his valvulotome to Alfred Blalock, Smithy would have liked to convince him to attempt the opening of his own aortic valve stenosis. Unfortunately he died of heart failure at the age of 34 before the intervention.

The first attempt at instrumental aortic commissurotomy was made in 1950 by Bailey using retrograde introduction via the carotid artery of a dilatator across the stenotic valve [10–12]. The later anterograde transventricular approach to the aortic valve using a cutting valvotome and then using an expanding dilatator to split the valve open induced regurgitations and was unsatisfactory and abandoned after 65 patients had undergone the operation [15–17].

The transaortic route was soon dogmatically stated as the "only route that should even be considered" [8].

The blindness had two consequences:

- It can be dangerous because of the risk of perforation of either the aorta or the cusp, inducing haemorrhage or regurgitation.
- It can be ineffective because of the resistance of the calcified tissue with residual stenosis.

These limitations of the closed techniques led surgeons to search for the possibilities of direct vision of the valve.

### 7.1.3 The Way Towards Open-Heart Procedures

The cross-clamping of the inflow procedure in normothermia developed as follows:

In 1907, Haecker [6] appeared to have been the first to use the technique of cardiac inflow occlusion to temporarily exclude the heart from the circulation for direct visualisation procedures on the dog. Later, Sauerbruck and Rehn [18] confirmed his work [2]. Laewen and Sievers demonstrated on a rabbit that inflow occlusion was better tolerated than outflow occlusion: as Kiser established, the over-distension of the heart was the primary cause of death with outflow obstruction [19].

On 10 April 1914, Carrel presented a lecture before the American Surgical Association on the "experimental operations on the orifices of the heart". He was the first to point out the necessity of direct vision to repair the aortic valve. After cross-clamping of the "pedicle" of the dog's heart following hyperventilation he could safely open the aorta to approach the aortic valve during the course of 2.5 half to 3 min. The venting of the air in the left ventricle was done by aspiration. He concluded that "it is not impossible that someday surgeons will be able to cauterise valvular lesions or repair them as we today in our experimental operations" [9].

It would appear that total inflow tract occlusion associated with open cardiotomy in normal dogs at normal temperature can be tolerated at essentially zero risk for 1.5 min.

### 7.1.4 The Importance of Hypothermia on Metabolism

The inner approach of the cardiac cavities and valves before the CPB era was possible thanks to the research into hypothermia carried out by Wilfred Gordon Bigelow (1913–2005) [20–22].

As a resident in Toronto, he amputated frozen fingers and toes during the Canadian winter and discovered a special interest in hypothermia. In 1947, he started his own research into hypothermia in the dog at the Banting Institute of the Toronto General Hospital.

He demonstrated the linear relationship between the drop in temperature and level of metabolism slowing down the heart rate. Consecutively, he realised successful open-heart surgery on the hypothermic dog (lower than 20 °C) stopping the circulation for 15 min with a 51 % mortality rate. It was the first time that man could observe the inside of a living heart with the animal still alive. In 1950, during the Denver's meeting of the American Surgical Association, he presented the results of his research: his film of the open heart was impressive and spectators had opinions that varied between "intense interest" and "strong doubts". In 1952 Bigelow promoted this technique, opening under direct visualisation the hearts of monkeys cooled at 18 °C: all the animals survived!

Impressed by Bigelow's communication, F. John Lewis started extensive experimentation using a canine model: with moderate hypothermia (26–28 °C) and a short bi-caval cross-clamping he could under direct vision create and close an atrial septal defect, reducing the problems of ventricular fibrillation owing to deep hypothermia and coronary air embolism.

The modified Bigelow's technique associating moderate hypothermia and inflow occlusion obtained a reduction in the mortality rate of the animals: out of 10 last operated on for a septal defect, 9 survived.

### 7.1.5 Possible Approach to the Valve Under Direct Vision in Humans

The timing of human application was justified: at Minnesota University, on 2 September 1952, F. John Lewis scheduled the closure of a broad atrial septal defect in a girl aged 5 years: it was the first successful operation under direct vision within an open human heart. Other procedures to treat congenital defects (VSD, pulmonary stenosis) were performed with success [20–29]. At the level of the aortic valve, the main fear of the surgeons was the possibility of air embolism in the coronary arteries. Swann et al. [30, 31] encouraged by the open approach to the pulmonary valve for isolated stenosis, performed in 24 cases without mortality with the technique of hypothermia and caval occlusion, decided that the direct vision of the pathological aortic valve was a new surgical target. The doubt concerning the coronary air embolism disappeared after experimentation on a series of seven animals. They were able to note: "the heart was beating slowly and regularly throughout, yet as one watched the blood–air interface visible in the mouth of the left coronary ostium, no tendency for this interface to recede into the artery was apparent…"

In 1956, Julian et al. reported two cases of aortic commissurotomy under direct vision using hypothermia and inflow occlusion: the first case in a live patient was performed on 10 October 1955 [27].

On November 17, 1955, Swann operated on a man of 29 years of age who suffered from post-rheumatic aortic valve stenosis. Diffuse calcification of the cusps was discovered. He described that "the manipulation consisted of attempting to cut with knife and scissors the two commissures on each side of the posterior valve cusp and to stretch these cuts with cervical dilatators…" The removal of the different clamps allowed the heart and aorta to fill and good venting to be obtained. Lewis et al. reported three cases of open aortic valvotomy, the first being operated upon on 2 December 1955 [28, 29]. Brock performed his first open aortic valvotomy on 26 January 1956 [8].

The imperfect results of the valvotomy for aortic valve stenosis even under direct vision, the absence of extra-corporeal support allowing a long period of cardiac arrest with coronary protection and the absence of aortic valve prosthesis to implant on the aortic ring led surgeons to imagine other devices, mainly to attempt to correct indirectly the aortic stenosis.

The high operative mortality and moderate improvement in patients who survived to the "direct attack" on the stenosed aortic valve led Sarnoff et al. [30, 32] to consider that the aortic stenosis could be indirectly effectively bypassed to induce a decrease in the left ventricular work load and increase the coronary perfusion.

They had chosen the connection between the ventricular apex and thoracic aorta using a "Y" shaped tube with interposition of a Hufnagel's valve. After insertion of a tube into the left ventricle apex, the two parts of the "Y" tube were inserted into the descending aorta. The aorta was closed by a nylon clip put in place on the ascending aorta immediately after the opening of the bypass to be sure that all blood flow would leave the ventricle apically. Ten of the 17 operations performed in dogs resulted in fatalities. The 7 surviving dogs lived well with good physical activity.

## 7.2 Aortic Insufficiency

### 7.2.1 The Extra-Aortic Aortoplasties for Aortic Regurgitation

In an effort to avoid using prosthesis in certain types of aortic regurgitation with annulus dilatation or shrinkage of a cusp, attempts to carry out plasties were described. The team of Lewis theorised the "bicuspidisation" of the aortic valve and described a simplified technique in animals: in 7–11 min of caval occlusion, the aorta was open and stitches were passed at the insertion of the non-coronary leaflet and across the aortic wall [31]. The excess of rings with regard to the non-coronary cusp and an ellipse of excess of the aortic wall were resected on a lateral cross-clamping and the longitudinal aortotomy closed by continuous suture. Out of ten operated dogs, there was no operative mortality, 1 of them died 6 days after surgery because of cardiac failure and the 9 remaining lived in order to undergo chronic study. A similar technique was also described by Hufnagel.

### 7.2.2 A Pericardial "Flap-Valve"

Brock, considering that in aortic insufficiency there is an axial stream of regurgitant blood, attempted to introduce a pericardial flap into the aorta in a series of animal experiments. The goal of these procedures was to use living tissues to try to obtain an accessory valve. He used in dogs a uni- or bipedicled flap. The death of the animals was due to the occurrence of fatal prolapse. Two patients were operated on and the two attempts ended fatally [33]. Brock concluded that the ideal would be a homograft of an aortic valve.

### 7.2.3 The Extra-Valvular Aortic Prosthesis

Jeger had performed the earliest attempt to treat aortic stenosis; not directly, but with a valvular biological bypass between the left ventricle and the aorta, on 11 December 1912, using a reinforced graft of a jugular vein he implanted this conductor from the left ventricle to the "innominate" artery [34]. The graft functioned for 3 days, but the animal died of haemorrhage on the fourth.

In 1944 Charles Hufnagel [34–37] began experimental work on animals to attempt to evolve a suitable valve for the treatment of aortic insufficiency. The initial experimental use of biological material (frozen pericardium, homologous valves, and veins stored at −70 °C) appeared to be unsatisfactory in the long term because of tissue failure.

As early as 1946 they renewed the investigations using some of the recent polymeric materials available: methyl methacrylate was chosen.

The first step was to probe the feasibility of the implantation and the tolerance of the synthetic material. A tube was machined from a block of polymer. The fixation of the rigid valve to the thoracic aorta was a problem: the circumferential ligature of the aorta around the tube induced necrosis of the aortic wall. Hufnagel conceived a semi-flexible ring of nylon devised with small teeth: the space between the teeth allowed maintenance of the perfusion of the wall, the juxta-position to the aorta was ensured and the tube remained patent and stable in place. This principle was termed "multiple point fixation".

The second step consisted of the realisation of the valve prosthesis: in the middle part of the tube was created a chamber into which a floating ball was inserted. The chamber provided an area around the ball for the passage of blood without pressure drop across the device. The efficiency and patency of the valve were demonstrated in the laboratory.

The first operation was performed in October 1952 with survival of the patient for many years.

After a short series of patients the hollow methacrylate ball was changed to one with a nylon core covered with a 5-mm layer of silicone elastomere. The goal was to reduce the noise and to maintain the specific gravity of blood for effectiveness and wearability. The interposition of a semi elastic Orlon cloth between the aorta and the ring permitted avoidance of clotting at this level. In the early experiment, 10 % of patients had had embolisation. The implantation was made by left thoracotomy and to avoid the total cross-clamping of the aorta which could be poorly tolerated by fragile patients a shunt was inserted if necessary between the subclavian artery and the distal aorta or femoral artery to provide a distal flow. The use of a valved shunt implanted using end-to-side anastomosis with partial aortic clamping followed by excision of the shunted aorta was the other possibility described by Hufnagel [38, 39].

### 7.2.4 The Beginning of the Concept of the Anatomical Aortic Valve

Hufnagel recognised that the position of this kind of valve on the descending aorta was safe, but did not attain the ideal of controlling all the insufficiency. He concluded that the ideal was the implantation of the prosthetic valve in a normal anatomical position [37]:

- The experimental implantation of modified ball valve prosthesis with an open chamber to permit reflux into the coronary vessels in the aortic valve position was carried out. It appeared that the important resistance due to the ball was not always adequate to permit flow without restriction.
- A type of thin-walled and flexible "cusp valve" was also constructed using silicone rubber. The cusps were held together only by a central ring. Easily experimentally implanted, they observed no embolisation or failure over a period of 6 months.
- One other type of original valve was described as the "spring valve". It was a helicoid spring that was open in systole by elongation and closed in diastole by retraction.

  Its implantation was easy by open way or using the multiple point fixations.

These procedures were only experimental. The beginning of the era of open heart surgery under cardio-pulmonary bypass led to changes in the concepts of the implantation of valves using classical sutures under view control.

## 7.3 Conclusion

As we can see in this retrospective study of the beginning of the aortic valve's conquest, many pioneers worked experimentally and clinically to lead the way to the repair or change. The main heroes of this adventure were the patients. History is always renewed in time: after the aortic valve replacement by conventional surgery under cardiac arrest with cardioplegia, nowadays the trans-arterial valve implantation represents a comeback for the old initial techniques and the problem of the way to approach the aortic annulus is again that of actuality: femoral anterograde approach, subclavian or trans-aortic or trans-carotid retrograde approach, etc.

It is with the experience of past and present that we can build the future.

## References

1. Billroth T (1882) Krankheiten der Brust. In: Pitha and Billroth (eds) Handbuch der allgemeiner und specieller chirurgie III. Emke, Stuttgart, pp 163–164
2. Rehn L (1907) Zur Chirurgie des Herzens und des Herzenbeutels. Arch Klin Chir 83:723
3. Lillehei CW, Varco RL, Cohen M, Warden HE, Patton C, Moller JH (1986) The first open-heart repairs of ventricular septal defect, atrio-ventricular communis and tetralogy of Fallot using extra-corporeal circulation by cross-circulation. A 30-year follow-up. Ann Thorac Surg 41:4–21
4. Brock RC (1951) Discussion on the surgery of the heart and great vessels. Proc R Soc Med 44(12):995–1003
5. Becker O (1872) Über die Sichtbaren Erscheinungen der Blutbewegen in der menschlichen Netzhaut. Graefes Arch Ophtalmol 18:208
6. Haecher R (1907) Experimentelle Studien zur Pathologie und Chirurgie des Herzens. Arch Klin Chir 84:1035

7. Tuffier T (1913) Etat actuel de la chirurgie intra-thoracique. Trans Internat Cong Med London, Sect 17, surg Part 2:246 9,19140
8. Brock R (1957) Surgical treatment of aortic stenosis. Br Med J 1:1019–1028
9. Carrel A (1914) Experimental operations on the orifices of the heart. Ann Surg 60:1
10. Bailey CP, Glover RP, O'Neill TJ, Redondo Ramirez HP (1950) Experiences with the experimental surgical relief of aortic stenosis; a preliminary report. J Thorac Surg 20(4):516–541
11. Bailey CP, Redondo Ramirez HP, Larzelere HB (1952) Surgical treatment of aortic stenosis. J Am Med Assoc 150(17):1647–1652
12. Bailey CP (1956) Surgical treatment of aortic stenosis. J Thorac Surg 31:375–441
13. Smithy HG, Pratt-Thomas HR (1947) Deyerle: experimental aortic valvulotomy: preliminary report. Surg Gynecol Obstet 84:625
14. Smithy HG, Parker EF (1947) Experimental aortic valvulotomy. Am J Med 3(4):502
15. Smithy HG, Pratt-Thomas HR, Deyerle HP (1948) Aortic valvulotomy; experimental methods and early results. Surg Gynecol Obstet 86(5):513–523
16. Smithy HG (1949) Aortic valvulotomy. South Med Surg 111(1):7
17. Uricchio JF, Litwak R, Cooley D, Goldberg H, Likoff W (1956) A medical appraisal of transaortic commissurotomy. Ann Intern Med 44(5):844–860
18. Uricchio JF, Bolton HE, Litwak R (1956) The surgical treatment of aortic stenosis. Conn State Med J 20(5):340–344
19. Uricchio JF (1958) The surgical treatment of mitral and aortic stenosis in patients over 55. Geriatrics 13(5):270–272
20. Sauerbruck F (1907) Die Verwendbarkeit des Unterdruckverfahrens bei Herzchirurgie. Arch Klin Chir 83:537
21. Laewen A, Sievers R (1908) Experimentelle Untersuchen über die chirurgish wichtigen Abklemmungen des grossen Gefässe in der Nähe des Herzens. Deutsche Ztschr f Chir 94:580
22. Bigelow WG, Callaghan JC, Hopps JA (1950) General hypothermia for experimental intracardiac surgery: the use of electrophrenic respirations, an artificial pacemaker for cardiac standstill and radio-frequency rewarming in general hypothermia. Ann Surg 132:531–539
23. Cookson BA, Neptune WB, Bailey CP (1952) Hypothermia as a means of performing intracardiac surgery under direct vision. Dis Chest 22(3):245–260
24. Bigelow WG (1984) Cold hearts and vital lessons. Closure of atrial septal defects with the aid of hypothermia; experimental accomplishments and the report of one successful case. Am Coll Surg Bull 69(6):12–20
25. Lewis FJ, Taufic M (1953) A device for the experimental creation of ventricular septal defects; preliminary report. Surgery 33(1):52–59
26. Taufic M, Lewis FJ (1953) Production and repair of experimental interventricular septal defects under direct vision with the aid of hypothermia. J Thorac Surg 25(4):413–416
27. Lewis FJ, Taufic M (1953) Closure of atrial septal defects with the aid of hypothermia; experimental accomplishments and the report of one successful case. Surgery 33(1):52–59
28. Shumway NE, Lewis FJ (1955) Experimental surgery of the mitral valve under direct vision using hypothermia. Surg Forum 5:12–16
29. Julian LC, Dye WS, Grove WJ (1956) Hypothermia in open heart surgery. Arch Surg 73:493
30. Swan H, Kortz AB (1956) Direct vision trans-aortic approach to the aortic valve during hypothermia; experimental observations and report of successful clinical case. Ann Surg 144(2):205–214
31. Swan H, Zeavin I (1954) Cessation of circulation in general hypothermia. III. Technique of intracardiac surgery under direct vision. Ann Surg 139:385
32. Sarnoff SJ, Donovan TJ, Case RB (1955) The surgical relief of aortic stenosis by means of apical-aortic valvular anastomosis. Circulation 11(4):564–575
33. Taufic M, Lewis FJ (1953) A technique for bicuspidization of the aortic valve. Surg Forum 4:67–72
34. Starzi TE, Cruzat EP, Walker BA, Lewis FJ (1959) A technique for bicuspidization of the aortic valve. J Thorac Cardiovasc Surg 38:262–270

35. Brock RC (1954) Mechanical principles in the surgery of aortic and mitral incompetence. Br Heart J 16(3):317–323
36. Küttner H (1923) Chirurgishe Operationslehre, vol 2, 5th edn. Barth, Leipzig
37. Hufnagel CA, Harvey WP, Rabil PJ, Mc Dermott TF (1989) Surgical correction of aortic insufficiency. Ann Thorac Surg 47:475–476
38. Fawcett AW, Dhillon BS (1956) Treatment of aortic insufficiency by the Hufnagel valve with four illustrated cases. Postgrad Med J 32:438–443
39. Hufnagel C, Vilkgas P, Nahas H (1958) Experiences with new types of aortic valvular prostheses. Ann Surg 147(5):636–644

# The History of Myocardial Revascularization Before the Advent of Cardiopulmonary Bypass

8

Marco Picichè

*Great spirits have always encountered violent opposition from mediocre minds.*

Albert Einstein

**Abstract**

The history of myocardial revascularization, as is often the case with medical progress, is replete with stories of visionary research surgeons and inspired, persevering, and self-sacrificing innovators—courageous men whose minds were open to serendipitous observation, and who were inured to failure, criticism, and skepticism. It may well be that earlier attempts to achieve myocardial revascularization constitute a fertile pool of ideas from which current and future researchers can draw to elaborate derivative strategies that employ the tools of modern technology. Prior to the advent of cardiopulmonary bypass, myocardial revascularization strategies fell into three categories: extracardiac procedures, cardiac operations on noncoronary artery structures, and direct coronary artery surgery.

The history of myocardial revascularization, as is often the case with medical progress, is replete with stories of visionary research surgeons and inspired, persevering, and self-sacrificing innovators—courageous men whose minds were open to serendipitous observation, and who were inured to failure, criticism, and skepticism. Remarkably, some alternative myocardial revascularization techniques attempted in recent years bear a resemblance to techniques tried and abandoned in the first half of the last century [1–8]. Today cardiovascular researchers are on the lookout for new myocardial revascularization methods to help the many patients suffering from diffuse coronary artery disease who may not benefit from conventional techniques. Since a certain level of morbidity and

M. Picichè (✉)
Cardiac Surgery Unit,
San Filippo Neri Hospital, Via Martinotti 20, 00135 Rome, Italy
e-mail: m.piciche@sanfilipponeri.roma.it; marcopiciche.history@libero.it

M. Picichè (ed.), *Dawn and Evolution of Cardiac Procedures*,
DOI: 10.1007/978-88-470-2400-7_8, 

mortality is still associated with direct surgical or endovascular coronary procedures [9, 10], the search is on for less invasive and less costly alternatives that ensure myocardial blood supply. It may well be that earlier attempts to achieve myocardial revascularization constitute a fertile pool of ideas from which current and future researchers can draw to elaborate derivative strategies that employ the tools of modern technology. Prior to the advent of cardiopulmonary bypass, myocardial revascularization strategies fell into three categories: extracardiac procedures, cardiac operations on noncoronary artery structures, and direct coronary artery surgery.

## 8.1 Extracardiac Surgery

### 8.1.1 Ligation of the Internal Thoracic Arteries

The history of myocardial revascularization began in 1880 when Langer [11] first described the existence of vascular communications between normal coronary artery circulation and the vascular supply of surrounding extracardiac structures. He observed small channels connecting the bronchial tree, pericardium, diaphragm, and esophagus with coronary circulation. These channels enter the heart through the pericardial reflections surrounding the pulmonary veins, the superior and inferior vena cava, the pulmonary artery, and the aorta, connecting with the vasa vasorum of the arterial wall. Also, the pericardiophrenic branch of the internal thoracic arteries (ITAs) constitutes a source of extracardiac anastomosis [6–8, 12, 13]. Nowadays we see indirect evidence of these connections in the course of cardiac surgery. Why is it that a patient with angiography-verified hyper-severe stenosis of the left main coronary artery and concomitant occlusion of the right coronary artery can still exhibit normal ventricular function? Why is it that during coronary artery operations, despite correct aortic cross-clamping and adequate venting, there may be an outpouring of arterial blood flow from the incised coronary artery? Why is it that when the aorta is opened during ascending aorta or aortic valve surgery, a variable amount of blood may leak from the coronary ostia? The answer lies with the heart's capacity for extracardiac anastomosis, which supports non-coronary collateral blood circulation. In 1939 an Italian surgeon named Fieschi suggested that bilateral ligation of the distal ITAs would shunt flow through branches of the pericardiophrenic arteries back to the heart. With the help of internal medicine physicians Zoia and Cesa-Bianchi, the procedure was successfully carried out and results were published in 1942 [14]. In 1955 Battezzati et al repeated the Fieschi procedure both experimentally and in humans. They injected blue methylene into the ITAs next to their origin from the subclavian artery after both distal and proximal ITA ligation, and observed blue areas that appeared on both the epicardium and within myocardial slices [15]. After this experimental demonstration, the Italian team operated on 304 patients under local anesthesia, using a small bilateral incision between the second and third ribs to access the ITAs [16]. The goal of ITAs ligation was to create a local hypertensive status above the obstruction and increase perfusion pressure in channels leading to the heart. Postoperative follow-up continued from 6 months to 4 years. Symptomatic improvement was observed in 288 cases (94.8 %) while no improvement was seen in 15 cases (4.9 %). In 14 patients (4.6 %), initial improvement was not sustained in the follow-up period. The operation itself was very safe, with no operative mortality. Of the 13 deaths that occurred at various intervals, 5 patients died from non-cardiac causes and 8 from cardiac disease. Moreover, in 195 cases (64.1 %) the electrocardiogram improved after surgery, although the authors did not observe in all cases the relationship between electrocardiographic and clinical improvement. Battezzati's papers, published in 1955 in Italian [15], and in 1959 in the *American Journal of Cardiology* [16], attracted the attention of an American pioneer in cardiac surgery, Robert P. Glover, former assistant to Charles Bailey at the start of the era of closed mitral commissurotomy. In Philadelphia he repeated the Italian procedure with similarly satisfying results [17–19]. Others started using the procedure, but with conflicting results, and indeed, some rejected it altogether, claiming the initial results to be a placebo effect [20–23]. Eventually, with the advent of cardiopulmonary bypass, ITA ligation fell into disuse, and Fieschi and Battezzati's publications were forgotten.

### 8.1.2 Cardiac Sympathectomy

In 1899 François-Franck suggested cardiac sympathectomy by resection of the upper thoracic ganglia to relieve angina [24]. Although he never did the procedure himself, his theory was adopted by Jonnesco, who performed the first sympathectomy in Bucharest in 1916 [25]. The incision ran from the mastoid tip to the clavicle, along the posterior border of the sternocleidomastoid muscle. He excised the first dorsal ganglia and the cervical sympathetic trunk and reported that denervation, which led to coronary vasodilation with enhancement in blood supply, was effective in relieving angina. An alternative denervation method performed by Mandl in 1925 involved paravertebral alcohol injection [26], and in 1929 Sussman suggested sympathectomy by paravertebral short wave radiation [27]. Nowadays, the denervation principle lives on with the use of left cardiac sympathetic denervation to treat long QT syndrome.

### 8.1.3 Partial and Total Thyroidectomy

In 1902 Theodor Kocher observed that a patient with angina became asymptomatic after total thyroidectomy [28]. This observation was uncovered 30 years later by Blumgart, Levine, and Berlin, who proposed that removal of the thyroid gland could be used to treat ischemic heart disease [29]. The rationale was based on the idea that the circulation rate decreases with diminishing basal metabolic demand. Partial resection brought only temporary relief, because as the gland regenerated, the former metabolic rate returned, and clinical improvement receded. Therefore, total resection was planned. On 14 December 1932, at the Peter Bent Brigham Hospital, the first total thyroidectomy was performed by Elliot Cutler and Max Schnitker [30]. They performed 53 operations between 1932 and 1934 to treat either congestive heart failure or angina pectoris. In the former case (24 patients), the underlying hypothesis was that a decrease in the body's demands on circulation allowed supply to come into equilibrium with metabolic demand. In the second group (29 patients) they considered that a reduction in metabolism by itself could not explain the immediate relief from angina. Indeed, a total thyroidectomy produced such a striking and immediate reduction in pain that it seemed disproportionate to the comparatively modest decrease in the basal metabolic rate. The relationship between the thyroid, adrenal, and sympathetic systems suggested that adrenal secretion played an important role in triggering angina pectoris. It was not known how total thyroidectomy shifts the adrenal effect, but their hypothesis was that since cardiac innervation was intact, and thyroidectomy did not decrease adrenaline output, the observed relief in angina was due to local effects that made the heart less sensitive to adrenaline.

## 8.2 Operations on the Epicardium, Myocardium, and Cardiac Veins

Despite the dogma that the heart was inaccessible, surgeons mustered the courage to approach it directly in the second era of research. The heart was assaulted in countless ways. In an effort to induce neovascularization, it was scarred, wrapped, implanted, perforated, and sutured to contiguous structures, and cardiac veins were ligated and arterialized. This era ran from the early 1930s into the early 1950s.

### 8.2.1 Beck's Experiments

Claude Schaeffer Beck, in Pennsylvania, read the paper published in 1932 by Moritz et al. [31] describing experiments on extracardiac anastomosis in which the coronary arteries of four hearts with pericardial adhesions, from human cadavers, were injected with a suspension of lamp black. Interestingly, they reported that the injection mass could be seen passing through vascularized adhesions from the epicardium to the parietal pericardium. The authors also observed, in humans dying from pericarditis, development of anastomoses between the coronary arteries and extracardiac structures, such as pericardial fat pads, internal thoracic arteries, and anterior branches of the thoracic aorta. These observations led Moritz and coworkers to believe that under certain conditions extracardiac anastomosis constituted an important source of blood supply to the heart. This idea was in keeping with a case reported by Thorel in 1903, in which autopsy results suggested that, throughout his life, a man with complete obliteration of both coronary arteries received blood supplied by numerous adhesions [32]. Throughout the 1920s Beck performed more than 1,200 experiments and observed that blood vessels extended between the heart and adherent scars [33]. Once, in surgery, he observed prolific bleeding while resecting a broad band of scar tissue extending from the base of the left ventricle to the parietal pericardium. This observation in a living patient demonstrated that a huge vascular connection between the heart and adherent tissues can exist in humans [34]. In many experiments the epicardium and a lining of the parietal pericardium were removed with a burr. The pericardium and pericardial fat were sutured to the abraded heart. Skeletal muscle flaps and the omentum, the latter brought up through an opening in the diaphragm, were sutured to myocardial muscle, and were also successful in creating vascular connections. In hearts with experimentally occluded coronary arteries, Beck observed that injected dye penetrated the myocardium through the collateral bed, and concluded that some noncoronary blood supply sources were possible. When normal blood supply to the heart was reduced and consequently a pressure-differential existed between extracardiac and cardiac vascular beds, anastomosis readily developed between skeletal and myocardial muscle. On the other hand, when coronary arteries were unobstructed, and there was no physiological need for an alternative blood supply, vascular neo-anastomosis was less evident or did not develop at all.

#### 8.2.1.1 Skeletal muscle flap (Beck's first method)

On 13 February 1935, J.K., a 48-year-old white male farmer, was operated on at Lakeside Hospital [34]. Gas-oxygen anesthesia was used. The insertion of the left pectoral muscle was incised for the purpose of mobilizing the muscle. The inferior portion of the muscle was incised for the purpose of making a pedicle graft. The pericardium was opened with a burr and roughened, and the epicardium was removed in shreds. The pedicle graft was divided longitudinally. Both pedicles were swung around to the circumflex area of the heart, and sutured laterally and posteriorly to the parietal pericardium. Seven months later the patient returned to work as a gardener with no pain. Beck successfully carried out the operation on five more patients.

#### 8.2.1.2 Epicardial abrasion, inflammatory agents, pericardial flap, and coronary sinus ligature (Beck's second method)

In the 1930s Louis Grosse and Lester Blom demonstrated that complete ligation of the coronary sinus in dogs could prevent death when a major coronary artery was occluded [35]. Congestion gradually subsided as collateral channels in the form of intercoronary arteriolar connections opened up. After the Mercier Fauteux operations, which involved ligation of cardiac veins, Beck switched from skeletal muscle and omental flaps to ligation of cardiac veins. In 1941 he described an operation that entailed abrasion of the pericardium and epicardium, application of an inflammatory agent to the pericardial cavity, partial occlusion of the coronary sinus, and suturing the mediastinal fat and pericardium to the myocardium [35].

Although this was chronologically Beck's second operation, it is usually known as the Beck I operation.

#### 8.2.1.3 Arterialization of the coronary sinus (Beck's third method)

At the end of the 19th century, Pratt suggested that the coronary venous system could be used to supply oxygenated blood to the ischemic heart [36]. This concept was then revived four decades later by various researchers, including Beck, and some six decades later by Walton Lillehi, who created the method of retrograde cardioplegia. In the 1940s Beck was among the authors who thought that blood flow and oxygenation could be achieved by retrograde flow through the coronary sinus. There were some experiments indicating that ischemic myocardium could be revascularized by joining a large artery to the coronary sinus or veins. In some experiments a glass cannula was anastomosed between the innominate or subclavian artery and the coronary sinus. This resulted in distension and pulsation of the coronary sinus, which had become arterialized. There were successful experiments in which, despite the coronary arteries being ligated, the myocardium continued to contract thanks to coronary sinus retrograde flow. On 27 January 1948, Beck applied this concept to a human [37]. The operation involved excising a brachial artery segment and joining it between the descending thoracic aorta and the coronary sinus. The operation was completed by ligation of the coronary sinus at its junction with the right atrium. This was a complex procedure, and Beck soon changed to a two-stage procedure where the graft was inserted first, then the coronary sinus partially ligated some weeks later. Operative mortality was 15–20 %, and the procedure was abandoned. Nonetheless, Beck concluded that arterialization was physiologically effective and that after anastomosis was established, it was possible to ligate a major coronary artery with little or no onset of myocardial infarction.

### 8.2.2 Cardio-Omentopexy and Cardiopneumopexy

In the "Carey Coombs Memorial Lecture" given in Britain in 1937, a young surgeon named Laurence O'Shaughnessy described his cardio-omentopexy technique [38]. The chest was entered through an incision along the fifth intercostal space, the fifth and sixth costal cartilages were divided, the pericardium was exposed, and the left leaf of the diaphragm was exposed and incised. The abdomen was then explored through the diaphragmatic incision, and a suitable portion of omentum was obtained and brought up into the chest. The pericardium was incised, and the omentum was sutured to the heart and pericardium. The dogs on which he performed experimental coronary occlusion and omental grafts recovered. In later operations he avoided suturing the myocardium by applying the omentum to the pericardium, using adhesive paste between the epicardium and omentum. In 1938 he reported that patients who survived more than 6 months experienced relief from angina. Unfortunately, World War II prematurely ended his research and his life at age 40, in Dunkirk. During those same years, in

Germany Albert Lezius introduced the technique of cardiopneumopexy—creating a firm heart–lung union [39]. In 1937, he painted acriflavine onto the epicardium via a pericardial window and sutured the lung to the heart. Injection studies were successful in demonstrating constant and consistent vascular neo-anastomosis between the two organs—in particular between the pulmonary artery and the coronary arteries. This approach was later used in the 1950s by others, after in vivo directional flow studies demonstrated that, as a result of a fall in coronary pressure, blood flow was diverted from the lung graft to the stenotic coronary arteries. Stomach (cardiogastropexy), jejunum (cardiojejunopexy), spleen (cardiolienopexy), and skin also served as viable grafts onto the heart, but results were not as impressive [40].

### 8.2.3 Chemical Pericarditis

Chemical pericarditis was a simple method for creating pericardial adhesions with neovessel formation. Several irritants were used: asbestos, powered beef bone, carborundum sand, kaolin, formaldehyde, alcohol, ether, iodine, iron fillings, kaolin, cotton, human skin, and water glass. In New York, Thomson used sterile talc and Novocain to prevent irritant-triggered ventricular fibrillation. He reported over years of observation that most patients experienced symptom relief. Dwight Harken used carbolic acid to remove the epicardium before instilling powdered talc [40]. However, it is possible that with some irritants nerve endings are destroyed; therefore, symptom relief was attributed to unintended denervation rather than to neovascularization.

### 8.2.4 Methods Involving Pulmonary Circulation

Other methods proposed using pulmonary circulation in various ways. Day and Lillehy experimentally created a shunt between the pulmonary artery and left atrium [41]. They considered this shunt to be a potent stimulus in the development of intercoronary anastomosis. Kownacki increased pulmonary collateral flow by ligating the lingular vein and then suturing the lingula to the epicardium [42]. Kline tried to improve myocardial flow by increasing bronchial artery collateral flow—achieved by occluding the left pulmonary artery and suturing parts of the lung to the epicardium denuded by silver nitrate [43].

### 8.2.5 Ligature of the Great Cardiac Vein and Pericoronary Neurectomy (Fauteux's Procedure)

The Canadian research surgeon Mercier Fauteux intensively studied the effects of cardiac vein ligation. In animals he demonstrated that after ligation of the great cardiac vein, circulatory re-adjustment occurred in the coronary system, which allowed the animals to survive subsequent ligation of the left anterior descending artery. Fauteux did not completely understand these compensatory mechanisms, but he observed that arterial pressure increased in the vascular field drained by the occluded vein. He thought that the rise in local arterial pressure might explain the circulatory re-adjustment within the myocardium. On 19 April 1939, a 54-year-old male patient with a 5-year history of angina underwent surgery [44]. An incision was made between the second and third ribs, the pericardium was exposed and incised vertically, and the great cardiac vein was identified and ligated. After the operation the patient was seen at frequent intervals and appeared to be free from pain. In 1946 Fauteux reported on further experiments in which great cardiac vein ligation was done with or without pericoronary neurectomy; or pericoronary neurectomy was done alone [45]. For the latter procedure, the thought was that by resecting pathways to and from the coronary arteries at the aortic root and at the origin of the coronary arteries, reflex effects would be blocked. This procedure was more than a sympathectomy, because vagal, sympathetic, and sensory branches were all resected to block reflex action. This combined procedure represented the melding of two different approaches for relieving angina: Francois Franck's idea (late 1800s) that resection of the sympathetic nerves in the neck might diminish angina pain, and Beck and O'Shaughnessy's attempts to bring a new blood supply to the heart.

### 8.2.6 Internal Thoracic Artery Implantation into the Myocardium (Vineberg's Procedure)

In Vineberg's procedure, the internal thoracic artery was placed within a tunnel in the myocardium [46]. Anastomoses were experimentally proven in over 200 experiments done on dogs using injection studies, radiographs, plastic casts, and serial sections. Anastomosis occurred in up to 75 % of the animals, and in these cases ligature of the left anterior descending artery was not followed by infarction or death. In man the left thorax was entered through the fifth intercostal space using an anterolateral approach. Despite the fact that an open vessel was embedded in the myocardium, there was usually no evidence of hemorrhage or intramural hematoma. In some patients ITAs remained patent through very long term follow-up. Marx and associates reported on a case of bilateral ITA implantation performed some 27 years earlier where both arteries showed good patency at follow-up [47]. In many patients angiography indicates a wide network of collaterals connecting the ITAs and coronary arteries. The first successful ITA implantation in humans was carried out in 1950. This procedure became popular over the next 20 years, until the aortocoronary bypass operation supplanted it.

## 8.3 Direct Operations on the Coronary Arteries

### 8.3.1 Alexis Carrel

Alexis Carrel was born in Lyon, France, in 1873 and attended medical school there. Withering under criticisms that he would never pass his surgical examination in France, he moved to Canada in 1904 and then to the United States, where he found many research opportunities [48]. Up until 1906 he was involved in a prolific experimental surgery partnership with the brilliant young physiologist Charles Claude Guthrie. Between 1901 and 1910, using experimental animals, he sutured arteries to arteries, veins to veins, and arteries to veins. He tested end-to-end, side-to-side, and end-to-side anastomoses. He used patch grafts, autografts, homografts, rubber, glass, metal, and absorbable magnesium tubes. He invented a new surgical trick to achieve end-to-end anastomosis, which he called "triangulation". This technique made suturing cut vessels much easier—he created three sutures, each one-third of the way around the circumference of the vessels to be joined, then by pulling two of the sutures in opposite directions the round junction was converted into three straight lines, enabling continuous suturing along those lines. Also, he preserved vessels, tissues, and organs by refrigerating them in Locke's solution. He transplanted the organs of laboratory animals and recognized that a homograft vessel, which he called a "homotransplant," served as a framework for new cell growth. He also noticed that when a vein was used to replace an arterial segment, the vein assumed arterial characteristics and became thick-walled, while when a segment of artery was used to replace a segment of vein, the arterial wall thinned and became more venous in nature. In the field of coronary surgery he was the first to perform an anastomosis on dogs between the descending aorta and left coronary artery [49]. This pioneering operation was also remarkable because of the nature of the graft, namely a long carotid artery preserved in cold storage. One end was implanted on the descending aorta, and the other end was passed through the pericardium and anastomosed to the coronary artery. Alexis Carrel won the 1912 Nobel Prize in Physiology and Medicine "in recognition of his work on vascular suture and the transplantation of blood vessels and organs" [50]. In 1954 Murray, building on Carrel's pioneering efforts, reported on his work using the internal thoracic, axillary, and carotid arteries to perform bypass grafting directly onto the coronary arteries of beating dog hearts [40].

### 8.3.2 Endarterectomy

At Hahnemann Hospital in Philadelphia on 29 October 1956, Charles Bailey performed the first human closed-coronary endarterectomy using a retrograde, distal, blind technique without cardiopulmonary bypass [40]. Also, working with dogs and cadavers, Absolon performed endarterectomies and coronary grafting, trying both end-to-end and end-to-side anastomoses using various types of arterial grafts [40]. In 1958 William Longmire published a description in the *New England*

*Journal of Medicine* of his technique of direct-vision coronary endarterectomy, where the heart is approached through a bilateral anterior thoracotomy without cardiopulmonary bypass [51, 52].

### 8.3.3 Vladimir Demikhov, Vasily Kolesov, and Robert Goetz

In the East there was a genius who, for too long, was unknown to medical scientists in the West. Demikhov's explorations were so far out "on the cutting edge of surgical research," as Igor Konstantinov put it [53], that they were not readily accepted in his lifetime. He created one of the earliest cardiac-assist devices, and he performed the first intra-thoracic heterotopic and orthotopic heart transplants, as well as the first isolated lung and heart–lung transplants in experimental animals, some of which survived for as long as 30 days. In July 1953 he performed a successful coronary bypass operation on a dog. To achieve coronary anastomosis, Demikhov adapted Payr's technique. This technique, described by the German surgeon Payr in 1900, consisted of a nonsuture anastomosis, using a ring around a vessel in order to make it possible to introduce a smaller vessel into a larger one. Of Demikhov's dogs, four survived for more than 2 years, and anastomotic patency was proven [53].

He also performed experiments in baboons and on cadavers. An adaptation of Payr's technique was also used by Robert Goetz, a German surgeon who courageously rejected Nazism and escaped to Switzerland, Great Britain, South Africa, and finally to the United States. On 2 May 1960, at the former Van Etten Hospital in the Bronx (now part of the Albert Einstein Medical Center), he successfully achieved anastomosis between the right internal thoracic artery and the right coronary artery by using a tantalum ring modification of Payr's technique. The patient remained free of angina for 1 year. As Konstantinov wrote [54], "Goetz was far ahead of his time. His work was too new for many to comprehend. The introduction of the coronary bypass operation created a great deal of anxiety. As it happened with most new procedures, the anxiety produced resistance." The operation performed by this great man, whose life was "full of mental torment and material adversity," had no support in his institution, and he was forced to stop coronary surgery [54]. Goetz is one of those unknown pioneers in cardiac surgery, woefully overlooked despite the fact that his operation [55] was really the first successful clinical coronary artery bypass grafting in the world! Two years later on 4 April 1962, Sabiston tried the first saphenous vein bypass, but the patient died 3 days later [56]. Then it was the moment of Kolesov, in Russia. Geniuses and revolutionary innovations are more often greeted with skepticism than support, and Demikhov's experiments were no exception, but he was undaunted by public criticism. However, Vasily Kolesov in Leningrad looked favorably on his work, and he commenced further experiments in the same "vein." On 25 February 1964, he performed the first successful operation using a suture technique to anastomose the left internal thoracic to the circumflex artery [57]. From February 1964 until May

1967, Kolesov's department of surgery was the only place in the world where coronary surgery was routinely performed. On 23 November 1964, Garret, Dennis, and DeBakey performed the first successful saphenous vein bypass—the patient did well for 7 years thereafter (the case was first reported in 1973) [58]. Believing that too much time was required for anastomosis, Kolesov created a stapling method, and on 22 March 1967, put the new method to the test by creating a LITA to coronary artery anastomosis; the patient was still well at the 3-year follow-up [59]. It was not until the late 1960s that Favaloro [60] and Green [61] successfully used the saphenous veins as a graft. Sadly and unjustly, Demikhov, Kolesov, and Goetz are unknown to most cardiac surgeons, despite the fact that their innovative work predated the achievements of much-renowned surgeons who are commonly considered pioneers in the field. A goal of the present chapter is to pay homage to these three pioneers of direct coronary surgery. In recognizing their work here, we accord them the honor they did not receive in their lifetime.

## References

1. Waltenberger J, Kranz A, Beyer M (1999) Neovascularization in the human heart is associated with expression of VEGF-A and its receptors Flt-1 (VEGFR-1) and KDR (VEGFR-2). Results from cardiomyopexy in ischemic cardiomyopathy. Angiogenesis 3(4):345–351
2. Krämer SC, Görich J, Beyer M, Merkle E, Gerber J, Rilinger N, Sokiranski R, Brambs HJ (2000) CT and arteriography in the evaluation of indirect myocardial revascularization with a free-muscle transplant: initial experience. Radiology 216(1):123–127
3. Beyer M, Kardiol Z (1997) Cardiomyopexy—current status of an indirect revascularization method. German 86(1):125–132
4. Beyer M, Beyer U, Mierdl S, Sirch J, von Behren H, Hannekum A (1994) Indirect myocardial revascularization—an experimental study in the dog. Eur J Cardiothorac Surg 8(10):557–562
5. Hughes GC, Biswas SS, Yin B, Baklanov DV, Annex BH, Coleman RE, DeGrado TR, Landolfo CK, Landolfo KP, Lowe JE (2002) A comparison of mechanical and laser transmyocardial revascularization for induction of angiogenesis and arteriogenesis in chronically ischemic myocardium. J Am Coll Cardiol 39(7):1220–1228
6. Picichè M, Kingma JJ, Fadel E, Dagenais F, Mathieu P, Simard D, Demaria RG, Voisine P (2011) Enhancement of non-coronary collateral blood flow from the internal thoracic arteries: the theoretical and practical basis of an alternative method of myocardial blood supply. J Cardiovasc Surg (Torino) 52(1):127–131
7. Picichè M, Kingma JG Jr, Voisine P, Dagenais F, Fadel E (2010) Angiogenesis and surgical or endovascular enhancement of noncoronary collateral circulation: a new research field. J Thorac Cardiovasc Surg 139(6):1675–1676; author reply 1676-1677
8. Picichè M, Kingma JG Jr, Fadel E, Dagenais F, Robillard J, Simard D, Voisine P (2010) Enhancement of noncoronary collateral circulation: the hypothesis of an alternative treatment for ischemic heart disease. Med Hypotheses 74(1):21–23
9. Rosamond W, Flegal K, Furie K, Go A, Greenlund K, Haase N et al (2008) Heart disease and stroke statistics—2007 update. A report from the American Heart Association Statistics Committee and Stroke Statistics Subcommittee. Circulation 117(4):25–146
10. Detre KM, Holmes DR Jr, Holubkov R et al (1990) Incidence and consequences of periprocedural occlusion. The 1985–1986 national heart, lung, and blood institute percutaneous transluminal coronary angioplasty registry. Circulation 82:739

11. Langer L (1880) Die Foramina thebesu in Herzen des Menschen. Sitzungsberichte Akad Wiss Wien 82:25–29
12. Hudson C, Moritz A, Wearn J (1932) The extracardiac anastomosis of the coronary arteries. J Exp Med 56:919–926
13. Bloor CM, Liebow AA (1965) Coronary collateral circulation. Am J Cardiol 16:238–252
14. Fieschi D (1942) Criteri anatomo-fisiologici per intervento chirurgico lieve in malati di infartondi cuore e di angina. Arch Ital Chir 63:305–310
15. Battezzati M, Tagliaferro A, De Marchi G (1955) La legatura delle due arterie mammarie interne nei disturbi di vascolarizzazione del miocardio. Minerva Med 46:1178–1188
16. Battezzati M, Tagliaferro A, Cattaneo AD (1959) Clinical evaluation of bilateral internal mammary artery ligation as treatment of coronary heart disease. Am J Cardiol 4(2):180–183
17. Glover RP, Davila JC, Khyle RH, Beard JC, Trout RG, Kitchell JR (1957) Ligation of the internal mammary arteries as a means of increasing blood supply to the myocardium. J Thorac Surg 34(5):661–678
18. Glover RP, Kitchell R, Kyle R et al (1958) Experiences with myocardial revascularization by division of the internal mammary arteries. Chest 33:637–657
19. Glover P (1957) A new surgical approach to the problem of myocardial revascularization in coronary artery disease. J Ark Med Soc 54(6):223–234
20. Sabiston DC, Blalock A (1958) Experimental ligation of the internal mammary artery and its effect on coronary occlusion. Surgery 43(6):906–912
21. Vansant JH, Muller W (1959) Experimental evaluation of the internal mammary artery ligation as a method of myocardial revascularization. Surgery 45(5):840–847
22. Hurley R, Eckstein RW (1959) Effect of bilateral internal mammary artery ligation on coronary circulation in dogs. Circ Res 7:571
23. Fish RG, Crymes TP, Lovell MG (1958) Internal mammary artery ligation for angina pectoris. Its failure to produce relief. N Engl J Med 259(9):418–420
24. Francois-Franck CA (1899) Signification physiologique de la résection du sympathique dans la maladie de Basedow, l'épilepsie, l'idiotie, et le glaucome. Bull Acad Med Paris 41: 565–594
25. Jonnesco T (1920) Angine de poitrine guérie par la résection du sympathique cervicothoracique. Bull Acad Med Paris 84:93102
26. Mandl F (1925) Weitere Erfahrungen mit der paravertebralen lnjektion bei der Angina pectoris. Wien Klin Wschr 38:759–760
27. Sussmann ML (1930) The treatment of angina pectoris by paravertebral short wave radiation. Am J Roentgenol 24:163–168
28. Kocher A (1902) Ueber morbus Basedowi. Mitt Grenzgeb Med Chir ix:1–13
29. Blumgart HL, Levine SA, Berlin DD (1933) Congestive heart failure and angina pectoris. The therapeutic effect of thyroidectomy on patients without clinical or pathologic evidence of thyroid toxicity. Arch Int Med 51:866–877
30. Cutler EC, Schnitker MT (1934) Total thyroidectomy for angina pectoris. Ann Surg 100(4):578–605
31. Moritz AR, Hudson CL, Orgain ES (1932) Augmentation of the extracardiac anastomoses of the coronary arteries through pericardial adhesions. J Exp Med 56:927–931
32. Thorel CH (1903) Pathologie der Kreislauforgane. Ergbn Allg Pathol Pathol Anat 9:1–559
33. Beck CS, Tichy VL, Moritz AR (1935) Production of a collateral circulation to the heart. Proc Soc Exp Biol Med 32:759–761
34. Beck CS (1935) Development of a new blood supply to the heart by operation. Ann Surg 102:801–813
35. Westaby S, Boscher C (1997) Surgery for coronary artery disease. In: Westaby S (ed) Landmarks in cardiac surgery. Isis Medical Media, Oxford, p 190
36. Pratt FH (1898) The nutrition of the heart through the vessels of Thebesius and the coronary veins. Am J Physiol 1:86–89
37. Beck CS (1948) Revascularization of the heart. Ann Surg 128(4):854–861

38. O'Shaughnessy L (1937) The pathology and surgical treatment of cardiac ischemia. Bristol Med Chir J 54:109–126
39. Lezius A (1937) Die kunstliche Blutversorgung des Herzmuskels. Arch Klin Chir 189: 342–346
40. Mueller RL, Rosengart TK, Isom WO (1997) The history of surgery for ischemic heart disease. Ann Thorac Surg 63:869–878
41. Day SB, Lillehei CW (1959) Experimental basis for a new operation for coronary artery disease. A left atrial-pulmonary shunt to encourage the development of interarterial intercoronary anastomosis. Surgery 45:487–495
42. Kownacki RJ, Kownacki VP, Kennel AJ, Imbriglia JE, Martin WL (1958) Collateral circulation to the heart by meant of cardiopneumonopexy and lingular vein ligation. AMA Arch Surg 76(1):106–112
43. Kline JL, Stern H, Bloomer WE, Liebow AA (1956) The application of an induced bronchial collateral circulation to the coronary arteries by cardiopneumonopexy. Am J Pathol 4: 663–693
44. Fauteux M, Palmer JH (1941) Treatment of angina pectoris of atheromatous origin by ligation of great cardiac veins. Can Med Assoc J 45:295–299
45. Fauteux M (1946) Surgical treatment of angina pectoris. Experiences with ligation of the great cardiac vein and pericoronary neurectomy. Ann Surg 1041–1046
46. Vineberg AM, Miller G (1951) Internal mammary coronary anastomosis in the surgical treatment of coronary artery insufficiency. Can Med Assoc J 64:543–549
47. Marx R, Jax TV, Kelm M (2001) Vineberg graft: flow reserve of bilateral implantation after 27 years. Ann Thorac Surg 71:341–343
48. Comroe JH (1979) Who was Alexis who? Cardiovasc Dis 6(3):251–270
49. Carrel A (1910) On the experimental surgery of the thoracic aorta and heart. Am J Surg 52:83–95
50. Carrel A (1967) Nobel lectures in physiology or medicine. Elsevier, Amsterdam, pp 437–466
51. Longmire WP, Cannon JA, Kattus AA (1958) Direct-vision coronary endarterectomy for angina pectoris. N Engl J Med 259(21):551–556
52. Picichè M Histoire de la chirurgie cardiaque. Site de la Société Française de Chirurgie Thoracique et Cardiovasculaire. Dossier. http://www.sfctcv.net/pages/college.php
53. Konstantinov IE (2009) At the cutting edge of the impossible: a tribute to Vladimir P. Demikhov. Tex Heart Inst J 36(5):453–458
54. Konstantinov IE, Robert HG (2000) The surgeon who performed the first successful clinical coronary artery bypass operation. Ann Thorac Surg 69:1966–1972
55. Goetz RH, Rohman M, Haller JD, Dee R, Rosenak SS (1961) Internal mammary–coronary artery anastomosis: a non suture method employing tantalum rings. J Thorac Cardiovasc Surg 41:378–386
56. Sabiston DC Jr (1974) The coronary circulation. Johns Hopkins Med J 134:314–329
57. Olearchyk AS, Olearchyk RM (1999) Reminiscences of Vasilii I. Kolesov. Ann Thorac Surg 67:273–276
58. Garrett HE, Dennis EW, DeBakey ME (1973) Aortocoronary bypass with saphenous vein graft. J Am Med Assoc 233:792–794
59. Konstantinov IE (2004) Circular vascular stapling in coronary surgery. Ann Thorac Surg 78:369–373
60. Favaloro RG (1968) Saphenous vein autograft replacement of severe segmental coronary artery occlusion-operative technique. Ann Thorac Surg 5:334–339
61. Green GE, Stertzer SH, Reppert EH (1968) Coronary arterial bypass grafts. Ann Thorac Surg 5:443–450

# 9 The History of Experimental Heterotopic and Orthotopic Heart Transplantation Before Cardiopulmonary Bypass

Tyson A. Fricke and Igor E. Konstantinov

*When I have fully decided that a result is worth getting I go ahead on it and make trial after trial until it comes.*

Thomas Edison

**Abstract**

Early experimental research in heart transplantation was conducted before the advent of the cardiopulmonary bypass. Carrel (1873–1944) was the first to perform a heterotopic transplant of the heart of a warm-blooded animal. Subsequently, Demikhov (1916–1998) performed the first orthotopic heart transplantation.

Advances in medicine and surgery come slowly. They are the result of the first creative and determined researchers and clinicians who strove to make a seemingly impossible idea a reality. Nowhere is this more evident than in the early history of cardiac transplantation. In the era before cardiopulmonary bypass, visionaries such as Carrel and Demikhov laid the foundations for later cardiac surgeons to achieve the once-thought improbable feat of transplanting a human heart. However, as is often the case, the names and achievements of these pioneers are mostly forgotten.

T. A. Fricke · I. E. Konstantinov (✉)
Cardiothoracic Surgery, Royal Children's Hospital, University of Melbourne, 50 Flemington Road, Melbourne, VIC 3052, Australia
e-mail: igor.konstantinov@rch.org.au

T. A. Fricke
e-mail: tafricke@gmail.com

M. Picichè (ed.), *Dawn and Evolution of Cardiac Procedures*,
DOI: 10.1007/978-88-470-2400-7_9, 

## 9.1 Alexis Carrel (1873–1944) and the First Experimental Extrathoracic Heart Transplant

A discussion of the early history of any type of organ transplantation invariably involves Carrel. This enigmatic and controversial father of transplantation, born near Lyon in 1873, was the first to develop a successful technique for vascular anastomosis. Vascular anastomosis, clearly a critical prerequisite for transplantation, had hitherto been met with failure [1]. Prior to 1902, only 21 successful arterial sutures had been reported [2, 3]. Carrel was to change all of this and the legend of the birth of his interest in this field is well-known. The story begins when Carrel was only a medical student in 1894. French president Sadi Carnot had been stabbed in the abdomen, which had resulted in a severed portal vein. Surgeons were unable to repair the vein and the French president subsequently bled to death. The young Carrel, however, had the belief that vascular anastomosis should be possible given the right technique [4]. It was after this experience that Carrel began working on his own technique of vascular anastomosis. His work was influenced by the work of Nikolai Eck. Eck was the first to attempt suturing of blood vessels and experimentally performed portacaval anastomosis in dogs, subsequently known as Eck's fistula [5]. However, the vascular anastomotic technique was truly revolutionized by Carrel. In 1902, Carrel first described his technique of triangulation, which enabled him to suture any vessel [6]. Carrel's technique was subsequently refined and published in 1906 [7]. It was during this time that Carrel met the American Charles Guthrie at the Hull Laboratory of Physiology at the University of Chicago and the vascular anastomotic technique of triangulation was born. Carrel and Guthrie's vascular anastomotic technique allowed them to transplant a variety of organs and, working with Guthrie, Carrel described many techniques of organ transplantation. Among his descriptions was included the first heterotopic heart transplant in which a heart was transplanted into the neck of a dog [8, 9]. Survival times for these dogs reached up to 2 h [3].

In recognition of his contribution to experimental transplantation, Carrel was awarded the Nobel Prize in Physiology or Medicine in 1912. He was only 39 years of age at the time. However, Carrel's work did not end there and was not confined to techniques of transplantation. His appreciation of the need to preserve organs in the period between harvest and transplantation led him to experiment in organ preservation [10] and later in the use of a perfusion pump with aviator and engineer Lindbergh [11]. His work on organ preservation, a major obstacle to transplant surgeons in the early 20th century, was years ahead of its time. He reported the use of hypothermia and Ringer solution to preserve parts of chick embryo spleen, skin and heart. His frustration with the limitations of these experiments led him to the development of a perfusion pump with Lindbergh, in which explanted feline hearts could be maintained for up to 12 h [1, 10].

In 1939 Carrel reached the age of mandatory retirement at the Rockefeller Institute where he had been working. In 1941 he returned to France, which was under German rule. He was appointed the director of the Carrel Foundation for the Study of Human Problems. His work there under the Vichy regime, along with his authoritarian beliefs, led to him being relieved of his position after the liberation of Paris in August 1944. He died shortly after in France on 5 November 1944. Despite being an obviously brilliant man, Carrel had ideas many believed were similar to those of Nazi fanaticism. He believed that society should be run by an intellectual elite that had to be protected from mixing with genetically inferior individuals. Many believe that, had he lived longer, he may have faced trial for his involvement in Nazi-occupied Paris.

After Carrel, experimental research in heart transplantation appeared to progress slowly over the subsequent years. Frank Mann and his colleagues from the Mayo Clinic published a report of two techniques of heterotopic heart transplantation into the neck of dogs in 1933. They were able to keep the donor heart alive for a maximum of 8 days. From their work on transplantation of other organs, Mann and his associates were some of the first to observe that "autotransplantation....is often successful, whereas homotransplantation....is rarely successful" [12]. Inadequate understanding of the rejection process was a major obstacle to the work of early transplant surgeons.

It took 18 years for experimental heart transplantation to again appear in the literature. In 1951, Marcus et al. [13] from the Chicago Medical School reported their experience with heterotopic transplantation into the neck of dogs. Their interesting technique involved the use of a third dog to support the circulation of the excised donor heart and was the first attempt at preserving a donor heart during transplantation.

Preserving the donor heart after it had been removed from the donor was clearly a challenge to early surgeons. As mentioned above, Marcus, Wong, and Luisada were the first to try and overcome the problem. Another approach was used by Wilford Neptune, Charles Bailey, and Brian Cookson of the Hahnemann Medical College in Philadelphia in 1953. Their idea was to use hypothermia for up to 30 min to prevent cell death in the donor heart [14]. Using this technique, they were able to achieve survival times of up to 6 h when transplanting both the heart and lungs into dogs. Their successful orthotopic heart–lung transplants were believed to be the first in the world. However, the Western medical community was unaware at the time of experiments performed by Demikhov, an unknown Soviet scientist and surgeon, who had already performed the world's first orthotopic heart and heart–lung transplants in dogs.

## 9.2 Vladimir Demikhov (1916–1998) and the First Experimental Intrathoracic Heart Transplant

Demikhov was born in 1916 to a peasant family in a Russian village. He was raised by his single mother who, despite being relatively uneducated herself, worked hard to provide her children with an education. At the age of 18, Demikhov went to Moscow to study biology at the University of Moscow. It was University policy that all new students bring a photograph of themselves wearing a white shirt and a tie. Unfortunately for Demikhov, he had neither the white shirt and the tie, nor the money to afford them! Luckily, the photographer was able to draw the required garments on to the photo [15]. It was an interesting twist of fate that this man from a rural area without a ruble to his name would one day be considered perhaps the most influential figure in experimental heart transplantation.

It did not take long for Demikhov to make his mark in the field of transplantation. By 1937 he had already designed the first mechanical assist device. For the first time in history, circulation was supported in an animal with the heart excised. The device could maintain a canine's circulation for 5.5 h [15]. He was still a student at the time.

Having graduated in 1940, Demikhov took up a position as an assistant in the university's department of physiology. He wasted no time, transplanting the hearts of cats into the inguinal region. However, his experiments led him to conclude that "because of its anatomical and physiological features the heart can only function actively when it is transplanted into the thorax….if it is transplanted to the vessels of the neck or into the inguinal region it cannot take an active part in the movement of the blood, and is a neutral organ, living on the recipient's blood" [15–17].

The next few years should have heralded breakthroughs in Demikhov's research, but World War II was to intervene. Demikhov was sent to combat zones where he served as a pathologist, in particular as a forensic expert. It was not until the end of 1945 that he was able to return to Moscow and continue his work.

Having returned home after the war, Demikhov performed the first heterotopic heart transplant into the thorax of an animal in 1946. That year he also performed the first heterotopic heart–lung transplantation. He was also the first to successfully accomplish an isolated orthotopic heart transplant in 1951. He was to complete this operation successfully 22 times between 1951 and 1955, achieving survival times of up to 15 h [9, 18]. These operations were, of course, before the arrival of the cardiopulmonary bypass and were a testament to Demikhov's ingenuity and technical skills.

Since Demikhov's research was published in Russian, it took a considerable amount of time for his achievements to become known to the Western world. It was not until 1962, when his work was translated and published in English [17], that the extent of his genius was revealed to the world. Overall, between 1946 and 1958 he performed 250 heart transplants in animals with no operative mortality and a longest survival of 30 days [2]. However, he was more well-known for his infamous head transplantation operation in which he transplanted the head of a dog on to the neck of another dog. The ethical arguments this raised and the criticism Demikhov received probably detracted from the legacy this man deserved as one of the great forerunners of heart transplantation. Many surgeons tried to visit his laboratory during the Cold War era. Christiaan Barnard was one of the few to be successful. In fact, Christiaan Barnard once remarked "if there is a father of heart and lung transplantation then Demikhov certainly deserves this title" [15, 19]. Before his death on 22 November 1998, Demikhov was honoured with the first "Pioneer award" awarded by the International Society for Heart and Lung Transplantation.

Early experimental heart transplant surgeons faced many problems in their work. Limited understanding and no treatment of allograft rejection, an inability to support the recipient's circulation after heart explantation and less than optimal perioperative care to name but a few. It makes one appreciate even more the significance of innovations achieved by Carrel and Demikhov. Both men suffered criticism, Carrel for his odd philosophical and political beliefs and Demikhov for his inexplicable canine head transplantation. Their eccentricities, or flaws depending on how they are viewed, were perhaps the price a mind pays for brilliance. Without the work of these early pioneers, heart transplantation may never have become what it is today.

## References

1. Dutkowski P, de Rougemont O, Clavien PA (2008) Alexis Carrel: genius, innovator and ideologist. Am J Transplant 8:1998–2003
2. Meine TJ, Russell SD (2005) A history of orthotopic heart transplantation. Cardiol Rev 13:190–196
3. Richardson RG (1970) The scalpel and the heart. Scribner, New York
4. Dente CJ, Feliciano DV (2005) Alexis Carrel (1873–1944)–Nobel Laureate, 1912. Arch Surg 140:609–610
5. Konstantinov IE (1997) Eck-Pavlov shunt: the 120th anniversary of the first vascular anastomosis. Surgery 121:640–645
6. Carrel A (1902) La technique operatoire des anastomoses vasculaires à la transplantation des viceres. Lyon Med 98:859–864
7. Carrel A, Guthrie CC (1906) Methode simple pour etablie une fistule l'eck. Compt Rend Soc Biol Par 60:1104
8. Carrel A, Guthrie CC (1905) The transplantation of veins and organs. Am Med 10:1101–1102
9. DiBardino DJ (1999) The history and development of cardiac transplantation. Tex Heart Inst J 26:198
10. Carrel A (1912) The preservation of tissues and its applications in surgery. JAMA 59:523–527
11. Lindbergh CA (1935) An apparatus for the culture of whole organs. J Exp Med 62:409–432
12. Mann FC, Priestley JT, Markowitz J, Yater WM (1933) Transplantation of the intact mammalian heart. Arch Surg 26:219–224
13. Marcus E, Wong SN, Luisada AA (1951) Homologous heart grafts: transplantation of the heart in dogs. Surg Forum 2:212–217
14. Neptune WB, Cookson BA, Bailey CP, Appler R, Rajkowski F (1953) Complete homologous heart transplantation. Arch Surg 66:174–178
15. Konstantinov IE (2009) At the cutting edge of the impossible a tribute to Vladimir P Demikhov. Tex Heart Inst J 36:453–458
16. Demikhov VP (1960) Transplantation of vital organs in experiments. Medgiz, Moscow
17. Demikhov VP (1962) Experimental transplantation of vital organs—authorized translation from Russian by Basil Haigh. Consultants Bureau, New York
18. Cooper DK (1968) Experimental development of cardiac transplantation. Br Med J 4:174–181
19. Konstantinov IE (1998) A mystery of Vladimir P. Demikhov: the 50th anniversary of the first intrathoracic transplantation. Ann Thorac Surg 65:1171–1177

# The History of Pediatric Cardiac Surgery Before the Introduction of Extracorporeal Circulation

# 10

Alessandro Frigiola

*Everything we did was because we thought it was right.*
Lyndon B. Johnson

**Abstract**

This chapter retraces the historical steps of cardiac surgery before the advent of extracorporeal circulation and highlights the great work done by physicians and researchers in laying the foundations for the development of cardiac surgery. Among the most significant figures quoted are Thomas Bevill Peacock and Maude Abbott who, with their studies on congenital malformations, revealed the anatomy of cardiopathies, and Vivien Thomas who, thanks to his manual dexterity, introduced the technique used later by Blalock to create the pulmonary systemic shunt. The chapter presents the most relevant surgical techniques created and developed by surgeons such as Robert Gross, who in 1938 successfully closed the first Botallo ductus and in 1952 closed the first atrial septal defect; Alfred Blalock, who made the first pulmonary systemic shunt and experimented with some techniques for aortic coarctation; Dammann, who made the first pulmonary artery banding; Blalock and Hanlon, who introduced the atrioseptectomy technique; Marc de Leval and Vishnevsky, who modified the technique of the Blalock–Taussig shunt, and Carlon, Glenn, and Darbinian, who introduced cavopulmonary anastomosis.

A. Frigiola (✉)
Cardiac Surgery Unit, I.R.C.C.S Policlinico San Donato,
San Donato Milanese, Italy
e-mail: alessandro.frigiola@grupposandonato.it; frigiola42@gmail.com

M. Picichè (ed.), *Dawn and Evolution of Cardiac Procedures*,
DOI: 10.1007/978-88-470-2400-7_10, 

## 10.1 Introduction

The knowledge of anatomy and physiology of the heart was very limited until the 19th century. It was during this period that many researchers devoted themselves to the study of congenital heart diseases, describing the characteristics of some of them. Henri-Louis Roger (1809–1891) described the characteristic murmur and thrill of VSD ("Bruit de Roger") and, in 1841, published a practical study on auscultation [1].

A special mention goes to a great scholar: Thomas Bevill Peacock (1812–1882). He was a general physician with a particular interest in pathology [2]. His main contributions were in cardiology, to which he added knowledge by keen observation, punctilious description, and illustration. His contribution on congenital heart disease remains one of the most important in this field. In 1846 he became a founder-member of the Pathological Society of London, of which he became president in 1864. Among numerous papers he published in 1858 his magnum opus, "On Malformations of the Human Heart" [3]. The paper was of great interest and became such a reference book that Maude Abbott in 1908 described it in the following way: "The first comprehensive study, covering the whole field and reviewing the earlier literature may be said to be Peacock's, which remains a classic and is still the leading authority in English upon the subject" [4]. Particularly interesting is the description of two cases of tetralogy of Fallot, published 42 years before the original report by Fallot.

Peacock in his work described the malformation in this way: "Malformation of the heart, consisting in contraction of the orifice of the pulmonary artery with deficiency at the base of the interventricular septum" [5].

But it was Maude Abbott (1869–1940) who made a comprehensive study of congenital anomalies of the heart (Fig. 10.1). In 1936 she published the comprehensive Atlas Of Congenital Cardiac Disease (American Heart Association) with critical analysis of more than 1,000 cases. Her work and her great knowledge of congenital heart disease have been a stimulus for the development of cardiac surgery.

In 1888 Etienne-Louis-Arthur Fallot (1850–1911) introduced important information about cyanotic heart disease describing the tetralogy that would later bear his name, explaining the mechanism of cyanosis [6].

As told before, scientists had slowly increased their interest in the human cardiovascular system during the previous centuries, but only at the beginning of the 20th century did they start to perform surgery for congenital heart disease. It had taken 3,000 years of experimentation to understand how the heart worked. The pioneers of cardiac surgery merged this knowledge with their new ideas and began experimenting with new surgical techniques. Our thanks are due to those pioneers who fought against the disbelief, diffidence, envy, and ignorance met from their more conservative colleagues. The 19th century medical reports did not mention congenital heart diseases because they were considered to be incurable diseases, and therefore not worth mentioning.

**Fig. 10.1** Maude Abbott

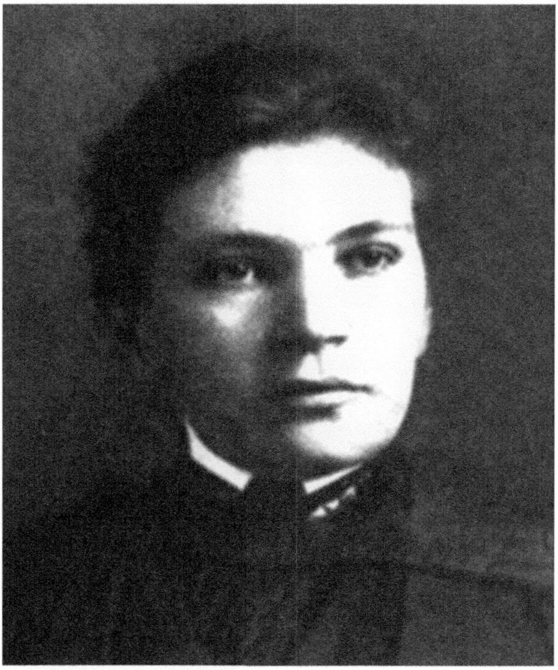

The 20 years from 1935 through 1955 represent the most important lapse of time for the birth of cardiac surgery. During this period the first closed heart surgery procedures were performed, which then led to modern cardiac surgery.

Physicians such as Gross, Blalock, etc., surely deserve to be mentioned. But as we are dealing with the history of cardiac surgery, it is important to remember that the results achieved by physicians are often a consequence of much lifelong research conducted by their predecessors, who have never become famous. Often new achievement in medicine comes from other similar previous achievement, maybe accomplished in different countries.

I would like to dedicate this chapter to those scientists that have spent many days, and often many nights, on research that has led other colleagues to new achievements in surgery and medicine.

The chronological history of paediatric cardiac surgery and its phases, before the introduction of extracorporeal circulation, are reported here.

## 10.2 Patent Ductus Arteriosus

The closure of the patent ductus arteriosus by means of ligation was first described in 1907 by John Munro, Professor of Surgery at Tuff's Medical School in Boston. He described ligating a persistent ductus in the cadaver of a newborn child [7]. The first surgical closure was instead performed by John Streider in Boston, in 1937,

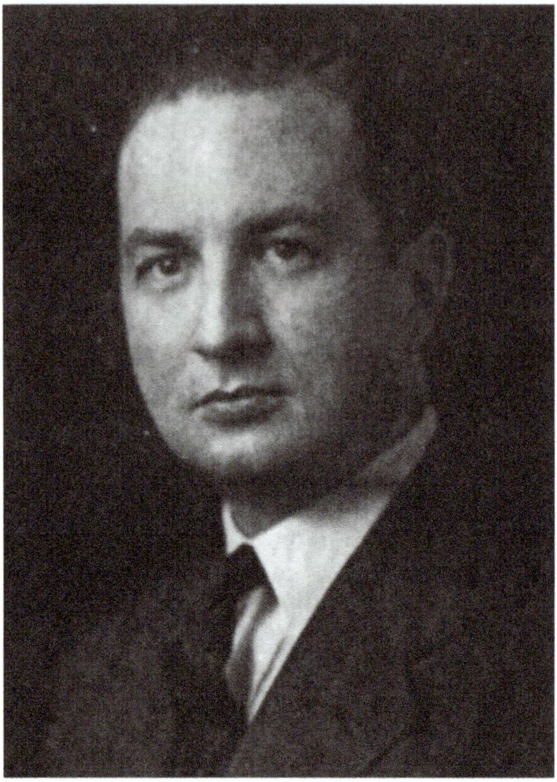

**Fig. 10.2** Robert Gross

in a 22-year-old woman with ductal endocarditis caused by *Streptococcus viridans*. Streider believed that once the ductus had been closed the infection would heal. The patient survived the intervention, but died 5 days later because of abdominal distension due to the infection [8].

Eighteen months later Robert Gross successfully ligated a ductus in a 7-year-old girl. This is why the year 1938 is frequently, although not universally, considered the starting point of modern cardiac surgery [9]. A curious story is reported about that intervention: although Gross was not allowed to perform the procedure, he was so certain of the result that, taking advantage of the absence of his chief, performed the ligation and succeeded (Fig. 10.2).

## 10.3 Aortic Coarctation

Aortic coarctation (AC) is a potentially life-threatening congenital heart syndrome. This condition, however, might be consistent with prolonged survival, even if untreated. Abbott and Coll reported an average survival of 36 years of age [10]. Since the 1940s, several researchers were focused on this matter in order to find a

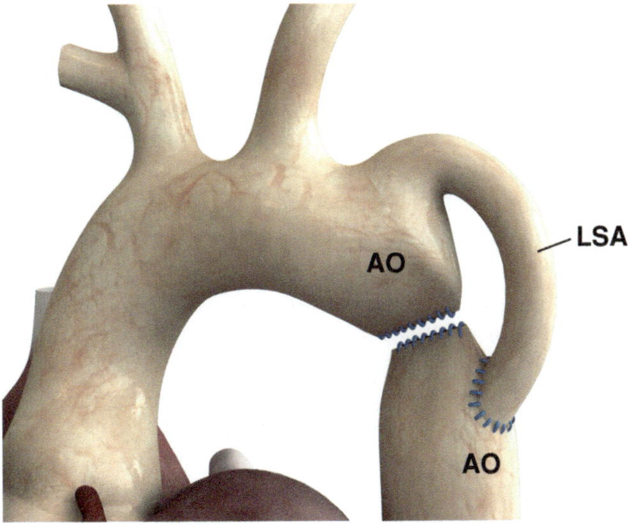


**Fig. 10.3** Experimental technique for aortic coarctation "subclavian turn-down". LSA left subclavian artery, AO aorta

surgical solution. Aortic cross-clamping was a main concern at that time because of the high incidence of the resulting paraplegia. Multiple surgical techniques were tested on animal models. In particular, the early 1940s, Blalock and Coll [11] experimentally induced an aortic stenosis condition by folding a rubber band around the aorta. Blalock and Park later described the "subclavian turn-down" surgical technique, performed by anastomosing the distal end of the transected subclavian artery to the descending thoracic aorta, thus bypassing the coerced segment (Fig. 10.3). A total of 43 procedures were performed on dogs. Only 10 of the 43 animals survived the operation for several months or longer. The predominating postoperative complication was paralysis of the posterior part of the body.

Blalock's footnotes and comments: "These experiments were undertaken with the idea of devising a mean for the surgical treatment of coarctation of the aorta. Some of the animals survived this procedure, and there was evidence of adequate blood flow to the posterior part of the body. The possible clinical application of these studies is discussed".

Unfortunately, because of the high mortality rate and the high incidence of paraplegia among the tested dogs, this technique was abandoned. But, once again, a prolonged experimental effort enabled future researchers to take advantage of past experiences and overcome previous drawbacks. As a matter of fact, in 1944 in Stockholm, Clarence Crafoord was the first surgeon to perform reconstructive surgery by cross-clamping the aorta, resecting the coerced segment, and restoring aortic continuity by a termino-terminal anastomosis. The first successful operation was soon followed by a second straightforward procedure [12].

Ever since, other surgeons have found specific solutions to different types of AC. Gross was the first surgeon to replace the resected segment of the coerced aorta with an aortic homograft in order to restore aortic continuity. That solution was necessary because of the extensive length of the coerced segment [13]. But there were still issues in the field, such as the high incidence of recoarctation. Several years needed to pass in order to understand that the ductal tissue around the anastomosis was a main determinant of recurrence. The "subclavian flap" technique, described by Waldhausen and Coll in 1966 [14], significantly reduced the rate of recoarctation.

Nowadays, many patients are treated by percutaneous dilatation (PTA) plus stenting procedure, but the surgical techniques described in the 1940s are still the only viable solutions for treating babies with AC.

## 10.4 Aorto-Systemic Shunt

Until the early 1900s congenital heart anomalies were merely autoptical findings and very few physicians could make a correct diagnosis on living individuals.

The "blue babies" were a significant diagnostic challenge and no suitable surgical solution was available.

Dr. Helen Taussig (Fig. 10.4) was the first physician to figure out a suitable surgical option for some specific congenital anomalies. She focused her attention on the so-called "tetralogy of Fallot," a congenital heart condition in which a ventricular septal defect is associated with right ventricular outflow tract obstruction and normal heart volumes. At that time Helen Taussig was testing hundreds of "blue babies" along with a heart surgeon, Dr. Blalock (Fig. 10.5). Helen Taussig suggested that those patients might be treated with an artificial conduit that Dr. Blalock had been testing at that time in his laboratories. Dr. Blalock himself emphasized Helen Taussig's role in this decision: "One of us has seen several infants with pulmonary stenosis in whom cyanosis was not apparent until the ductus arteriosus closed. It was an appreciation of this fact, together with an extensive experience with the experimental use of large arteries for the purpose of conducting blood to sites not usually supplied by such vessels, that led to the clinical work recorded in this paper" [15].

The successful outcome of the Blalock operation was also down to Vivien Thomas (Fig. 10.6) who played an important role in structuring and accomplishing the shunting surgical procedure [16]. Vivien Thomas, son of a Louisiana carpenter, had to give up medical school when his savings for tuition disappeared following the October stock market crash. He found a job as lab technician at Vanderbilt University, working with Dr. Blalock. When Dr. Blalock moved to Hopkins University, he asked Thomas to follow him. Together with the Blalock team and the cardiologist Helen Taussig, Thomas played a critical role in structuring the "blue-baby operation". The aim was to increase the blood flow to the lungs in order to improve oxygenation. Thomas had gifted hands and he was known as "the man with hands blessed by God". For over 2 years they worked in the

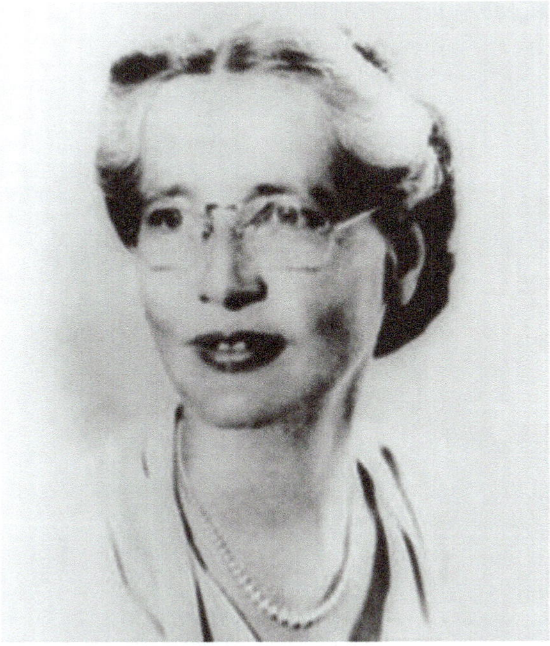

**Fig. 10.4** Helen Taussig

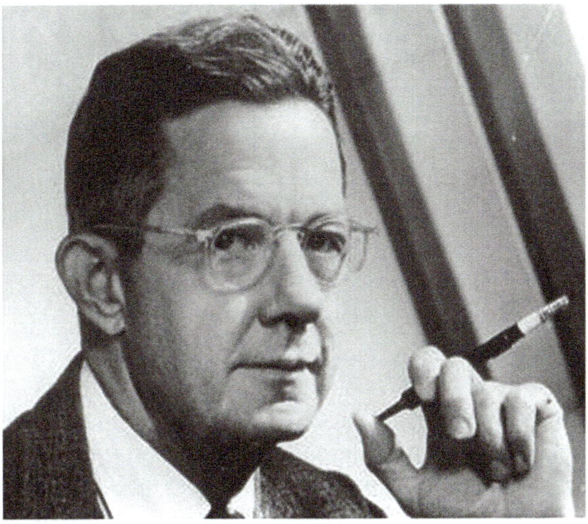

**Fig. 10.5** Alfred Blalock

Blalock lab to arrange the technique known as the "Blalock–Taussig shunt." He also created new surgical instruments specifically designed to perform the shunting technique. Thomas himself supervised the first successful "subclavian-pulmonary anastomosis" on 29 November 1944. The operation was performed by cutting the subclavian artery distally, reversing its course, and achieving an end-to-side anastomosis to the pulmonary artery (Fig. 10.7). Thomas was a key partner in

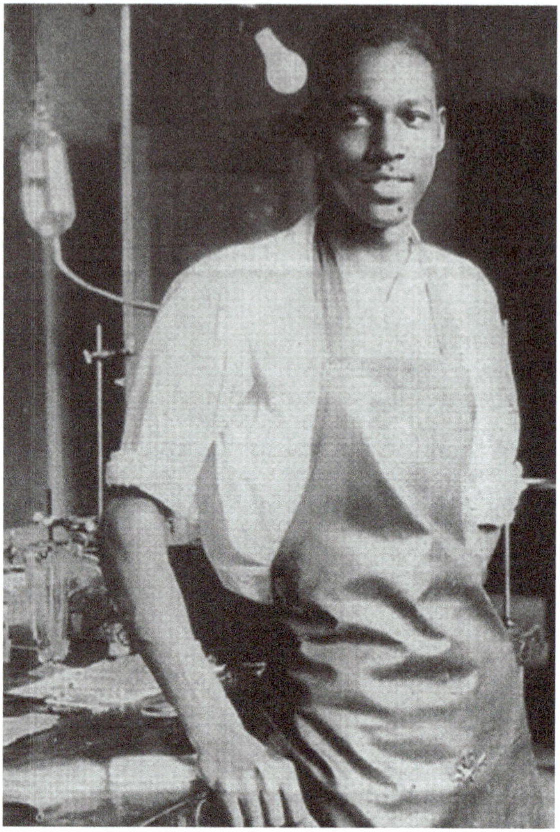

**Fig. 10.6** Vivien Thomas

hundreds of "blue-baby operations." This operation represents a milestone in the history of medicine, but, because sometimes the anatomy does not fit the Blalock–Taussig shunt, some other surgeons were looking for either alternatives or modified shunting procedures.

In 1946 in Chicago, Willis Potts arranged a new "shunt operation" by performing a side-to-side anastomosis between the pulmonary artery and the descending thoracic aorta just distal to the left subclavian artery [17]. The Potts shunt was a viable option but had several drawbacks such as uneasy assessment of the size of the anastomosis in order to prevent pulmonary blood overflow and technical issues in tearing down the shunt. Because of all these issues this technique did not find support. Another technique was introduced in 1964 by Waterstone in London who performed a direct anastomosis between the ascending aorta and the right pulmonary artery [18]. This technique was also abandoned because of the same disadvantage. Other cardiac surgeons dedicated themselves to finding a solution, which could modify the original Blalock–Taussig shunt. In 1948 Robert Gross introduced an arterial homograft as a means of extension of the short subclavian artery [19]. In 1957 Vishnevsky, a surgeon at the Institute of

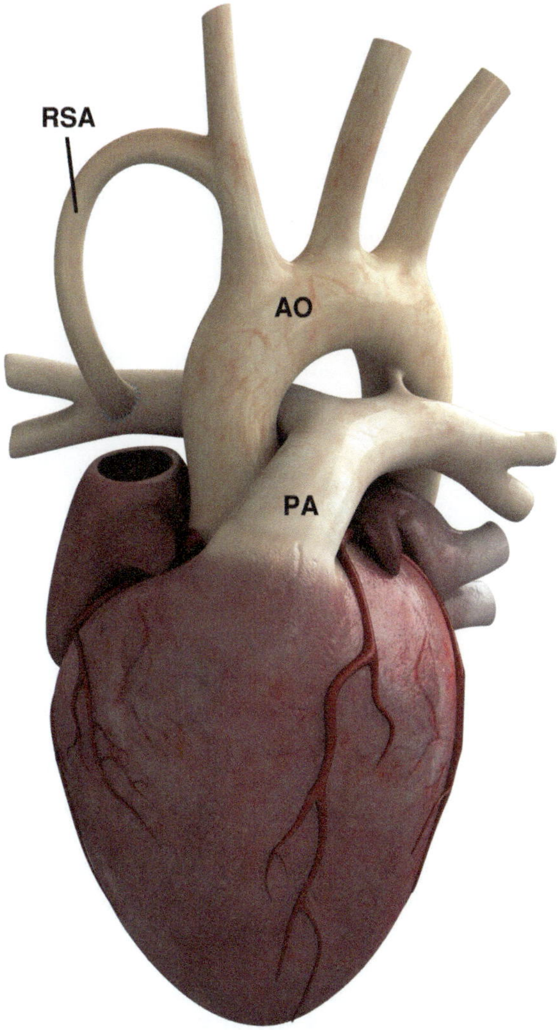


**Fig. 10.7** Blalock–Taussig aorto-pulmonary shunt. RSA right subclavian artery, AO aorta, PA pulmonary artery

Surgery in Moscow, published an article in which he described the use of an arterial homograft while performing a Blalock–Taussig shunt in 31 patients. In that series three of the patients died. It was peculiar that Vishnevsky did not interrupt or ligate the subclavian artery, but simply inserted the arterial homograft between the subclavian artery and the pulmonary artery, thus diverting the blood flow from the subclavian artery into the pulmonary artery [20]. Following this concept, in 1981 Marc Roger de Leval from the Great Ormond Street Hospital in London (Fig. 10.8) used a Dacron graft as a bridge between the subclavian artery and the

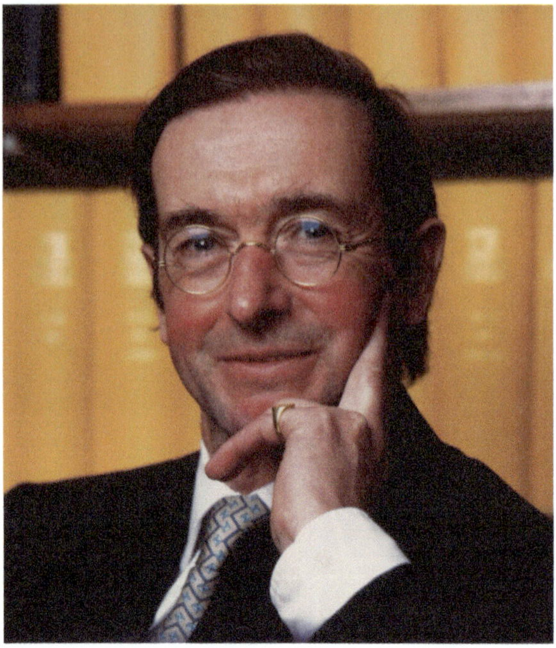

**Fig. 10.8** Marc de Leval

pulmonary artery in 13 patients and a Goretex graft in 83 patients [21]. The critical benefit of this new procedure was the adaptability of the Goretex conduit, available in different sizes, which could be anchored to any segment of the ascending aorta, the anonymous trunk, and the subclavian artery. It was also easy to dismantle at the time of the ultimate correction.

The Blalock–Taussig operation modified by de Leval still remains the procedure of choice for any condition which might benefit from increased blood flow to the lungs (Fig. 10.9).

## 10.5 Atrial Septectomy and Atrial Septostomy

In the 1950s transposition of great arteries (TGA) was one of the most significant determinants of death among all congenital heart anomalies (20 % of all deaths) [22]. It was mandatory to find at least a palliation to allow these babies to survive. A surgically-induced atrial septal opening appeared to be the right choice to prolong survival.

Thus, in 1950, Blalock and Hanlon [23] introduced the atrioseptectomy technique, which implies a surgical breach in the atrial septum performed with a beating heart by placing a clamp between the right pulmonary veins and the right atrium, along the Waterston sulcus (Fig. 10.10). This procedure represented the only surgical option until 1966, when Rashkind introduced the atrioseptostomy technique using a balloon catheter [24].

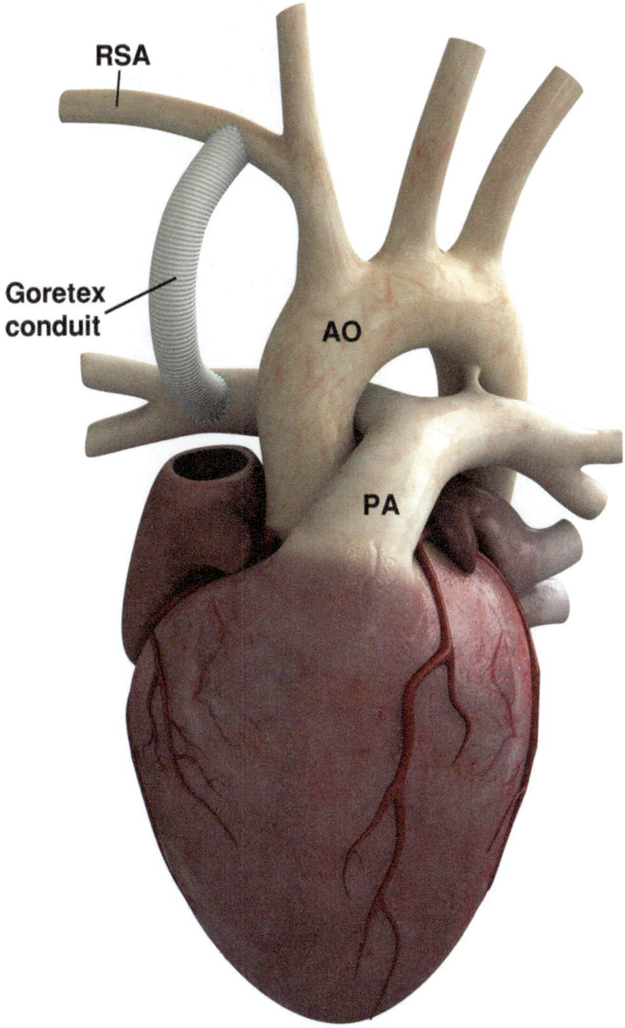


**Fig. 10.9** Modified Blalock–Taussig shunt with Goretex conduit. RSA right subclavian artery, AO aorta, PA pulmonary artery

William Rashkind was not a surgeon but a pediatric cardiologist at the Children's Hospital in Philadelphia. Besides the balloon atrial septostomy he also developed other devices to close atrial septal defects and persistent patent ductus arteriosus.

The Rashkind technique is routinely used nowadays in all neonates with TGA.

## 10.6 Pulmonary Artery Banding

Another surgical technique developed in the 1950s is pulmonary artery banding, performed in 1952 by Muller and Dammann [25].

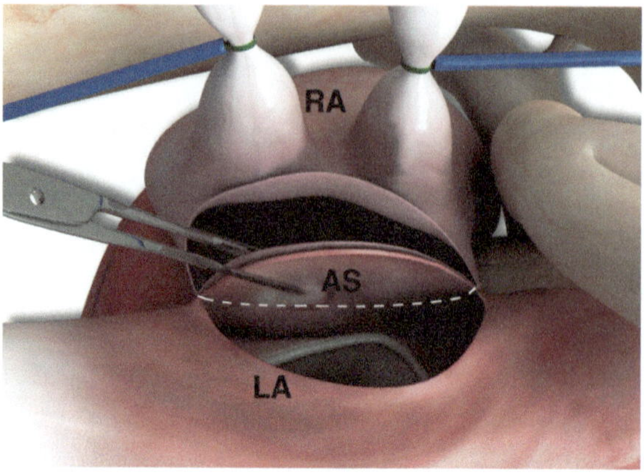


**Fig. 10.10** Blalock and Hanlon atrial septectomy. RA right atrium, AS atrial septum, LA left atrium

This is a valid alternative to extracorporeal circulation correction for pulmonary overflow when open heart surgery is not possible or is burdened by a high surgical risk. It is used in the case of newborns or infants with multiple interventricular defects, double outlet right ventricle or univentricular heart without pulmonary stenosis. The banding was a great idea that saved thousands of children and made a major contribution to pediatric cardiac surgery.

The technique developed by Muller and Dammann differs greatly from the one used today, and I think it is quite interesting to quote the original description. The first operation took place on 11 July 1951 on a 5-month-old infant who weighed 3.74 kg (Fig. 10.11).

Between 1951 and 1955 Muller and Dammann operated on 25 patients and in their original paper, published in 1955, they present the results of those early interventions [26]. There were nine deaths of which five occurred in the operating room before the artery was banded. This shows how difficult it was to follow the road of innovation and how the negative results could influence the decisions of surgeons to continue implementing their ideas. But the conviction to do the right thing luckily almost always prevailed, and most surgeons continued in their hard work.

Nowadays, banding of the pulmonary artery represents a valid alternative to correction, especially in those centers or countries where cardiac surgery is at the beginning and open heart surgery in the first months of life represents a high mortality risk.

## 10.7 Atrial Septal Defect

The atrial septal defect is an intracardiac disease and, like all the other intracardiac diseases, was systematically cured only after 1953 with the introduction of extracorporeal circulation. Until 1952 it was very difficult to imagine the treatment of an intracardiac disease such as atrial septal defect.

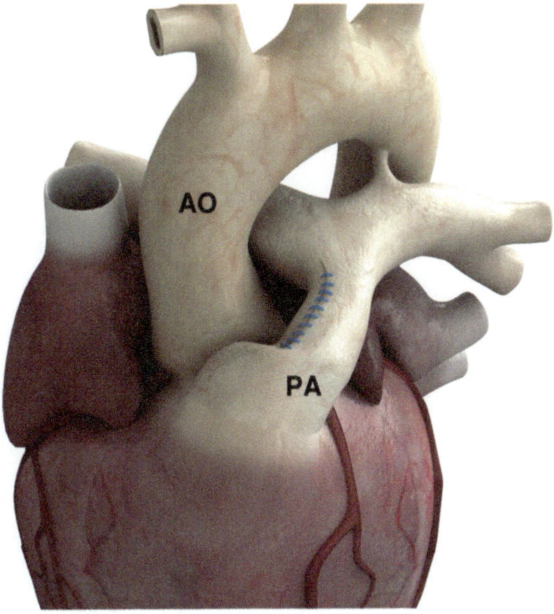


**Fig. 10.11** Pulmonary artery banding. AO aorta, PA pulmonary artery

It was Robert Gross who in 1952 carried out a successful closure of an atrial septal defect without the use of extracorporeal circulation. Before Gross' successful intervention, various methods were suggested or were actually used in the attempt to close atrial septal defects. Murray passed mattress sutures of silk or strips of fascia through the heart, attempting to place these in the plane of the septum [27]. Swan et al. inverted the right and left auricular appendages in this coapted position with mattress stitches passed through them [28]. Cohn suggested pushing into the right auricular wall to plug a septal opening, suturing the inverted wall to the septum [29]. No reports of the successful use of these methods have been published; each of the methods enumerated above presented serious technical disadvantages, and none of them had a more than limited usefulness.

Gross' idea was instead rather successful, and, in 1952, he described it as follows: "Pursuing a somewhat different line of thought, we considered it possible to attach temporarily some sort of coneshaped rubber bag (open at the top) to the right auricular wall so that the auricle could be opened and blood allowed to rise up into the rubber well. Through this column of blood, it might be possible to pass the operator's fingers down into the auricle, to find the septal opening and to close it either by direct suture or by the onlay of a piece of flat substance (such as a plaque of fascia, pericardium or plastic)".

A series of 114 dogs were used to develop proficiency in the techniques of applying a well to an auricle.

After extensive trials with the use of auricular wells in experiments on animals, it was considered justifiable to attempt closure of defects of the interauricular septum in man. And so, in 1952, Gross performed the first intervention on a patient [30].

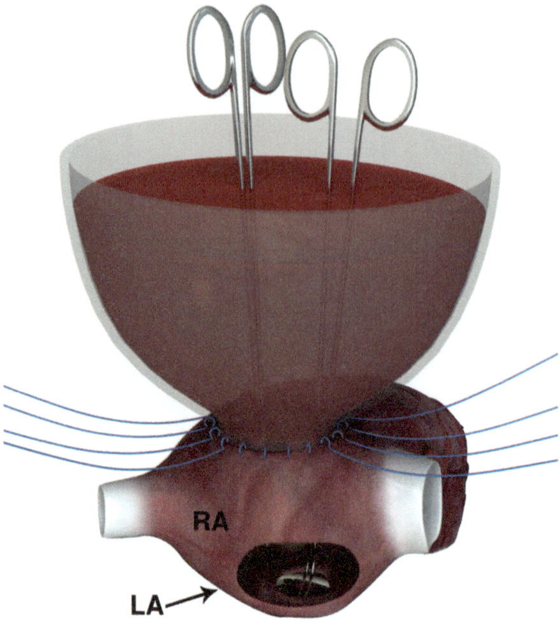


**Fig. 10.12** Atrial well. RA, right atrium, LA left atrium

In order to work on human beings, a rubber well was constructed with a height of 15 cm, an upper orifice diameter of 13 cm, and a lower orifice diameter of 4 cm (Fig. 10.12).

One year later the first intervention in extracorporeal circulation was made by Gibbon: the closure of an atrial septal defect. It was the beginning of "on pump" open heart surgery [31].

## 10.8 Cavopulmonary Anastomosis

The history of cavopulmonary anastomosis is characterized by the work of many researchers who, at different times and in different locations, however, had been working on a common goal: to find an alternative solution to the pulmonary systemic shunt in cases of pulmonary hypoperfusion by connecting the superior vena cava to the pulmonary artery.

Although the pulmonary anastomosis bears the name of Glenn who performed the first clinical application in 1958 [32] in a 7-year-old child suffering from single ventricle and pulmonary stenosis (Fig. 10.13), this technique had already been described by other surgeons who performed it on 11 dogs, and for some of them the intervention was successful.

A special contribution was made by the Italian Carlon, Professor of Surgery at the University of Padua Medical School, who first described the concept of the cavopulmonary shunt.

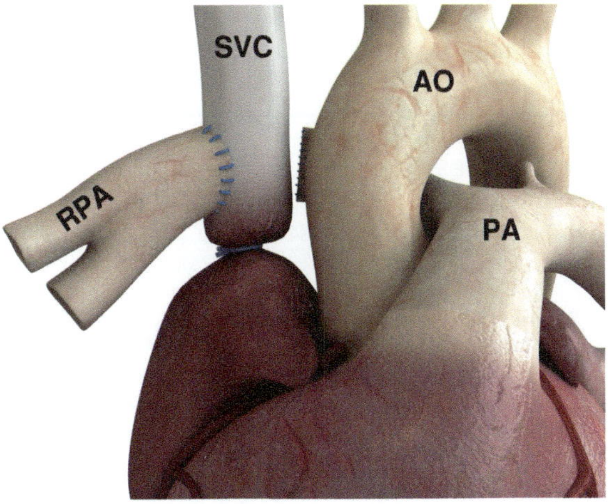


**Fig. 10.13** Cavopulmonary anastomosis (Glenn operation). RPA right pulmonary artery, SVC superior vena cava, AO aorta, PA pulmonary artery

Carlon's intervention was thus described in the paper published in 1950 [33]: "the superior vena cava is tied short of its opening into the right auricle and the blood from the superior part of the body flowing into the right lung and returning to the left side of the heart through the right pulmonary veins, avoids the right side of the heart."

Also in the early 50s, independently from Carlon's work, many other surgeons were continuing their research into cavopulmonary anastomosis, for example, Francis Robicsek from Hungary [34], Jose Patino and William Glenn in the USA [35], and Tigran Darbinian and Nikolai Galankin in Russia [36].

Furthermore, in the decade 1950–1960, Schumacker [37], Robicsek, and Sanger [38] made other significant contributions to understanding the physiology of the advantages and disadvantages of this type of procedure. We cannot forget the contribution of Gaetano Azzolina, who, in 1972, developed the concept of a bidirectional shunt [39].

In the same year in Russia Meshalkin was carrying out important work on cavopulmonary anastomosis both in dogs and in humans and in 1956 he finally took advantage of his great experience, operating on 24 children with 21 successes [40].

Cavopulmonary anastomosis is surely still one of the most frequently used surgical procedures in the world and it also represents one of the most valid solutions of increased pulmonary flow in the case of hypoperfusion.

## 10.9 Conclusions

This presentation of the historical milestones in the pre-extracorporeal circulation era highlights the relevance of teamwork and collaboration and makes us realize how it is very hard, in the research field, to say who was the first. Very often, the publication of a new technique is the outcome of the work of other researchers, each of them contributing to the realization of the final idea. The pioneering contributions of many surgeons are strictly connected.

## References

1. Barth JB, Roger HL (1841) Traité pratique d'auscultation; ou, Exposé methodique des diverses applications de ce mode d'examen à l'état physiologique et morbide de l'économie; suivi d'un précis de percussion. Béchet et Labé, Paris, p 515
2. Porter JH (1962) The ninetheenth-century physician and cardiologist Thomas Bevill Peacock (1812–1882). Med Hist 1962 6(3):240–254
3. Peacock TB (1858) On malformation of the human heart. Churchill, London p 204
4. Abbott ME (1908) Congenital cardiac disease. In: William O (ed) Modern medicine, vol 4. Lea and Febiger, Philadelphia
5. Peacock TB Malformation of the heart, consisting in contraction of the orifice of the pulmonary artery with deficiency at the base of the interventricular septum. Trans Pathol Soc London 1846–1848, 1, 52
6. Fallot ELA (1888) Contribution à l'anatomie pathologique de la maladie bleue (Cyanose cardiaque). Marseille médical, 25:77–93, 138–158, 207–223, 341–354, 370–386, 403–420
7. Munro JCM (1907) Ligation of the ductus arteriosus. Ann Surg 46(3):335–338
8. Streider J (1937) Discussion of Blalock A, Levy SE. Tuberculosis pericarditis. J Thorac Surg 7:132–152
9. Gross RE, Hubbard JP (1939) Surgical ligation of a patent ductus arteriosus. Report of first successful case. JAMA 112:729–731
10. Abbott ME (1931) Congenital heart disease. Nelson Loose Leaf Living Medicine. vol. 4, Thomas Nelson and Sons, New York
11. Blalock A, Park EA (1944) The surgical treatment of experimental coarctation (atresia) of the aorta. Ann Surg 119:445–456
12. Crafoord C, Nylin G (1945) Congenital coarctation of the aorta and its surgical treatment. J Thorac Surg 14:347–361
13. Gross RE, Hufnagel CA (1945) Coarctation of the aorta. Experimental studies regarding its surgical correction. N Engl J Med 223:287–293
14. Waldhausen JA, Nahrwold DL (1966) Repair of coarctation of the aorta with a subclavian flap. J Thorac Cardiovasc Surg 51:532–533
15. Blalock A, Taussig HB (1945) The surgical treatment of malformations of the heart in which there is pulmonary stenosis or atresia. JAMA 128:189–202
16. Damon M, Kennedy DO (2005) In search of Vivien Thomas. Tex Heart Inst J 32(4):477–478
17. Potts WJ, Smith S, Gibson S (1946) Anastomosis of the aorta to a pulmonary artery. JAMA 132:627–631
18. Waterston DJ (1962) Treatment of Fallot's tetralogy in children under one year of age. Rozhl Chir 41:181
19. Gross R, Bill AJ, Pierce E (1949) Methods for preservation and transplantation of arterial grafts. observations on arterial grafts in dogs. report of transplantation of preserved arterial grafts in 9 human cases. Surg Gynecol Obstet 88:689–701
20. Alexi-Meskishvili VV, Konstantinov IE (2005) Pioneering contributions of Alexander A. Vishnevsky and his team to cardiac surgery. J Card Surg 20:569–573
21. De Leval M, McKay R, Jones M et al (1981) Modified Blalock-Taussig shunt. Use of subclavian artery as flow regulator in prosthetic systemic-pulmonary artery shunts. J Thorac Cardiovasc Surg 81:112–119
22. Keith JD et al (1953) Transposition of the great vessels. Circulation 7:830–838
23. Blalock A, Hanlon CR (1950) The surgical treatment of complete transposition of the aorta and the pulmonary artery. Surg Gynecol Obstet 90:1–15

24. William J, Rashkind MD, William W, Miller MD (1966) Creation of an atrial septal defect without thoracothomy. JAMA 196(11)991–992
25. Muller WH Jr, Dammann JF Jr (1952) The treatment of certain congenital malformations of the heart by the creation of pulmonic stenosis to reduce pulmonary hypertension and excessive pulmonary blood flow. Surg Gynecol Obstet 95:213–219
26. Muller WH Jr, Dammann JF Jr (1956) Results following the creation of pulmonary artery stenosis. Ann Surg 143:816–821
27. Murray G (1948) Closure of defects in cardiac septa. Ann Surg 128:843–852
28. Swan H, Maresh G, Johnson ME, George W (1950) The experimental creation and closure of auricular septal defects. J Thorac Surg 20:542–551
29. Cohn R (1947) An experimental method for the closure of interauricular septal defects in dogs. Am Heart J 33:453–457
30. Gross RE (1952) Surgical closure of defects of the interauricular septum by use of an atrial well. N Engl J Med 247:455–460
31. Gibbon JH (1954) Application of a mechanical heart and lung apparatus to cardiac surgery. Minn Med 37:171–177
32. Glenn WWL (1958) Circulatory bypass of the right side of the heart. IV. Shunt between superior vena cava and distal right pulmonary artery—report of the clinical application. N Engl J Med 259:117–120
33. Carlon CA, Mondini PG, De Marchi R (1951) Surgical treatment of some cardiovascular diseases. J Int Coll Surg 16:1–10
34. Robicsek F, Temesvari A, Kadar RL (1956) A new method for the treatment of congenital heart disease associated with impaired pulmonary circulation. Acta Med Scand 154:151–161
35. Glenn WWL, Patino GF (1954) Circulatory bypass of the right heart. I. Preliminary observations on the direct delivery of vena cava blood into the pulmonary arterial circulation: azygos vein-pulmonary artery shunt. Yale J Biol Med 27:147–151
36. Galankin N, Darbinian T (1956) Anastomosis between superior vena cava and the right pulmonary artery. Eksp Khirurgiia 1:54–57
37. Schumacker HB (1955) Rationale of anastomosis of right auricular appendage to pulmonary artery in the treatment of tricuspid atresia. J Thorac Surg 30:503–512
38. Sanger PW, Robicsek F, Robicsek LK, Gallucci V (1965) The clinical application of cavopulmonary anastomosis. Dis Chest 48:145–153
39. Azzolina G, Eufrates S, Pensa PM (1972) Tricuspid atresia: experience in surgical management with a modified cavopulmonary anastomosis. Thorax 27:111–115
40. Meshalkin EN (1956) Anastomosis of the superior vena cava with the pulmonary artery in patients with congenital heart disease with blood flow insufficiency in the lesser circulation: experiment. Eks Khir 1:3–10

# Part II

# Research on the Cardiopulmonary Bypass Machine

# On the Path to Cardiopulmonary Bypass: From Le Gallois' Experiments to Brukhonenko's Machine

# 11

Matthew S. Yong, Stephen B. Horton and Igor E. Konstantinov

> *But if the place of the heart could be supplied by injection—and if, for the regular continuance of this injection, there could be furnished a quantity of arterial blood, whether natural, or artificially formed, supposing such a formation possible—then life might be indefinitely maintained in any portion; and consequently, after decapitation, even in the head itself, without destroying any functions peculiar to the brain. Not only life might thus be kept up both in the head and in any other portion separated from the body of an animal, but might also be re-produced after its entire extinction. It might be restored likewise to the whole body, and thereby a complete resurrection be performed in the full extent of the word.*
>
> César Julien Jean Le Gallois

**Abstract**

The success and achievements in the field of cardiac surgery are attributed to the discovery of cardiopulmonary bypass techniques. The pioneering work of nineteenth century scientists, physicians, and engineers in experimental animal organ perfusion laid the foundations for artificial oxygenation techniques (film, bubble, and isolated lung) and closed circulation circuits. The first half of the twentieth century featured the work of Brukhonenko, Crafoord, Björk, Jonblogbloed, and Gibbon in refining perfusion methods in search of achieving

M. S. Yong
Cardiac Surgery Unit, Royal Children's Hospital, University of Melbourne, Melbourne, Australia

S. B. Horton
Department of Perfusion, Royal Children Hospital, University of Melbourne, Melbourne, Australia

I. E. Konstantinov (✉)
Cardiac Surgical Unit, The Royal Children's Hospital, Flemington Road, Parkville, Melbourne 3052 Australia
e-mail: igor.konstantinov@rch.org.au

M. Picichè (ed.), *Dawn and Evolution of Cardiac Procedures*,
DOI: 10.1007/978-88-470-2400-7_11, 

clinical application in humans. They assembled heart–lung machines intended for use age during cardiovascular operations. The first clinical application of the heart–lung machine was recorded in 1951, heralding a new era in cardiac surgery.

## 11.1 The Beginning

The origin of the extracorporeal circulation is attributed to the early work of César Julien Jean Le Gallois (1770–1814). In 1813, Le Gallois' experiments [1] led him to suggest that an artificial circulation could sustain the function of a body part. In 1858, Eduard Brown-Séquard [2] injected blood into the limbs of beheaded prisoners. His perfusion experiments demonstrated that a neural response could be preserved by early maintenance of oxygenated blood supply.

Ernst Bidder [3], in continuing Loebell's study on urine secretion [4], assembled one of the first continuous perfusion apparatuses in 1862. In these early days, mechanical circulatory pumps had not yet been devised; thus, perfusion pressure was created using a cylinder filled with mercury. The cylinder was connected to a basin of blood and pressure could be varied according to the level of mercury. Arterial blood was drawn from a living animal. The blood was filtered and anti-coagulated by stirring before perfusion into animal kidneys. Ludwig and Schmidt [5, 6], from the Physiological Institute at Leipzig, developed an apparatus for artificial perfusion into an isolated organ. In 1868, they reported on experiments with dog kidneys and muscle tissue. Their rudimentary oxygenation technique involved whisking blood in normal air. Ludwig and Schmidt observed the potential of perfusion methods in conserving "the viability of muscles and nerves" [6].

## 11.2 From Pulsatile to Continuous Perfusion

Early perfusion techniques required interruption of the blood flow to oxygenate the venous blood and to return oxygenated blood back into the arterial reservoir. In 1885, at the Physiological Institute in Leipzig, Max von Frey and Max Gruber revolutionised perfusion techniques by designing the first closed artificial circulation system [7]. In the following years, many others incorporated this method of perfusion into their experiments [8–13]. Elements essential to this system included a method of blood oxygenation and a reliable pump mechanism. Von Frey and Gruber's initial apparatus comprising an injection syringe capable of achieving a pulsatile flow [7]. Earlier perfusion techniques utilised continuous flow in their experiments of organ perfusion. In contrast, Von Frey and Gruber's double-action pump system was designed to imitate the heart action and they described, "as a result of the swinging movement of blood elements and through the constant change of vessel diameter, obstructions occurred less frequently and resolved quicker" [7]. In 1890, Jacobj produced pulsatile perfusion by incorporating a rubber balloon, which was intermittently compressed, into his pump mechanism [8]. The role of pulsatile flow was further emphasised by the work of others [13–15]. The early continuous perfusion experiments relied on gravity as a driving force, which proved insufficient for the closed circulation system [16]. Thus, basic pumps [7, 8, 14] were developed for usage in closed circulation systems. Eventually, these were superseded by the introduction of electrically powered syringe pumps in 1907 [17]. Further modification led to the development of the rotary pump for closed circuit perfusion [18]. The first roller pumps were patented in 1855 [19], but were not used for organ perfusion experiments until 1927 by von Issekutz [20].

## 11.3 First Oxygenators

A key component of an artificial circulation is replacement of the lungs' function of oxygenating blood. Over a century ago, perfusion experiments were utilising three different systems, in particular, the bubble oxygenator, the film oxygenator and the lung oxygenator. Von Frey and Gruber, after their invention of the closed circulation system, developed the first film oxygenator. Published in 1885, they described the possibility of oxygenating blood, in the form of a thin film, as it flowed through a rotating cylinder [21]. The blood would be spread across a large surface area and exposed to air, thus allowing gas exchange. Furthermore, Von Frey and Gruber's apparatus was amongst the first to include preheater and temperature-measuring devices. In their experiments, they maintained perfusion to the rear end of a dog after cannulation of the aorta and vena cava [21]. From the beginning of the 20th century, scientists had attempted the use of rotating discs, plates or spirals [22–25] to improve film oxygenation. Further work in refining the film oxygenation technique was described by Borstein [26] in 1926, Straub [27] in 1931 and Gregory in 1939 [28].

Von Schroder was the first to describe the method of bubble oxygenation in 1882 [29]. In his experiments in organ perfusion, oxygenation was achieved by contact of blood with directed air currents. The problems that plagued this technique in the early years were already apparent, as von Schroder described: "Because of the rapid air current passing through the blood, foaming often occurs quite heavily" [29]. Several years later in Strasburg, Carl Jacobj [8], developed what was termed a "hematisator". Drawing from the previous technique described by von Schroder, he combined the principle of bubble oxygenation with a closed circulatory perfusion system. In 1903, Brodie's apparatus included a reciprocating pump and achieved oxygenation by blood with air mixing [9]. From his experiments, he observed, "If too much air is admitted a great deal of frothing occurs in most cases". These methods enabled rapid blood oxygenation, but the complication of foaming would remain unsolved until revisited in 1950. Alcohol was shown to reduce foaming by both Clark [30] and Brukhonenko [31], although the side effects of intoxication rendered it impractical. Clark made the break-through when he discovered that the introduction of silicone prevented foam formation [30]. This paved the way for application in future heart–lung machines.

In a further modification of his "hematisator", Jacobj in 1895 [32], accomplished blood oxygenation by utilising the harvested lungs of dogs or pulmonary lobes of pigs. Jacobj was spurred on in search of "a way which resembles the natural way..." to avoid the foaming that occurred during the direct blood–gas contact of bubble oxygenators. This method required two organs to be perfused in parallel. The ventilated donor lung served as a physiological oxygenator for the de-oxygenated blood. This technique was later used in the extracorporeal experiments of Brukhonenko [33] and others [10, 34].

## 11.4 First Machine for Total Body Perfusion

The early innovators, in developing oxygenators and pump mechanisms, had laid the foundation towards achieving a clinically applicable "cardiopulmonary bypass machine". However, researchers still only remained successful in the experimental perfusion of isolated organs. Carrel and Lindbergh were amongst the first in "realizing the concept of Le Gallois" as they perfused hearts, kidneys and ovaries outside the body [35, 36]. It was not until Brukhonenko reported his experiments in 1927 that the concept and possibility of total body perfusion was first established [37].

After graduation from the University of Moscow, Sergei Sergeyevich Brukhonenko was assigned as a junior doctor to an infantry regiment [38]. During the First World War, he witnessed many fatal injuries to the heart, lungs and great vessels. Thus, he searched for methods of supporting life during surgical repair of these injuries. In 1926, working with Tchetchuline [33], he designed a machine for "artificial circulation with blood of warm-blooded animals". The machine, termed the "autojector", incorporated two parallel mechanical diaphragm pumps along with a valve system. Lungs of a donor animal were artificially ventilated and functioned as an oxygenator. The first pump delivered de-oxygenated blood into the animal lungs, whilst the second pump perfused the systemic circulation [33]. Suramin, a drug capable of producing an "artificial haemophilia" [39], was used to anti-coagulate the blood. On 1 November 1926, in the first experiment of its kind, the circulation of a dog was maintained for 2 h after arresting the heart [33, 40, 41]. Further experiments on isolated organs and total perfusion ensued [33, 40, 41]. Brukhonenko presented his work at the 3rd Physiology Congress of the Soviet Union, June 1928, to an audience of international delegates [42]. Subsequently, using his machine, Brukhonenko demonstrated perfusion of a severed dog's head to visiting correspondents, scientists and the Russian Minister of Education [40]. The isolated head apparently reacted to environmental stimulation and swallowed a piece of cheese [40]. On 11 October 1928, he wrote, with foresight, suggesting a possible application of his machine in cardiac surgery: "Would not this method, duly perfected, be useful in clinical medicine; notably in those cases where it would be essential to replace, if only for a time, the work of the failing human heart? Without going more deeply into this question we can state as a result of the present work that in principle artificial circulation is applicable to man not only clinically, but perhaps also for certain operations on the temporarily arrested heart…The solution of the problem of the artificial circulation of the whole animal opens the door to the problem of operations on the heart, for example on the valves [42]."

Subsequently, on 29 November 1928, he applied for a patent on his machine [38].

By 1931, Brukhonenko had begun utilising deep hypothermia in his perfusion experiments. Cardiac arrest was achieved after the dogs were cooled down to 3 °C. Brukhonenko was able to demonstrate normal cardiac function and survival after rewarming [43]. Using Brukhonenko's machine, Nikolai Terebinski performed many successful open-heart operations on dogs from 1926 to 1937 [44, 45]. The first operations on cardiac valves were amongst the results of more than 260 experimental open-heart surgeries published by Terebinski [44, 45]. At this stage, the machine depended on donor lungs for oxygenation. Thus, it was suitable only for experimental open-heart surgery. This was overcome in 1936, with the introduction of a bubble oxygenator by Brukhonenko. The device comprised a double-wall glass vessel where the inner vessel was used for blood oxygenation and the outer for heating. The oxygen passed from the bottom of the inner vessel and alcohol was used to suppress the production of foam. In 1939, he demonstrated the success of his heart–lung machine in resuscitating 12 out of 13 animals after circulatory arrest [31]. Terebinski and Brukhonenko were close to achieving clinical application of the heart–lung machine. However, the beginnings of the Second World War halted their experiments. They resumed their experiments in 1950 and trialled the machine for resuscitation after sudden death [38]. Although Brukhonenko was the first to predict a future of extracorporeal circulation in cardiac surgery [46], his work remained unfinished until his death on 20 April 1960. Instead, Gibbon's success in implementing the heart–lung machine into clinical practice overshadowed the early work of Brukhonenko [38].

In 1930, John Heysham Gibbon began constructing a heart–lung machine after witnessing the death of a patient from a pulmonary embolism. In his device, venous blood entered into a vertical rotating cylinder where the blood was arterialised by the film oxygenation method. The oxygenated blood was pumped into the systemic circulation by the action of pulsatile pumps. Gibbon used heparin for anticoagulation. He reported the ability of his experimental machine to replace the function of the heart and lungs in cats for 25 min after occlusion of the pulmonary artery [47]. After success of his earlier bypass experiments, Gibbon further improved his machine's oxygenation ability [48] and replaced the pulsatile system with roller pumps [49].

As other organs were able to tolerate longer periods of reduced perfusion, the success of any future open-heart surgery would be limited by ischaemic damage to the brain [50]. Thus, the other scientists of the time, such as Crafoord [51] and O'Shaughnessy [52], focused on optimizing perfusion to the brain. Crafoord learnt, from observing Gibbon's experiments, the method of gas exchange with a thin blood film over a large surface area [53, 54]. He created a heart–lung machine consisting of 40 discs mounted on a central axis [55]. With each rotation, a thin layer of blood was spread over the discs' surfaces. Using Crafoord's machine, Bjork reported 30 min of isolated perfusion to the brains of dogs [55]. In contrast, Jongbloed sought to perfuse the entire body [56]. Inside the oxygenator, gas exchange occurred at a thin blood film along several rotating synthetic tubes arranged in a spiral fashion. Using modified pumps, Jongbloed was able to achieve gas exchange up to a rate of 4.2 L of blood per minute [56]. This system was close to replicating baseline cardiac output in humans. His work was published in 1949 [56] and the transition to clinical application appeared to be reaching its conclusion.

## 11.5 First Clinical Application of the Heart–Lung Machine

On 5 April 1951, at a University of Minnesota hospital, a 6-year-old girl was due to undergo correction of an inter-atrial defect. As reported by Clarence Dennis [57], this landmark case represented the first application of the heart–lung machine. The case was complicated by excessive blood loss and despite the poor outcome, the authors were optimistic and suggested: "This apparatus appears to have a place in further development of the surgery of cardiac abnormalities" [57]. That same year, the Italian team consisting of Dogliotti and Constantini [58, 59] successfully placed a 49-year-old male on partial cardiopulmonary bypass. A planned excision of a mediastinal tumour was complicated by the patient's in-theatre deterioration [58, 59]. The heart–lung machine was instituted in the hope of augmenting and improving the patient's circulation. Remarkably, the situation improved, enabling completion of the surgical procedure.

The first successful open-heart surgery occurred only one year later. The team in Minneapolis, using hypothermia and inflow occlusion, successfully closed an atrial septal defect in a 5-year-old girl [60]. Two years later, on 6 May 1953, the work of Gibbon [61] and the earlier pioneers of the heart–lung machine culminated into the first successful use of total cardiopulmonary bypass. An 18-year-old patient had a large atrial septal defect repaired with he support of a cardiopulmonary bypass. The success of Gibbon's heart–lung machine marked the end of over a century of experimentation and development. Thus, this occasion heralded the dawn of a new era in cardiac surgery. The achievements of both past and present cardiac surgeons were made possible due to the invention, work and foresight of these pioneers from Le Gallois to Brukhonenko.

## References

1. Le Gallois JJC (1813) Experiments on the principle of life, and particularly on the principle of the motions of the heart, and on the seat of this principle: including the report made to the first class of the Institute, upon the experiments relative to the motions of the heart. M. Thomas, Philadelphia, pp 130–131
2. Brown-Séquard E (1858) Recherches expérimentales sur les propriétés physiologiques et les usages du sang rouge et du sang noir et leurs principaux éléments gazeux, l'oxygène et l'acide carbonique. J de la Physiologie De l'Homme et des Animaux 1:95–122, 353–367, 729–735

3. Bidder E (1862) Beiträge zur Lehre von der Function der Niere. Inaugural Dissertation Dorpat
4. Loebell CE (1849) De conditionibus quibus secretiones in glandulis perficiuntur. Dissertatio Inauguralis Marburg, Marburg
5. Schmidt A (1867) Die Athmung innerhalb des Blutes. Zweite Abhandlung—Aus dem physiologischen Institute zu Leipzig. Vorgelegt von dem wirkl. Mitgliede C. Ludwig. Berichte über die Verhandlungen der Königlich Sächsischen Gesellschaft der Wissenschaften zu Leipzig. Mathematisch–Physische Classe 19:99–130
6. Ludwig C, Schmidt A (1868) Das Verhalten der Gase, welche mit dem Blut durch den reizbaren Säugethiermuskel strömen. Berichte über die Verhandlungen der Königlich Sächsischen Gesellschaft der Wissenschaften zu Leipzig, mathematisch–physische Classe 20:12–72
7. Von Frey M, Gruber M (1885) Untersuchungen über den Stoffwechsel isolierter Organe. Ein Respirationsapparat für isolierte Organe. Archiv für Anatomie und Physiologie. (Fortsetzung des von Reil, Reil u. Autenrieth, J. F. Meckel, Joh. Müller, Reichert u. Du Bois-Reymond herausgegebenen Archives). Physiologische Abtheilung Leipzig 9:519–532
8. Jacobj C (1890) Apparat zur Durchblutung isolirter überlebender Organe. Archiv für experimentelle Pathologie und Pharmakologie (Naunyn/Schmiedeberg) 26:388–397
9. Brodie TG (1903) The perfusion of surviving organs. J Physiol 29:266–272
10. Embley EH, Martin CJ (1905) The action of anaesthetic quantities of chloroform upon the blood vessels of the bowel and kidney; with an account of an artificial circulation apparatus. J Physiol 32:147–158
11. Friedmann E (1910) Zur Technik der Durchströmung überlebender Organe. Biochemische Zeitschrift 27:87–96
12. Neubauer O, Groß W (1910) Zur Kenntnis des Tyrosinabbaus in der künstlich durchbluteten Leber. Hoppe-Seyler's Zeitschrift für Physiologische Chemie 67:219–229
13. Hooker DR (1910) A study of the isolated kidney: the influence of pulse pressure upon renal function. Am J Physiol 27:24–45
14. Hamel G (1889) Die Bedeutung des Pulses für den Blutstrom. Zeitschr Biologie 25:474–495
15. McMaster PD, Parsons RJ (1938) The effect of the pulse on the spread of substances through tissues. J Exp Med 68:377–400
16. Kermack WO, Lambie CG (1925) An automatic perfusion apparatus. J Physiol 60:24–25
17. Bock J (1907) Ein Apparat zu Infusionsversuchen. Naunyn0Schmiedebergs Arch Exp Pathol Pharmakol 57:177–182
18. Fröhlich A (1913) Eine Vorrichtung für Dauerdurchströmungen von Kaltblüterorganen mit kleinen Flüssigkeitsmengen. Zentralbl Physiol 27:1011–1013
19. Cooley DA (1987) Development of the roller pump for use in the cardio-pulmonary bypass circuit. Texas Heart Inst J 14:113–118
20. von Issekutz B (1927) Beiträge zur Wirkung des Insulins. II. Mitteilung: Insulin-Adrenalin-Antagonismus. Biochem Zeitschr 183:283–297
21. von Frey M (1885) Versuche über den Stoffwechsel des Muskels. Arch Physiol 9:533–562
22. Hooker DR (1915) The perfusion of the mammalian medulla: the effect of calcium and of potassium on the respiratory and cardiac centers. Am J Physiol 38:200–208
23. Bayliss LE, Fee AR, Ogden E (1928) A method of oxygenating blood. J Physiol 66:443–448
24. Cruickshank EWH (1934) A magnetic blood oxygenator. J Physiol 82:26–32
25. Evans CL, Grande FYHF (1934) Two simple heart-oxygenator circuits for blood-fed hearts. Q J Exp Physiol 24:283–287
26. Bornstein A (1926) Über Durchblutungsversuche an der überlebenden Hundeextremität. Naunyn-Schmiedebergs Arch Exp Pathol und Pharmakol 115:367–374
27. Staub H (1931) Methode zur fortlaufenden Bestimmung des Gaswechsels isoliert durchströmter Organe im geschlossenen System. I. Mitteilung: Über Leberstoffwechsel. Naunyn-Schmiedebergs Arch Exp Pathol Pharmakol 162:420–51
28. Gregory RA (1939) A new oxygenator for blood-perfused hearts. J Physiol 95:49P–51P

29. Von Schröder W (1882) Ueber die Bildungsstätte des Harnstoffs. Arch Exp Pathol Pharmakol 15:364–400
30. Astrup P, Severinghaus JW (1986) The history of blood gases, acids, and bases. Munksgaard, Copenhagen, pp 281–284
31. Brukhonenko SS (1964) Artificial circulation. Nauka, Moscow
32. Jacobj C (1895) Ein Beitrag zur Technik der künstlichen Durchblutung überlebender Organe. Arch Exp Pathol Pharmakol 31:330–348
33. Brukhonenko SS, Tchetchuline S (1929) Experiences avec la tête isolée du chien. J Physiol Pathol Gen 27:31–45
34. Dale HH, Schuster EHJ (1928) A double perfusion-pump. J Physiol 64:356–364
35. Carrel A, Lindbergh CA (1935) The culture of whole organs. Science 81:621–623
36. Lindbergh CA (1935) An apparatus for the culture of whole organs. J Exp Med 62:409–433
37. Brukhonenko S (1929) Circulation artificielle du sang dans l'organisme entier d'un chien avec coeur exclu. J Pathol Pathol Gen 27:257–272
38. Konstantinov IE, Alexi-Meskishvili VV, Sergei S (2000) Brukhonenko: the development of the first heart–lung machine for total body perfusion. Ann Thorac Surg 69:962–966
39. Brukhonenko S, Steppuhn O (1927) Experimentelles zur Anwendung von "Germanin" (Bayer 205) bei Bluttransfusionen. Munchener Med Wochenschr 74:1316–1317
40. Brukhonenko SS, Tchechulin SI (1928) Experiments on isolation of dog's head. Trudi Nauchnogo Khimiko-Pharm Inst 20:7–43
41. Brukhonenko SS (1928) Artificial circulation of the whole body of a dog with arrested heart. Trudi Nauchnogo Khimiko-Pharm Inst 20:44–72
42. Probert WR, Melrose DG (1960) An early Russian heart–lung machine. Br Med J 1:1047–1048
43. Shaw GB (1929) Shaw will sich kopfen lassen, wenn ... Berliner Tageblatt 130:1
44. Alexi-Meskishvili VV, Potapov EV, Beyer EA, Hetzer R (1998) Nikolai Terebinski: a pioneer of the open valve operation. Ann Thorac Surg 66:1440–1443
45. Terebinski N (1938) Experimental stenosis of the atrioventricular valves of the heart and their repair. Khirurgia 12:36–43
46. Richardson RG (1979) Scalpel and heart. Scribner, New York, p 223
47. Gibbon JH (1937) Artificial maintenance of circulation during experimental occlusion of pulmonary artery. Arch Surg 34:1105–1131
48. Gibbon JH (1939) An oxygenator with a large surface-volume ratio. J Lab Clin Med 24:1192–1198
49. Gibbon JH (1939) The maintenance of life during experimental occlusion of the pulmonary artery followed by survival. Surg Gynecol Obstet 69:602–614
50. Boettcher W, Merkle F, Weitkemper HH (2003) History of extracorporeal circulation: the conceptional and development period. J Extra Corpor Technol 35:172–183
51. Crafoord C (1949) Some aspects of the development of intrathoracic surgery. Surg Gynecol Obstet 89:629–637
52. O'Shaughnessy L (1939) Future of cardiac surgery. Lancet 2:969–971
53. Crafoord C (1958) Operationen am offenen Herzen mit Herz-Lungen-Maschine (Stockholmer Modell). Langenbecks Arch Klin Chir 289:257–266
54. Crafoord C (1965) The development of cardiovascular surgery. J Cardiovasc Surg 6:1–12
55. Björk VO (1948) An artificial heart or cardiopulmonary machine. Performance in animals. Lancet 260:491–493
56. Jongbloed J (1949) The mechanical heart–lung system. Surg Gynecol Obstet 89:684–691
57. Dennis C, Spring DS, Nelson GE et al (1951) Development of a pump-oxygenator to replace the heart and lungs; An apparatus applicable to human patients and application in one case. Ann Surg 134:709–721
58. Dogliotti AM (1952) Clinical use of the artificial circulation with a note on intra-arterial transfusion. Bull Johns Hopkins Hospital 90:131–133

59. Dogliotti AM, Constantini A (1951) Primo caso di applicazione all'uomo di un apparecchio di circulazione sanguigna extracorporea. Minerva Chir 6:657–659
60. Lewis FJ, Taufic M (1953) Closure of atrial septal defects with the aid of hypothermia; experimental accomplishments, and the report of one successful case. Surgery 33:52–59
61. Gibbon JH (1954) Application of a mechanical heart and lung apparatus to cardiac surgery. Minnesota Med 37:171–187

# Research on Cardiopulmonary Bypass in North America

# 12

Manon Caouette

*The difference between the impossible and the possible lies in a man's determination.*

Tommy Lasorda


**Abstract**

The second half of the 20th century witnessed the emergence of cardiovascular surgery. The world recognized that this breakthrough began with the development of the heart–lung machine. In the mid-1950s, numerous teams around the world shared a common goal to build a machine to take over the function of the heart and lungs during open heart surgery. Among them, five investigators working in different academic centres in North America were actively engaged each with a different idea of how it should function. John Gibbon of Philadelphia was the person with the longest commitment to the development of a heart–lung machine. He finally performed the first intracardiac repair using a pump oxygenator in 1953. This achievement stimulated rapid development of the knowledge base and equipment necessary for the accurate diagnosis and successful intracardiac operation worldwide.


The history of cardiac surgery is fairly recent, with important developments starting at the end of the Second World War. Sad as it is, we must recognize that the war brought significant advances in the fields of surgery and medicine. In the United States intensive efforts were put into scientific research and the development of cardiovascular surgery. That era brought about the evolution of new technologies, the discovery of penicillin and the improvement of anaesthesia and blood transfusions technology [1]. Major progress in cardiac surgery allowed the limitations of closed heart surgery to be overcome with the use of hypothermia, and led to the present day techniques of open heart surgery with the extracorporeal heart–lung machine [2].


M. Caouette (✉)
Perfusion, IUCPQ, 2725 chemin Sainte-Foy, Québec, QC G1V4G5, Canada
e-mail: manoncaouette2008@hotmail.com



M. Picichè (ed.), *Dawn and Evolution of Cardiac Procedures*,
DOI: 10.1007/978-88-470-2400-7_12, © Springer-Verlag Italia 2013

The history of open heart surgery has been the making of many talented and dedicated pioneers. Between 1950 and 1955, all were actively engaged in the development of a pump-oxygenator apparatus, each with a different idea of the ideal design. The purpose of this chapter is to remember some of the courageous medical investigators in North America who had the vision and dedication needed for the development of the cardiopulmonary bypass machine, which, ultimately, gave birth to open heart surgery as we know it today.

## 12.1 Before the Second World War

The individual with the longest commitment to the development of a heart–lung machine was Dr John Gibbon from Jefferson Medical College. His interest in constructing an artificial heart–lung machine was sparked one night in 1931 while working as a surgical research fellow under the direction of Dr Churchill in the Anaesthesia Laboratory and Department of the Harvard Medical School at the Massachusetts General Hospital, Boston.

On that night, Dr Gibbon was on duty recording the vital signs of a young woman who was dying of massive pulmonary embolism following complication of a cholecystectomy. Should the patient status become hopeless, Dr Churchill was planning, as a last resort, to attempt a Trendelenburg operation (pulmonary embolectomy). During that night-long vigil, Dr Gibbon came to realise that in order to be able to surgically remove the pulmonary embolus, a new apparatus was needed. That new apparatus would drain venous blood from patients, bypassing their heart and lungs, then oxygenating it before returning it to the patient's arteries. Unfortunately, there was no such machine at that time and the patient did not survive the pulmonary embolectomy performed the following morning. This tragic clinical experience had a profound and long-lasting effect on Gibbon. From that day on, he dedicated his life to developing a heart–lung machine. He returned to Philadelphia and spent the following 3 years practising surgery and reviewing previous work in this field. He discussed his ambition with colleagues who showed no interest in the project, doubting its feasibility [3].

In 1934, Dr Gibbon returned with Dr Churchill for a second year of research fellowship. Together with his new wife Mary Hopkinson (who was Dr Churchill's laboratory assistant), they finally assembled the first heart–lung machine. The extracorporeal circuit contained a vertical rotating cylinder type oxygenator in which a film of blood coated the inner surface of the cylinder while being exposed to oxygen. The blood pumps were of the Dale–Shuster type in which positive and negative pressures were alternately exerted to propel the blood contained within a rubber finger cot. In full operation, the machine could oxygenate 500 ml of blood per minute [4]. His early experiments were performed on cats, which were often in short supply. Dr Gibbon wrote: "when our supply ran short, I can recall prowling around Beacon Hill at night with some tuna fish as bait and a gunny sack to catch any of the numerous stray alley cats which swarmed over Boston in those days" [5].

During these experiments, they encountered a great number of problems such as foaming, hemolysis, production of vasoconstrictor substances in the blood from mechanical agitation and excess blood loss, since the antagonist of heparin, protamine sulphate, was not yet available. However, by the end of the year, Dr Gibbon and his wife demonstrated the feasibility of supporting cats with occluded pulmonary arteries for up to 171 min. Gibbon's work was interrupted by 4 years of military service in the Second World War. Afterwards, he was appointed chief of surgery at the Thomas Jefferson Medical College in Philadelphia. There, he resumed clinical work in the morning and research work in the laboratory in the afternoon, developing the heart–lung machine [3].

## 12.2 After World War II

### 12.2.1 Clarence Dennis

Meanwhile, other groups were also working intensively to build their own version of heart–lung machines. Among them was Dr Clarence Dennis, a surgeon at the University of Minnesota. His interest in the heart–lung machine began in 1945, a few months after the end of the Second World War. It all started when Dr Owen Wangensteen and Maurice B. Visscher, chair of Surgery and chairman of the Department of Physiology at the University of Minnesota respectively, approached their younger faculty member Dr Clarence Dennis to work on the creation of a pump oxygenator that would allow direct vision repairs of intracardiac lesions [6]. Seeking advice from colleagues in the country, Dr Dennis met and befriended Dr Gibbon who was flattered and delighted to finally meet someone interested in working on his project. Over years of research, the two exchanged information between their respective laboratories to speed up the development of the machine [7].

By early 1951, Dr Dennis and his colleague Dr Karl Karlson finally assembled a workable apparatus using a modified Dale–Shuster pump and a revolving disk multiple screens oxygenator. Although the system had achieved nearly 100 % survival in dogs, the trials on the first two patients were unsuccessful. The first patient was thought to have an atrial septal defect, but turned out to have a complex atrioventricular canal, a lesion that was not successfully handled by surgeons at that time. While the machine worked as it should, the attempted repair was untreatable and the patient died in the operating room. The operation was the first attempt to perform intracardiac surgery with total heart–lung bypass in a human subject. The second operation, also performed to repair an atrial septal defect was successful. Unfortunately, towards the end of the surgery, the operator of the apparatus inadvertently pumped air into the patient, who died in the operating room of a gaseous embolism. The same year, Dr Dennis moved to Brooklyn, where he accepted a position as chief of the Department of Surgery at Downstate Medical Center. There, he resumed his work on cardiopulmonary bypass in an abandoned funeral home converted into a laboratory. Over subsequent years,

Dr Dennis's research interest focussed on other topics such as the development of synthetic heart valves [6, 8].

### 12.2.2 Forest Dodrill

During the same period, Dr Forest Dodrill, a surgeon at Wayne State University Harper Hospital and President of the Michigan Heart Association, was confident that a machine could be developed to temporarily replace the human heart's blood pumping function and make open heart surgery possible. Dodrill's plan was to divert blood from the right or the left side of the heart and use the patient's lung as the oxygenator. Dr Dodrill and his medical team used a mechanical blood pump developed by engineers from General Motors Research Laboratories. After extensive experimental work on animals for univentricular, biventricular or cardiopulmonary bypass, it was decided that the first clinical application would be a left heart bypass since it was not associated with the profound hypotensive reflex seen with the other forms of bypass. In July 1952 Dodrill successfully performed the first surgery on a human subject using the Dodrill-GMR Mechanical Heart pump to support the left side of the heart while he repaired a mitral valve. The surgery lasted 80 min and the mechanical heart kept the patient alive for 50 min while his own heart was being repaired. In October of the same year, he performed the first successful right-sided heart bypass in a 16-year-old boy with congenital pulmonary stenosis. Between July 1952 and December 1954, Dr Dodrill performed approximately 13 procedures on the heart and thoracic aorta using the Dodrill-GMR pump with at least 5 hospital survivors. The development of partial bypass was a landmark in the field of cardiac surgery, but the technique was limited to repair defects of the pulmonary and mitral valves. For this and various other reasons, no further clinical work was reported [9, 10].

### 12.2.3 John H. Gibbon

After the Second World War, Dr John Gibbon resumed his research. His immediate problem was to build an artificial lung with a better oxygenation capacity so that the heart–lung machine could be used on animals larger than cats and on human subjects. He was soon introduced to Mr Thomas Watson, who was then the Chairman of the Board of the International Business Machine (IBM) Corporation. He explained his idea and that he was looking for engineering assistance to develop a larger heart–lung machine. Mr Watson was fascinated by Gibbon's work and promised to help. Shortly afterwards, six IBM engineers were sent to built the Model I of the heart–lung machine, a model similar to Gibbon's earlier machine. It contained modified DeBakey rotary pumps and a rotating vertical cylindrical oxygenator. The blood pumps were designed to minimize hemolysis and the oxygenator was designed to prevent small air bubbles. The entire apparatus had the capacity to maintain the cardiorespiratory function of larger experimental animals [3].

Gibbon successfully used this new machine for intracardiac surgery on small dogs and had several long-term survivors, but the blood oxygenator was insufficient for patients [3]. In the late 1940s, Thomas Stokes and John Flick, two surgical residents in Gibbon's laboratory, found a solution to that problem. They realized that when the blood flow on the smooth inner surface of the revolving cylinder was more turbulent, it increased the efficiency of oxygenation. They lined the surface with six stainless screens, and found that the efficiency of oxygen uptake increased by 800 %. The model II IBM heart–lung machine was finally designed and built (Fig. 12.1) [11].

In 1952, after many trials in the laboratory, Dr Gibbon was able to achieve almost 90 % survival in dogs for periods of over 30 min on the new heart–lung machine. The device functioned splendidly and oxygenation with the new vertical screens oxygenator was sufficient for perfusion in human patients [12]. Dr Gibbon and his laboratory group had full confidence that it was time to move to clinical application. To initiate the use of this device in humans, the heart–lung machine needed to be sterilized by first filling the machine with zephiran solution followed by repeated flushes with saline prior to priming the machine with a large volume of whole fresh heparinised blood, which was donated from many donors, mostly medical students who lined up in the hallway to donate blood on the morning of the surgery [13].

The first patient was treated in February 1952, a 15-month-old girl with severe congestive heart failure. The preoperative diagnosis was an atrial septal defect, but during the surgery, no atrial defect was found. Her condition rapidly deteriorated and she died. The autopsy revealed a huge patent ductus arteriosus. The second patient was an 18-year-old college student with congestive heart failure. Her cardiac catheterization revealed a large atrial septal defect with a left-to-right shunt. She had been hospitalized with right ventricular failure three times in the 6 months prior to the operation. The surgery was performed on 6 May 1953 [12]. After being placed on cardiopulmonary bypass, the large atrial septal defect was found. However, an inadequate dose of heparin led to blood clotting on the oxygenator screens and Gibbon was forced to quickly close the defect with continuous suture and to end the bypass as quickly as possible [14]. The patient had her ASD successfully closed with 45 min of partial bypass and 26 min of total bypass. She had an uneventful recovery with no adverse effects. She was catheterized 2 months later and the defect remained completely closed [3]. This operation marked the world's first successful use of a heart–lung device for intracardiac operations.

John Gibbon studied and worked tirelessly on this project for 23 years before the first successful application. His work in general was well received, but it garnered surprisingly little enthusiasm among cardiac surgeons and cardiologists. This was probably due in part to the fact that he has never been able to repeat his one success of closure of an ASD. After two more unsuccessful operations, Dr Gibbon became upset at these failures, decided to end all open heart surgeries for a year until more work could be done to solve the problems causing the deaths. It was also believed that the "sick human heart" could not tolerate the magnitude of

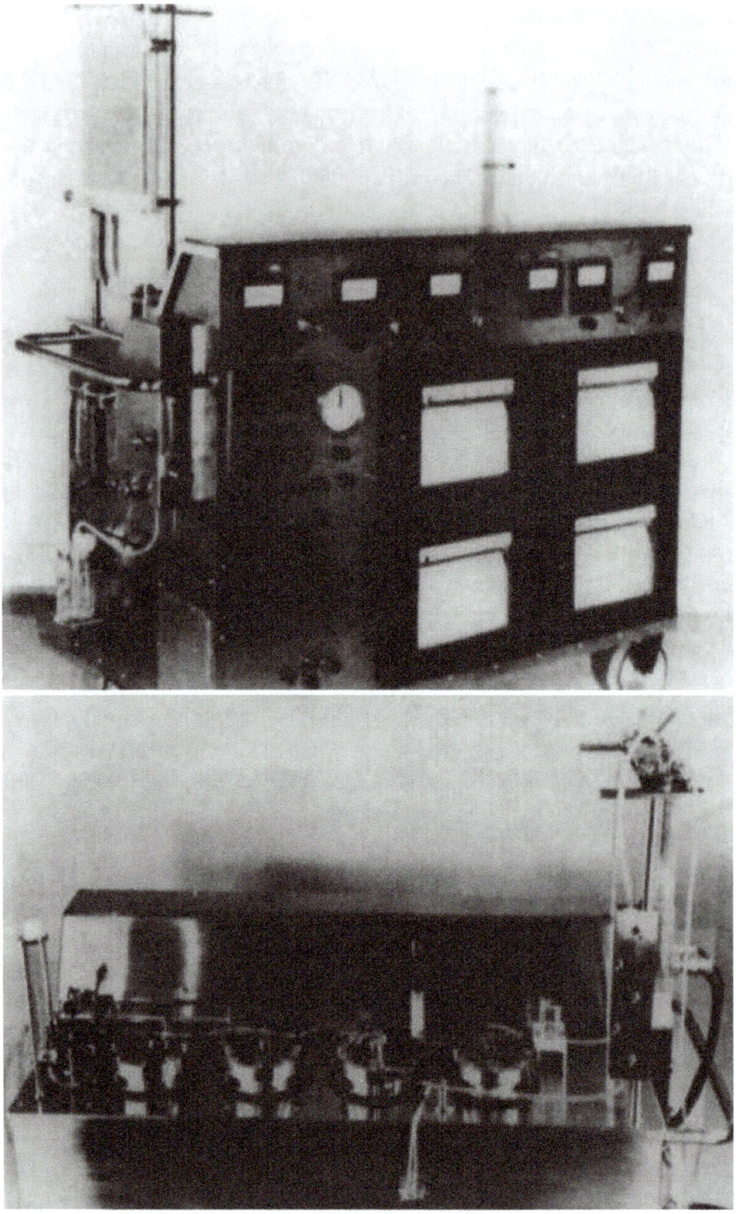

**Fig. 12.1** The Gibbon–IBM heart–lung machine model II. *Top* the oxygenator screens at the top on the left. *Bottom* the roller pumps. (Reprinted from Miller et al [25], with permission)

the operation required and then recover immediately the same way the healthy dogs' hearts were recovering when the same machine and techniques were applied. Another reason may have been that some surgeons believed that the hypothermia and inflow obstruction technique to close the ASD held more promise than mechanical support. Gibbon never performed open-heart surgery again. He did maintain a research interest in the development of subsequent models of the heart–lung machine and returned to the active practice of general thoracic surgery [14, 15].

### 12.2.4 The Principle of Controlled Cross Circulation

Progress and fundings in open heart surgery research totally stopped thereafter, and many surgeons lost all confidence of ever being able to correct complex intracardiac defects [15]. Fortunately, the situation changed in 1954 when Dr Walton Lillehei and his two associates, Herbert Warden and Marley Cohen, developed a technique called "controlled cross circulation".

The idea came one evening while the team, including Cohen whose wife was pregnant, was discussing blood circulation of a placenta. They realized that the mother was the oxygenator for the placenta. That led them with the plan of using the patient's parent as the heart–lung machine in which blood circulation at low flow of the genetic parent was temporarily used while the patient heart was stopped and opened [16]. This low flow was based on a study published by Andreasen and Watson that demonstrated that dogs survived on 10 % of their basal cardiac output without damage [17].

The technique consisted of taking blood flow from the patient's caval system to the parent's femoral vein and lungs, where it was oxygenated and returned to the patient's carotid artery. They used a single Sigmamotor pump to precisely control the reciprocal exchange of blood between the patient and donor (Fig. 12.2).

After successful experimentations done on dogs, Dr Lillehei and his colleagues planned to use this technique on human subjects. The first surgery with the controlled cross circulation was to correct a ventricular septal defect in a 1-year-old boy. The operation was performed in March 1954. The father served as the oxygenator. The cardiac defect was repaired with a total pump time of 19 min; unfortunately, the patient died several days later of pneumonia. A month later, the second operation was performed on a 4-year-old boy with a ventricular septal defect, again using the boy's father as the donor. They closed the defect without difficulty and this time the patient survived. This was the first successful open heart operation performed with cross circulation. During a 1-year period, Dr Lillehei operated on 45 patients using controlled cross circulation, including 27 patients with ventricular septal defects, 10 patients with tetralogy of Fallot, and 5 with an AV canal. The operations were mostly successful, with 28 of the 45 patients surviving and no donor mortality [15, 18].

Although cross circulation was a stepping stone in the development of cardiac surgery, it was not adopted for widespread use. It was pointed out that the technique carried serious risks for both the recipient and the donor. One critic even said that "this operation could have 200 % mortality" [19]. Another major problem was that flow rates were far too low for use in adults. An artificial oxygenator was needed to progress to larger children and adults [14].

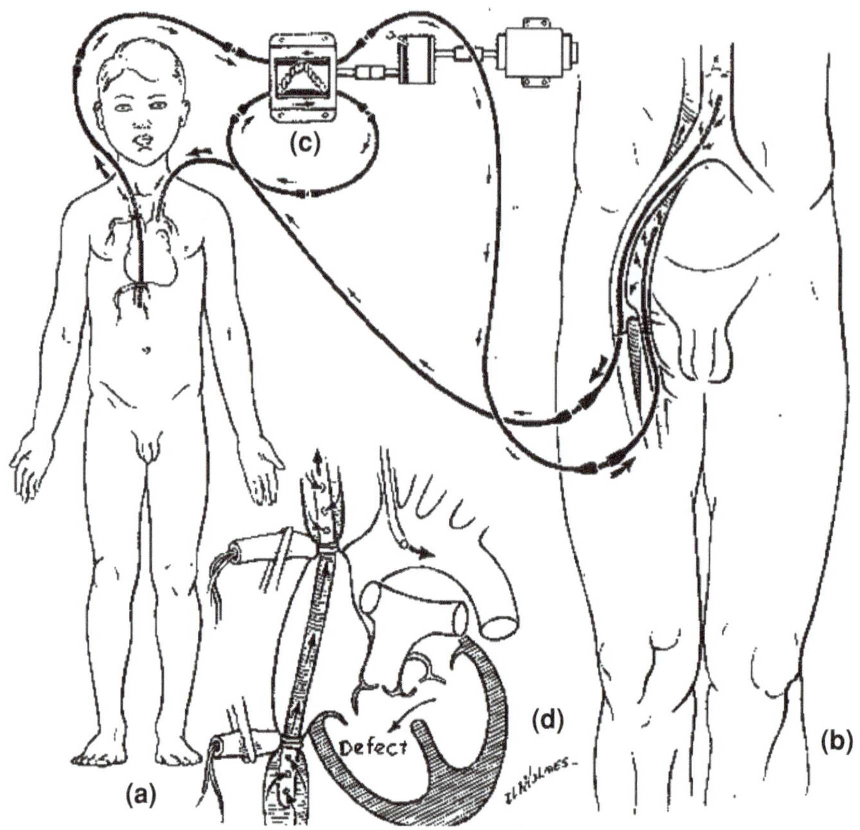


**Fig. 12.2** Diagram of the cross circulation technique used by Walton in 1954–1955. Either the mother or the father of the patient was a donor. (Reprinted with permission from Lillehei et al. [15])

### 12.2.5 The Mayo Clinic

Meanwhile, progress in heart–lung bypass was also being made at the Mayo Clinic, only 145 km away from Dr Lillehei's laboratory [20]. There, Dr John Kirklin assembled a multidisciplinary team including a physiologist, a cardiologist, a pathologist and an anaesthesiologist, among others, to develop a cardiac surgical program for the clinical application of a mechanical pump-oxygenator.

Instead of designing an entirely new machine, they decided to visit a number of groups working on potential devices, such as the Gibbon–IBM pump oxygenator and the Dodrill–GMR Mechanical Heart. After reflection, they opted for the Gibbon–IBM pump despite criticism among the medical community. Dr Kirklin persuaded the Mayo Clinic to let them build a pump oxygenator similar to the Gibbon machine, but with additional refinements and modifications. Dr Gibbon graciously shared the plan of his machine and his hard-earned expertise.

After 2½ years of research, the Mayo Clinic engineers finally developed a pump oxygenator based on Gibbon's pump design with new safety features, an oxygenator with 14 wire-mesh screens and an occluding mechanism to control the source of the blood flow to the oxygenator [20, 21]. It was a relatively expensive machine and quite complex to set up and manage. It required 6 units of blood to prime, a separate operating room to prepare the machine, and extensive cleaning after each use [14].

By the winter of 1954–1955, they had 9 surviving dogs out of 10 cardiopulmonary bypass runs. The team judged that it was time to proceed with clinical application. They decided to begin the clinical trials on 8 patients with the understanding that they would treat all 8 cases regardless of the outcomes. Families were informed about the risks and possible benefits of this new unproven surgical treatment. The first procedure involved closure of a ventricular septal defect in a 5-year-old child, which was performed successfully with five silk sutures in March 1955. The patient recovered completely and she was discharged from the hospital after 10 days. Two months later they had operated on all 8 children with various types of ventricular septal defects and 4 were hospital survivors [19, 22].

In their report published in May 1955 in the Proceedings of the Staff Meetings of the Mayo Clinic, Kirklin and his group described patients being on cardiopulmonary bypass for 20–73 min and flows were maintained at 100 ml/kg/min [21]. Although the mortality was 50 %, this relatively successful series of open heart surgery using a heart–lung machine was a world premiere. From that time, Lillehei at the University of Minnesota abandoned the cross circulation technique and started using the DeWall pump and his personally-designed bubble oxygenator device developed at the University of Minnesota [20]. By the fall of that year, over a period of 12–18 months, these two institutions were the only ones in the world performing open heart surgery with mechanical heart–lung machines [22]. Kirklin's group having treated 40 patients, with 93 % survival among their last 14 ventricular septal defect cases [23], and Lillehei's group having treated 36 patients with 89 % survival in their last 19 cases [24]. Finally, the mystery of open heart surgery had been solved and pushed universities from all over the world to launch open-heart programs.

## 12.3 Conclusion

During the 10 years following the first surgery using a cardiopulmonary bypass machine, the risk of death rapidly decreased as cardiac surgery progressed, bringing today's operative mortality near 1 % for some operations. The technology of the heart–lung machine continues to be refined and to evolve, and is becoming safer while being operated by dedicated, trained health professionals, called perfusionists.

The creation of the heart–lung machine changed the world of cardiothoracic surgery. Almost 60 years ago it was just a dream, today 1 million cardiac operations are performed worldwide each year. John Gibbon deserves major credit for his dedication, which led to the first successful open heart surgery with his heart–lung machine on 6 May 1953.

## References

1. Franco A, Diz JC (2000) Wars stimulated the development of anaesthesia. Curr Anaesth Crit Care 11:137–140
2. Lewis FJ, Taufic M (1953) Closure of atrial septal defects with the aid of hypothermia: experimental accomplishment and the report of one successful case. Surgery 33:52–59
3. Gibbon JH (1968) Development of the artificial heart and lungs extracorporeal blood circuit. JAMA 206:1983–1986
4. Gibbon JH (1937) Artificial maintenance of circulation during experimental occlusion of pulmonary artery. Arch Surg 34:1105–1131
5. Gibbon JH (1963) The gestation and birth of an idea. Philadelphia Med 59:913–914
6. Dennis C (1985) Perspective in review one group's struggle with development of a pump-oxygenator. Trans Am Soc Artif Intern Organs XXXI:1–11
7. Dennis C (1989) A heart-lung machine for open- heart operations. How it came about. Trans Am Soc Artif Intern Organs 35:767–777
8. Dennis C, Spreng D et al. (1951) Development of a pump-oxygenator to replace the heart and lungs; an apparatus applicable to human patients and application to one case. Ann Surg 134:709–721
9. Stephenson LW (2002) Forest Dewey Dodrill: heart surgery pioneer, Michigan Heart, part II. J Card Surg 17:247–257
10. Dodrill F, Hill E et al (1952) Temporary mechanical substitute for the left ventricle in man. JAMA 150:642–644
11. Stokes TL, Flick JB (1950) An improvement vertical cylinder oxygenator. Proc Soc Exp Biol Med 73:528–529
12. Gibbon JH (1954) Application of a mechanical heart and lung apparatus to cardiac surgery. Minn Med 37:171–180
13. Miller BJ (2003) Laboratory work preceding the first clinical application of cardiopulmonary bypass. Perfusion 18:145–154
14. Stoney WS (2009) Evolution of cardiopulmonary bypass. Circulation 119:2844–2853
15. Lillehei CW, Varco RL, Cohen M et al (1986) The first open-heart repairs of ventricular septal defect, atrioventricular communis, and tetralogy of Fallot using extracorporeal circulation by cross-circulation: a 30-year follow-up. Ann Thorac Surg 41:4–21
16. Dewall RA (2003) Origin of the helical reservoir bubble oxygenator heart-lung machine. Perfusion 18:163–169
17. Andreason AT, Watson F (1952) Experimental cardiovascular surgery. Br J Surg 39:548–551
18. Lillehei CW (1955) Controlled cross circulation for direct-vision intracardiac surgery: correction of ventricular septal defects, atrioventricularis communis and tetralogy of Fallot. Postgrad Med 17:388–396
19. Rainer WG (2003) Cardiac surgery before cardiopulmonary bypass. Perfusion 18:13–144
20. Stephenson LW (2008) History of cardiac surgery. In: Cohn LH (ed) Cardiac surgery in the adult. McGraw-Hill, New York, pp 3–28
21. Jones RE, Donald DE, Swan JC et al (1955) Apparatus of the Gibbon type for mechanical bypass of the heart and lungs. Proc Staff Meet Mayo Clin 30:105–113

22. Kirklin JW (1989) The middle 1950s and C. Walton Lillehei. J Thorac Cardiovasc Surg 98:822–824
23. Kirklin JW, Donald DE, Harshbarger HG et al (1956) Studies in extracorporeal circulation. I. Applicability of Gibbon-type pump-oxygenator to human intracardiac surgery: 40 cases. Ann Surg 144:2–8
24. Lillehei CW, Dewall RA, Read RC et al. (1956) Direct vision intracardiac surgery in man using a simple, disposable artificial oxygenator. Dis Chest 29:1–8
25. Miller BJ, Gibbon JH, Fineberg C (1953) An improved mechanical heart and lung apparatus; its use during open cardiotomy in experimental animals. Med Clin North Am 37:1603–1624

# From Research on Hibernation and Hypothermia to Recent Advances in Cardiopulmonary Bypass

**13**

Isabelle Plamondon and Edoardo Gasparotto

*I was taught that the way of progress was neither swift nor easy.*
Marie Curie

*I do not think that the practice of science can be separated from courage.*
Berthold Brecht

**Abstract**

For many years, progress in cardiac surgery were limited by the inability to operate within the empty heart under direct vision. There have been several methods devised in the effort to obtain intracardiac exposure with a dry field. The early models of heart-lung machines developed were not widely applicable with safety to the human patient. The other avenue of approach has been the attempt to reduce the metabolic demand until circulation can be interrupted for periods of time long enough without recourse to extracorporeal pumps. General hypothermia has been investigated as a means of reducing the oxygen requirements of the body to allow deliberate and extensive intracardiac maneuvers.

Since the early days of surgery, operations on the heart have been hampered by the difficulty of creating a "bloodless field." Many innovative closed-vision procedures within the beating heart have been developed, but the limitations of closed, indirect-vision intracardiac surgery were obvious. To enable further progress in the field of cardiac surgery, it became necessary to obtain intracardiac exposure with a dry field. The early models of heart–lung machines needed tedious preparation before being used, and were cumbersome, complex, and expensive. General hypothermia has been investigated as a way of reducing the oxygen requirements

I. Plamondon (✉)
Critical Care Division, Institut Universitaire de Cardiologie et de Pneumologie de Québec, Hôpital Laval, 2725 chemin Sainte-Foy, Québec, QC G1V 4G5, Canada
e-mail: i_plamondon@videotron.ca

E. Gasparotto
Cardiac Surgery Unit, Department of Cardiovascular Science, San Bortolo Hospital, Via Rodolfi 37, Vicenza 36100, Italy
e-mail: edoardo.gasparotto@libero.it

M. Picichè (ed.), *Dawn and Evolution of Cardiac Procedures*,
DOI: 10.1007/978-88-470-2400-7_13, 

of tissue to a fraction of normal to temporarily remove the heart from the circulation, enabling intracardiac surgery under direct vision. Brief periods of complete arrest of the circulation had been previously used in the warm subject, but the period of time available, 1.5–3 min, was too short to allow elaborate intracardiac procedures. If the blood flow was interrupted for a longer period of time, irreversible damage to the brain and other vital organs occurred.

## 13.1 Hibernation and Hypothermia

In the late 18th century, James Currie attempted to cure patients afflicted by a variety of illnesses with the use of cold temperatures. Temple Fay and Lawrence Smith reported the effects of cooling on cancer growth in 1938. They termed general reduction of body temperature "hibernation" while local cooling of a tumor was called "refrigeration", the term hypothermia coined by J.H. Talbott in 1941 [1, 2]. At this time, the principal conditions treated were intractable pain, cancer, morphine addiction, leukemia, and schizophrenia.

Bigelow and Lindsay [3] and Penrod [4] found that cold temperatures reduced the metabolism and oxygen consumption of the tissues, increasing the resistance to anoxia. It was reported that newborn mammals can survive lower body temperatures that adults of the same species and that the lethal temperature that could be endured increased with age [5, 6]. Many workers tried to find the substance secreted by the so-called "hibernating gland" which would allow some animals to enter into winter sleep.

Prec et al. [7] and Bigelow et al. [8] published the results of their studies showing that blood pressure, pulse rate, respiratory rate, oxygen consumption and cardiac output decrease as cooling becomes more intense. Peripheral vasoconstriction occurs concomitantly to compensate for the decreased cardiac output.

### 13.1.1 Application to Cardiac Surgery

From 1938 to 1952, hypothermia was being applied in order to decrease the complications and mortality of anesthesia for cyanotic congenital heart disease [9]. Aortic–pulmonary anastomoses, subclavian–pulmonary anastomoses and closed pulmonary valvulotomies were performed with concomitant hypothermia. Surface cooling was used to obtain a moderate hypothermia used as an adjunct to closed surgical techniques.

Investigative studies on hypothermia as a mechanism for performing cardiac surgery were begun more than a decade after efforts to design a heart–lung machine were initiated. Wilfred Bigelow et al. [8] and Ite Boerema et al. [10] were the first to experiment induced hypothermia for intracardiac surgery under circulatory arrest, independently for one other. While the body temperature is low and the oxygen needs of the tissues are reduced, it is possible to occlude the blood flow for a longer period of time than is tolerable at normal temperatures, allowing time to carry out surgery in an open, dry field while the blood flow is interrupted. Hypothermia was utilized not as an adjunct to closed cardiac surgery, but as a means of correcting more difficult cardiac anomalies under direct vision. With more severe hypothermia, the heart could be temporarily deprived of its blood by inflow stasis, i.e. occlusion of both venae cavae for about 6–8 min. However, caval occlusion is not the same thing as absolute cardiac arrest, as there is still a small residual circulation maintained by the left side of the heart as demonstrated by a continual flow of blood from the coronary sinus.

Bigelow et al. published reports of experiments in which they utilized hypothermia during production of circulatory arrest by occlusion of cardiac inflow for 15 min, during which time the left atrium could be opened and then closed [8]. Longer procedures with complete arrest of circulation were tolerated by the heart and brain of the surviving animals. Unfortunately, the survival rate was only 15 %, ventricular fibrillation or cardiac arrest occurring during occlusion of the cavae or shortly after relief of caval occlusion. Furthermore, 70 % of the animals revived to normal temperature died of shock in the first 12 h. The problems and complications involved in the production and maintenance of lower levels of hypothermia were not noted with moderate hypothermia. Cookson and colleagues modified Bigelow's procedure and obtained 80 % survival of their animals after 12 min of occlusion of cardiac inflow [11]. Because of all the changes to the protocol, the fundamentals of the fibrillation did not emerge.

Lewis and Taufic [12] reported their successful application of this method to one patient who survived to the closure of an atrial septal defect. However, with this technique, if the diagnosis was in error and a primum defect or another defect was found instead of a secundum defect, the time allowance was inadequate and the surgeon had to switch to perfusion at short notice or abandon the operation and start afresh another day [13]. Swan devised an operation for correcting isolated pulmonary stenosis under direct vision during hypothermia [14] and Lewis used hypothermia in a similar fashion to operate upon stenosed aortic valve under direct vision [15].

Various methods [16] have been tried to reduce the body temperature. Surface cooling by immersion in ice water, a draught of cold air or refrigerating blankets were used to decrease the patient's temperature after induction of anesthesia controlled at such a depth as to prevent shivering. However, it may take a long time in adults to obtain sufficient hypothermia and it is difficult to control the temperature level because the temperature may continue to fall after surface cooling has been stopped. Moreover, immediate detection and treatment of cardiac arrest and arrhythmia were difficult. Several surgeons, notably Swan, used the immersion technique. A large bath of water and ice was brought alongside the patient who was immersed with the anesthetizing apparatus attached, EKG leads, intravenous drips, and intra-arterial needle. The patient was again immersed at the end of the surgery, this time in warm water, with a wound and drainage tubes. Blades and Pierpont proposed intrapleural cooling for the production of hypothermia, their technique consisting of directly cooling the circulating blood by allowing cold physiological saline to bathe the pulmonary vascular bed of the lung, aorta, and the pleura, the overflow being siphoned off [17].

Another method, introduced by Delorme [18] and Boerema et al. [10], was to create an artificial arterio-venous fistula to cool the blood during its passage through the fistula. Originally, a cannula was inserted into an artery and blood flowed through a coil immersed in ice-cold water and returned into a vein. Brock and Ross modified the method, whereby both venae cavae were cannulated via the right atrial appendage and the blood circulated through a cooling chamber by means of a simple hand pump [19].

An "artificial hibernation technique" induced by a combination of drugs was evoked by Laborit, Huguenard, and others [20]. The "lytic cocktail" was thought to have a direct depressant action on the temperature-regulating mechanism, but everyone agreed later that the drug mixture did not induce a real state of hibernation.

### 13.1.2 Drawbacks to Hypothermia

A number of practical problems in the management of hypothermia had to be faced by the anesthetist such as the type of anesthesia needed, the enhanced effect of certain drugs, the deliberate over-ventilation of the patient throughout the procedure to prevent the occurrence of respiratory acidosis and the difficulty in estimating the blood pressure clinically in the cold patient [21].

The cooling technique became safer with the development of an electrical defibrillator for the heart and a method of supplying the heart with an electrical pacemaker for standstill. As the main danger of hypothermia was ventricular fibrillation, many teams addressed the problem. Fibrillation occurring in the hypothermic state had proved to be largely refractory to the usual methods of resuscitation, but immediate rewarming proved valuable. Swan has emphasized the changes in potassium metabolism under hypothermia and its role in ventricular fibrillation [22]. The recognition that ventricular fibrillation was a consequence of air embolism in the coronary circulation and excessive cooling reduced operative mortality considerably. Other studies investigated the use of an artificial pacemaker, electrophrenic respiratory stimulation, and radio-frequency rewarming [23].

The use of hypothermia in cardiovascular surgery had both its dedicated proponents and its avid critics, although hypothermia has been described as the single most important component of myocardial protection. The major drawback to hypothermia was the short interval of time afforded to the surgeon to correct the anomaly, leading to the development of extracorporeal circulation for open cardiotomy. A wider range of operative procedures are possible with a longer time interval. In spite of all the improvements made in the efficiency of the heart–lung machines, hypothermia found a lasting place in clinical medicine as deep hypothermic circulatory arrest with cardiopulmonary bypass (CPB) is still indicated for complex surgical operations in adult patients involving the aortic arch, thoraco-abdominal aorta, cerebral vasculature, and tumors extending into the vena cava and heart.

## 13.2 Research into Cardiopulmonary Bypass After the 1970s

After research on hypothermia and application to CPB and cardioplegia, research turned in part to biocompatibility. Since the late 1970s, great attention was paid to the physiological reactions of blood following contact with the surfaces of the CPB circuit. The concept of "biomaterial" appeared, meaning a material with the highest level of biofunctionality and biocompatibility. The hallmark of biomaterial was to contain drugs or biological active agents, so that the interaction with the blood was no longer inert but active. Biocompatible surfaces for circuits and oxygenators became commercially available in the 1980s [24]. The first biocompatible treatments were based on heparin bonding, either ionic or covalent. Many different kinds of biocompatible treatments became available for clinical use and despite some differences among them, all mimicked the normal endothelial surface [25]. This was achieved by coating circuits and oxygenators with different types of molecules, such as heparin, phosphorylcholine, poly2-methoxyethylacrylate, siloxane/caprolactone, polyethylene oxide chains, and sulfate/sulfonate groups. The expected results were a decrease in the systemic inflammatory reaction, of hemostatic system activation, and of platelet depletion, due to a decrease in platelet activation and adhesion [24–28]. However, clinical studies conflicting results offered with respect to the real efficacy of biocompatible treatments. Vacuum-assisted venous drainage (VAVD) was a further research field, aimed at the improvement of venous return and at the achievement of a lowering priming volume by eliminating the need to prime the venous line [29]. Adopted from mid-1990s, VAVD was expected to allow the use of smaller venous cannulae, and to achieve higher hemoglobin levels and a lower transfusion rate. Despite this innovation, which was revealed to be useful in both pediatric and adult cardiac surgery, in some clinical situations VAVD was seen to enhance CPB-induced hemolysis, and to be a source of increased microembolism [30]. To reduce the disadvantages of CPB, research turned also to miniaturized systems (mini-CPB). This innovation consisted of a mini-circuitry that allowed priming and hemodilution to be reduced, resulting in a better hematocrit. Biocompatible surfaces were adopted allowing a reduction in heparinization. Mini-CPB was studied to be a closed system, namely without a reservoir, separated from field suctions, which allowed a reduction in the area of contact between blood and the surfaces and the elimination of air–blood contact [31]. Another research field has been leukocyte-depleting filters. These filters were studied to reduce circulating leukocyte counts, as was seen in most studies, but failed to produce convincing evidence of clinical benefit [32]. From pumps to heat exchangers, form filters to cardiotomy reservoirs, from oxygenators to hemoconcentrators and perfusion monitors [33–36], research into CPB advanced restlessly after Gibbon's first open heart operation, which is currently still true.

## References

1. No authors listed (1941) Treatment by hypothermia. Br Med J 2(4206): 231–232
2. Talbott JH (1941) The physiologic and therapeutic effects of hypothermia. N Engl J Med 224(7):281–288
3. Bigelow WG, Lindsay WK et al (1950) Oxygen transport and utilization in dogs at low body temperatures. Am J Physiol 160(1):125–137
4. Penrod KE (1949) Oxygen consumption and cooling rates in immersion hypothermia in the dog. Am J Physiol 157(3):436–444
5. Adolph EF (1951) Responses to hypothermia in several species of infant mammals. Am J Physiol 166(1):75–91
6. Bigelow WG, Mcbirnie JE (1953) Further experiences with hypothermia for intracardiac surgery in monkeys and groundhogs. Ann Surg 137(3):361–365
7. Prec O, Rosenman R, Braun K, Rodbard S, Katz LN (1949) The cardiovascular effects of acutely induced hypothermia. J Clin Invest 28(2):293–300
8. Bigelow WG, Lindsay WK, Greenwood WF (1950) Hypothermia; its possible role in cardiac surgery: an investigation of factors governing survival in dogs at low body temperatures. Ann Surg 132(5):849–866
9. Baffes TG (1958) Hypothermia in cardiovascular surgery. J Natl Med Assoc 50(6):426–428
10. Boerema I, WildschutI A, Schmidt WJ, Broekhuysen L (1951) Experimental researches into hypothermia as an aid in the surgery of the heart. Arch Chir Neerl 3(1):25–34
11. Cookson BA, Neptune WB, Bailey CP (1952) Hypothermia as a means of performing intracardiac surgery under direct vision. Dis Chest 22(3):245–260
12. Lewis FJ, Taufic M (1953) Closure of atrial septal defects with the aid of hypothermia; experimental accomplishments and the report of one successful case. Surgery 33(1):52–59
13. Sellors JH (1967) The genesis of heart surgery. Br Med J 1(5537):385–393
14. Swan H, Zeavin I, Blount SG Jr, Virtue RW (1953) Surgery by direct vision in the open heart during hypothermia. J Am Med Assoc 153(12):1081–1085
15. Lewis FJ (1956) Hypothermia in surgery. J Natl Med Assoc 48(5):317–322
16. No authors listed (1953) Hypothermia. Br Med J 2(4848):1256–1257
17. Blades B, Pierpont HC (1954) A simple method for inducing hypothermia. Ann Surg 140(4):557–563
18. Delorme EJ (1952) Experimental cooling of the blood-stream. Lancet 2(6741):914–915
19. Brock R (1956) Hypothermia and open cardiotomy. Proc R Soc Med 49(6):347–352
20. Smith A, Fairer JG (1953) Hibernation anaesthesia in major surgery; a report of 36 cases. Br Med J 2(4848):1247–1248
21. Lucas BG (1956) Discussion on the application of hypothermia to surgical procedures. Proc R Soc Med 49(6):345–347
22. Swan H, Zeavin I, Holmes JH, Montgomery V (1953) Cessation of circulation in general hypothermia. I. Physiologic changes and their control. Ann Surg 138(3):360–376
23. Shumacker HB (1992) The evolution of cardiac surgery. Indiana University Press, Bloomington
24. Gravlee GP, Davis RF, Kurusz M, Utley JR (2000) Cardiopulmonary bypass: principles and practice, 2nd edn. Lippincott Williams & Wilkins, Philadelphia
25. Ranucci M, Balduini A, Ditta A, Boncilli A, Brozzi S (2009) A systematic review of biocompatible cardiopulmonary bypass circuits and clinical outcome. Ann Thorac Surg 87:1311–1319
26. Mahoney CB (1998) Heparin-bonded circuits: clinical outcome and costs. Perfusion 13:1892
27. Ranucci M, Mazzucco A, Pessotto R et al (1999) Heparin-coated circuits for high-risk patients: a multi-center prospective randomized trial. Ann Thorac Surg 67:994
28. DeSomer F, VanBelleghem Y, Cases F et al (2002) Phosphorylcholine coating offers natural platelet preservation during CPB. Perfusion 17:39

29. Taketani S, Sawa Y, Massai T et al (1998) A novel technique for cardiopulmonary bypass using vacuum system for venous drainage with pressure relief valve: an experimental study. Artif Organs 22:337
30. La Pietra A, Groggi EA, Pua BB et al (2000) Assisted venous drainage presents the risk of undetected air microembolism. J Thorac Cardiovasc Surg 120:856
31. Biancari F, Rimpiläinen R (2009) Meta-analysis of randomised trials comparing the effectiveness of miniaturised versus conventional cardiopulmonary bypass in adult cardiac surgery. Heart 95(12):964–969
32. Gu YJ, de Vries AJ, Voa P et al (1999) Leukocyte depletion during cardiac operations: a new approach through the venous bypass circuit. Ann Thorac Surg 67:604
33. Hessel EA II (2001) Cardiopulmonary bypass equipment. In: Estafanous FG, Barash PG, Reves JG (eds) Cardiac anesthesia: principles and clinical practice, 2nd edn. Lippincott Williams & Wilkins, Philadelphia, p 335
34. High KM, Williams DR, Kurusz M (1995) Cardiopulmonary bypass circuits and design. In: Hensley FA Jr, Martin DE (eds) A practical approach to cardiac anesthesia, 2nd edn. Little, Brown, Boston, p 465
35. Stammers AH (1998) Monitoring controversies during cardiopulmonary bypass: how far have we come? Perfusion 13:35
36. Baraka A, Barody M, Harous S et al (1990) Continuous venous oximetry during cardiopulmonary bypass: influence of temperature changes, perfusion flow and hematocrit level. J Cardiothorac Anesth 4:35

# Cardiac Anaesthesia

**14**

Fabio Guarracino and Rubia Baldassarri

> *If I would be a young man again and had to decide how to make my living, I would not try to become a scientist or scholar or teacher. I would rather choose to be a plumber or a peddler in the hope to find that modest degree of independence still available under present circumstances.*
>
> A. Einstein

**Abstract**

Anaesthesia was developed in the middle of the 19th century with the discovery of the anaesthetic effects of nitrous oxide, ether and chloroform. Ether and chloroform were used for many years to induce unconsciousness and relieve pain during surgery. Anaesthesia improved slowly, and did not achieve its own identity as a specific branch of medicine for many years; thus, it was administered by either surgeons or nurses. Only later did it become a medical specialty. As heart surgery expanded, it became clear that cardiac anaesthesia required a specific skill set: the cardiac anaesthetist had to manage induction and maintenance of anaesthesia, problems associated with thoracic wounds and the opening of the chest, massive bleeding from cardiac chambers and major blood vessels, and haemodynamic instability.

## 14.1 Cardiac Anaesthesia Before the Advent of Cardiopulmonary Bypass (CPB)

Anaesthesia was developed in the middle of the 19th century with the discovery of the anaesthetic effects of nitrous oxide, ether and chloroform [1]. Ether and chloroform were used for many years to induce unconsciousness and relieve pain during surgery (Fig. 14.1). Anaesthesia improved slowly, and did not achieve its own identity as a specific branch of medicine for many years; thus, it was administered by either surgeons or nurses (Fig. 14.2) [1–4]. Only later did it

F. Guarracino (✉) · R. Baldassarri
Anesthesia and Intensive Care Department,
Azienda Ospedaliero Universitaria Pisana, Pisa, Italy
e-mail: fabiodoc64@hotmail.com

M. Picichè (ed.), *Dawn and Evolution of Cardiac Procedures*,
DOI: 10.1007/978-88-470-2400-7_14, © Springer-Verlag Italia 2013

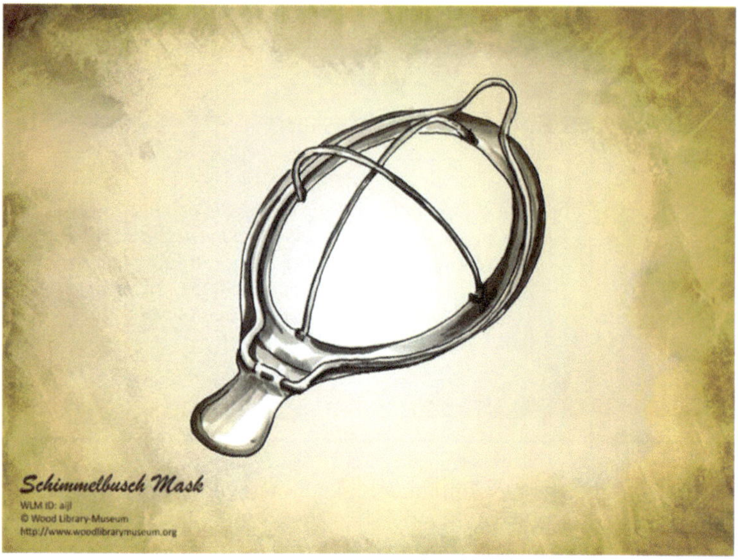


**Fig. 14.1** Mask to provide ether and chloroform anaesthesia

**Fig. 14.2** Anaesthesia was performed by nurses and surgeons: anaesthesia was far from becoming a subspecialty

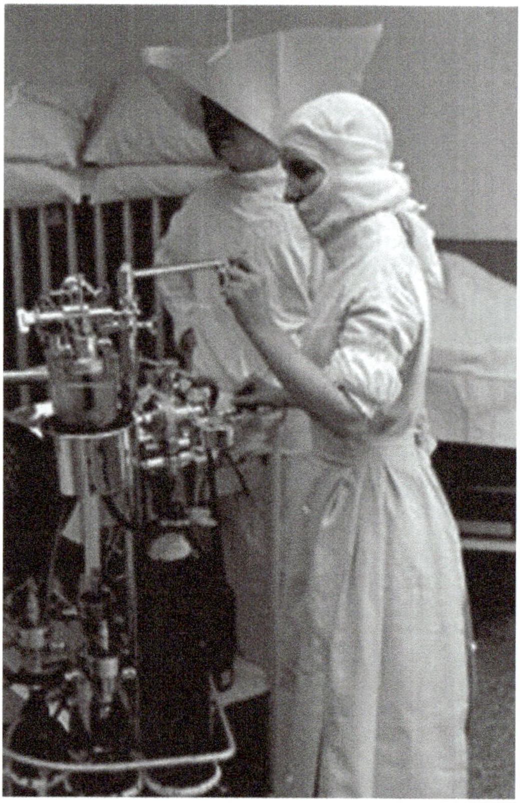

become a medical specialty. As heart surgery expanded, it became clear that cardiac anaesthesia required a specific skill set: the cardiac anaesthetist had to manage induction and maintenance of anaesthesia, problems associated with thoracic wounds and the opening of the chest, massive bleeding from cardiac chambers and major blood vessels, and haemodynamic instability.

Cyclopropane was adopted in 1933. Because of its high degree of inflammability, it was replaced by halothane in the 1950s. Two years later, the invention of the copper kettle (Fig. 14.3), which provided a more precise dosage of the anaesthetic gas, and the advent of temperature-compensated (TEC) agent-specific vaporisers made the management of cardiac anaesthesia safer and more adequate for heterogeneous cardiac procedures. The introduction of thiopental in 1934 and curare in 1942 improved the anaesthesiological management and laid the foundation for modern cardiac anaesthesia [5–7]

One of the considerable challenges concerned the ventilation of patients with open chests, as the techniques that were used prior to the advent of mechanical ventilation were hazardous and experimental. Brauer in 1904 and Murphy in 1905 placed patients' heads in a box where positive pressure was delivered, whereas Sauerbruch in 1904 placed the patient in a negative pressure chamber and left the patient's head outside of this chamber [8]. The solution was endotracheal ventilation. Although the first one was performed in 1878 by the Scottish surgeon W. Macewan and the first mechanical ventilators appeared at the beginning of 1900s, the combination of these two techniques was not routinely used until the late 1950s [9] (Fig. 14.4, 14.5).

In the 1950s, anaesthesia management for cardiac surgery benefitted from intravenous cannulae, endotracheal intubation and mechanical ventilation. The first to-and-fro carbon dioxide absorber was introduced in 1924 by Waters, while in the mid-1950s, a new system for the removal of respiratory carbon dioxide became available and improved patient ventilation. Basic haemodynamic monitoring with the use of electrocardiogram (ECG), non-invasive blood pressure and peripheral oxygen saturation measurements were available but not always used. Moreover, the majority of the anaesthetic drugs were used both to induce and to maintain general anaesthesia throughout the procedure [9, 10].

The first open-heart surgeries were performed in children with severe cyanotic congenital heart defects. Although little was reported in literature about the anaesthesia techniques, the majority of patients were given heavy premedication with opioids (morphine) and scopolamine, which was followed by routine general anaesthesia performed with the most commonly available anaesthetic drugs [10].

Papers of that time described an absence of haemodynamic monitoring. Common intraoperative adverse events such as bleeding, fatal arrhythmias, and cardiogenic shock were very difficult to treat. Papers that were published between 1951 and 1955 regarding the first interventions for heart valve diseases recommended the use of very light anaesthesia to reduce cardiac depression that would occur at the induction of anaesthesia. Some authors reported beneficial effects provided by the associations between different anaesthetic drugs, while others adopted extreme measures to decrease the haemodynamic effects of anaesthesia, such as providing a mild sedation that left the patients almost awake during the operation [1, 6–9].

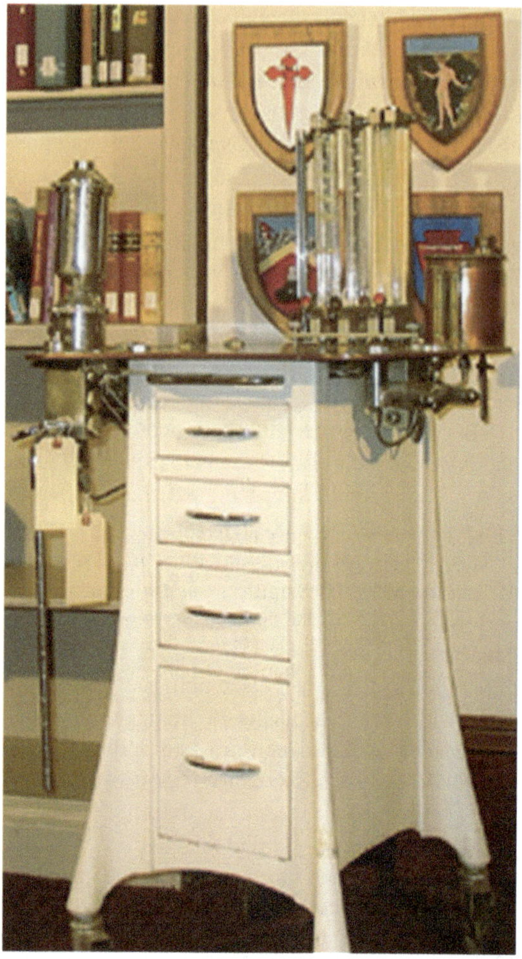

**Fig. 14.3** An image of a copper kettle

During the early phases of open-heart surgery, the direct visualisation of the cardiac lesion being operated on was greatly limited either because the heart was still beating or because the blood was still flowing through the cardiac chambers. Clamping the cardiac inflow vessels provided the surgeon with a few minutes of a bloodless surgical field that improved the operating conditions. Before the advent of CBP, temporary suppression of heart perfusion was one of the most critical components of surgical procedures. Experiments on animals had demonstrated that mild hypothermia could protect the brain from hypoperfusion injury for approximately 10 min [11]. Because hypothermia provided both a reduction in body metabolism and oxygen consumption, the brain could resist longer periods without oxygen. Hypothermia also allowed the surgeons to work in better surgical conditions (arrest of circulation, empty heart, extreme bradycardia) for a longer time. The method adopted by Swan [12] was the most widely used: body temperature was progressively reduced by immersion in a cold water bath, and the patient was

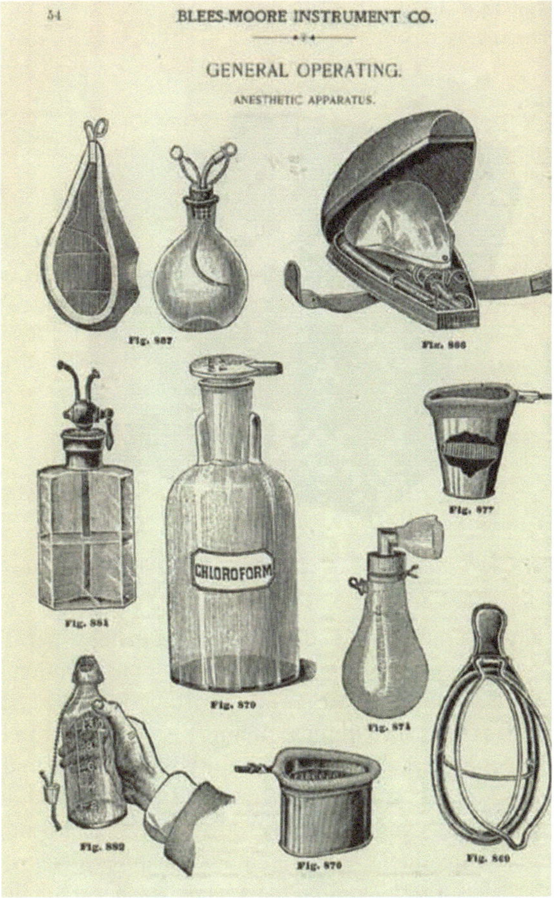


**Fig. 14.4** Instruments for endotracheal anaesthesia administration

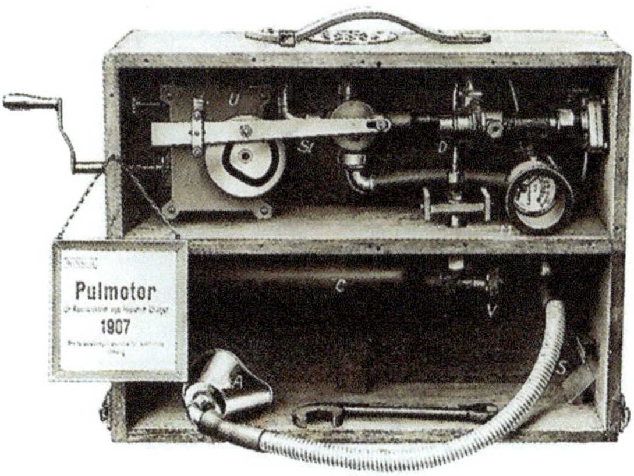


**Fig. 14.5** Pulmotor

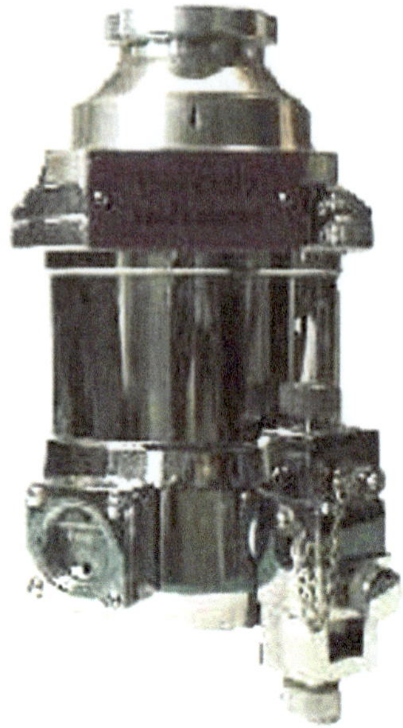

**Fig. 14.6** Volatile anaesthesia vaporizer

subsequently rewarmed by immersion in hot water. The anaesthesia management of hypothermic patients required the consideration of important metabolic and haemodynamic effects resulting from significant variations in body temperature, such as fatal arrhythmias, clotting disturbances, bleeding, and neurological injuries. Hypothermia was successfully used on a 5-year-old girl to repair an atrial septum defect in 1952, and in general it was first applied during heart surgery in children affected by cyanotic diseases [13]. However, hypothermia alone was not sufficient for the treatment of more complex cardiac defects. At this point in its evolution, cardiac surgery required the advent of a new technical approach.

## 14.2 Cardiac Anaesthesia After the Advent of CPB

The introduction of the heart–lung machine represented the fundamental step in the evolution of cardiac surgery and anaesthesia [5].

In the beginning, extracorporeal circulation was performed with unsafe experimental systems. Between 1950 and 1955, several prototypes of heart–lung machines were proposed and used by different surgical teams, with many technical and clinical limitations. The majority of these patients died or reported significant morbidity [5].

Although the anaesthetist was progressively assuming an emerging role in the cardiac surgery team anaesthesia was still not considered to be a subspecialty, and the anaesthetist was not a physician expert specifically in anaesthesia.

Almost all anaesthetic agents available induced myocardial depression. The introduction of curare in 1942 and halothane in 1956 improved anaesthesia [1, 7]. The use of curare for muscle relaxation allowed for a lighter plane of anaesthesia with less haemodynamic impairment, especially during the induction of anaesthesia and endotracheal intubation. In addition, with the advent of vaporisers, halothane could be safely administered and quickly managed (Fig. 14.6).

Since the beginning it was clear that cardiac anaesthesia was not "ordinary" anaesthesia. The advent of extracorporeal circulation revealed important pathophysiological alterations that influenced the anaesthetic management of patients undergoing CPB. The anaesthetist had to become an expert in haemodynamic management.

In the beginning, cardiac surgery only dealt with congenital defects. Subsequently, the field evolved to include heart valve surgeries followed by coronary artery surgeries [3]. The cardiac anaesthetist had to be well-versed in managing these more complex surgeries, the new technology available, and the performance of CPB. This progressive improvement in cardiac anaesthetists led to the foundation of the modern concept of cardiac anaesthesia [14].

The concept that cardiac surgery patients needed postoperative monitoring, was first considered when coronary artery surgery became effective in the 1960s. In those years, intensive care units were established to monitor the coronary surgery patients for the early postoperative hours. Although the measurements of both arterial blood pressure and central venous pressure have been available since the late 1950s, it was not until the 1970s that the introduction of the Swan–Ganz catheter allowed for the percutaneous catheterisation of the pulmonary artery. This catheter allowed for measurement of the pulmonary artery pressure and the left atrial pressure. Furthermore, with the application of the thermodilution technique, the door was opened to the monitoring of cardiac output [15].

Although cardiac anaesthetists are still debating the effective role of the PAC, the revolutionary role played by the Swan–Ganz catheter in advancing haemodynamic monitoring is undeniable [16]. It was in the early 1980s that transoesophageal echocardiography (TOE) was introduced into the clinical practice to evaluate cardiac function and to assess haemodynamic status. TOE has progressively become a fundamental diagnostic or monitoring device [17, 18]. The increasing number of less-invasive procedures, such as percutaneous coronary angioplasty and percutaneous heart valve treatment, namely transcatheter aortic valve implantations and percutaneous mitral valve repair, have altered the way cardiac anaesthetists approach a patient. These patients require well-rounded perioperative management, including a proper preoperative evaluation and intraoperative safe monitoring: when surgery becomes less invasive, anaesthesia and postoperative care cannot be less invasive [19–22]. Conversely, the expanded role of the extremely invasive procedures, such as extracorporeal assistance (ECMO) and the ventricular assist devices (VAD), have imposed complexities on the ICU management of these cases. Pulmonary artery catheterization is still considered the gold standard for CO monitoring, nevertheless the introduction of less-invasive CO monitoring systems has changed the clinical approach to critically ill patients. These methods are based on the pulse contour wave form analysis and provide a good measurement of either the CO or other haemodynamic parameters [23, 24].

## References

1. Keown KK (1982) A brief history of anaesthesia and surgery of the heart and great vessels. Can Anaesth Soc J 29(4):325–329
2. Cleland WP (1983) Historical review. The evolution of cardiac surgery in the United Kingdom. Thorax 38:887–896
3. Kobak MW (1968) The history of cardiac valve surgery before the advent of repair under vision. Angiology 19(2):80–94
4. Hessel EA II (2001) History of cardiac surgery and anesthesia. In: Estafanous FG, Barash PG, Reves JG (eds) Cardiac anesthesia: principles and practice, Lippincott Williams & Wilkins, Cleveland, pp 17–28
5. Stoney WS (2009) Evolution of cardiopulmonary bypass. Circulation 119:2844–2853
6. Rink EH (1950) Anaesthesia for cardiac surgery. Ann R Coll Surg Engl 7(2):151–158
7. Lyons SM (1998) The advance(s) of cardiac surgery and anaesthesia. Ulster Med J 67 [Suppl 1]:15–17
8. Brodsky JB, Lemmens HJ (2007) The history of anesthesia for thoracic surgery. Minerva Anestesiol 73(10):513–524
9. Elsberg CA (1911) III. Experiences in thoracic surgery under anaesthesia by the intratracheal insufflation of air and ether: with remarks on the value of the method for general anaesthesia. Ann Surg 54(6):749–757
10. Denson JS, Joseph S, Miller H (1953) Anesthesia in cardiac operations. Calif Med 78(5):450–452
11. Bigelow WG, Mustard E (1954) Some physiologic concepts of hypothermia and their application to cardiac surgery. J Thorac Surg 28:463
12. Swan H, Zeawn I, Blount SG Jr, Virtue RW (1953) Surgery by direct vision in the open heart during hypothermia. J Am Med Assoc 153:1081
13. Lewis FJ, Taufic M (1953) Closure of atrial septal defects with aid of hypothermia: experimental accomplishments and the report of one successful case. Surgery 33:52–59
14. Cohn LH (2003) Fifty years of open-heart surgery. Circulation 107:2168–2170
15. Chatterjee K (2009) The Swan-Ganz catheters: past, present, and future. A viewpoint. Circulation 119(1):147–152
16. Pugsley J, Lerner AB (2010) Cardiac output monitoring: is there a gold standard and how do the newer technologies compare? Semin Cardiothorac Vasc Anesth 14(4):274–282
17. Hutteman E (2006) Transoesophageal echocardiography in critical care. Minerva Anestesiol 72:891–913
18. Guarracino F, Baldassarri R (2009) Transesophageal echocardiography in the OR and ICU. Minerva Anestesiol 75(9):518–529
19. Guarracino F, Covello RD, Landoni G, Baldassarri R, Stefani M, Cariello C, Ruggeri L, Franco A, Gerli C, Pappalardo F, Zangrillo A (2010) Anesthetic management of transcatheter aortic valve implantation with transaxillary approach. J Cardiothorac Vasc Anesth 25(3):437–443
20. Sellevold OF, Guarracino F (2010) Transcutaneous aortic valve implantation: recent advances and future. Curr Opin Anaesthesiol 23(1):67–73
21. Yuksel UC, Kapadia SR, Tuzcu EM (2011) Percutaneous mitral repair: patient selection, results, and future directions. Curr Cardiol Rep 13(2):100–106
22. Goldberg SL, Feldman T (2010) Percutaneous mitral valve interventions: overview of new approaches. Curr Cardiol Rep 12(5):404–412
23. Ranucci M (2006) Which cardiac surgical patients can benefit from placement of a pulmonary artery catheter? Crit Care 10 [Suppl 3]:S6
24. Guarracino F, Stefani M, Lapolla F, Cariello C, Doroni L, Danella A, Baldassarri R (2007) Monitoring cardiac output with Flo Trac Vigileo. Br J Anaesth 99(1):142. Author reply 142–143

# Part III

# Research on Interventional Cardiology and Cardiac Surgery After the Advent of Cardiopulmonary Bypass

# The History of Research on Coronary Angiography and Coronary Angioplasty

# 15

Luigi La Vecchia

*In the field of scientific observation chance favors the prepared mind.*

Louis Pasteur

**Abstract**

The history of coronary angiography and intervention begins with the first human heart catheterization performed in 1929, continues with a series of progressive technical and cultural developments, such as selective coronary angiography, direct needle vascular puncture, pre-shaped dedicated coronary catheters, refinement of radial access, and merges into the new exciting field of endovascular intervention, thanks to the pivotal work of C. Dotter and, above all, A. Gruentzig, who set the pace for one of the most rapidly growing and challenging branches of modern medicine. This chapter briefly takes the reader along the path of this adventure.

## 15.1 Introduction

Mr. C.A, an 82-year-old gentleman, was taken to the Catheterization Laboratory of our Department at 08.00 a.m. on a Monday morning. This patient, who had suffered an acute myocardial infarction in 1977 and was subsequently treated with

L. La Vecchia (✉)
Catheterization Laboratory, Department of Cardiovascular Medicine,
San Bortolo Hospital, Viale Rodolfi 37 Vicenza, Italy
e-mail: luigilavecchia@libero.it

M. Picichè (ed.), *Dawn and Evolution of Cardiac Procedures*,
DOI: 10.1007/978-88-470-2400-7_15, 

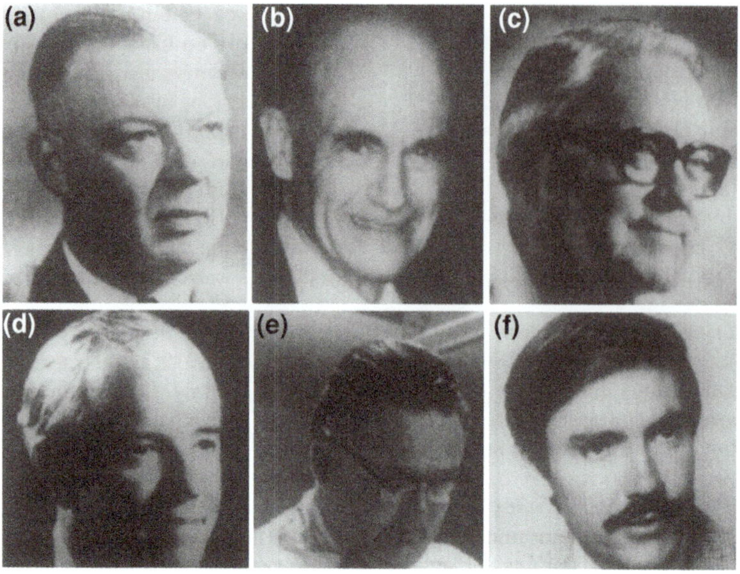


**Fig. 15.1** Major contributors to the development of invasive cardiovascular medicine, **a** Werner Forssman; **b** Charles T. Dotter; **c** Sven I. Seldinger; **d** Mason F. Sones; **e** Melvin P. Judkins; and **f** Andreas R. Gruentzig. For details, see text

coronary artery bypass grafting for triple vessel disease in 1986, had been experiencing recurrence of chest pain for the last 2 months. Coronary angiography revealed a 90% stenosis of the left anterior descending coronary artery distal to left internal mammary anastomosis and severe disease of the saphenous vein graft for the right coronary artery. The patient received successful percutaneous treatment of both lesions and was discharged 2 days later.

The story of Mr. C.A., apparently unremarkable, encompasses the evolution of coronary angiography and intervention showing surprising coincidences. First, this gentleman was born in 1929, when Forssmann performed on himself the first human catheterization. Second, he sustained a myocardial infarction in 1977, when Gruentzig performed the first coronary angioplasty on a patient. Third, he received coronary artery bypass surgery in 1986, the year when the first coronary stent was implanted, a radial approach for coronary angiography was first attempted, and the first monorail balloon catheter was presented to the medical community.

From these observations, we can clearly appreciate that the history of coronary angiography and intervention parallels the lifespan of those elderly patients that we see today in our laboratories and who survived to an old age thanks to the developments of cardiovascular medicine over the past decades.

If our parents today and, ourselves in the future, benefit from the prodigious advances of intervention we all must be aware that a long, complex and thwarted process of experiments, achievements and failures was stubbornly brought about by pioneer researchers (Fig. 15.1) who dedicated their intuitions, reasoning, and efforts to the development of the technologies that we now handle with confidence for our patients.

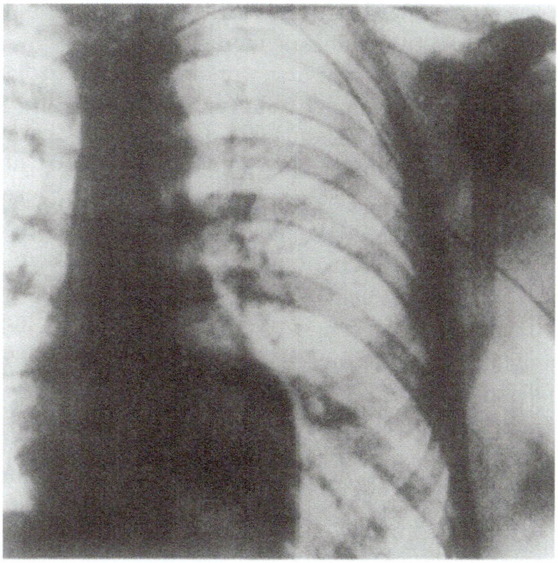

**Fig. 15.2** X-Ray documentation of self-right heart catheterization performed by W. Forssman in 1929

## 15.2 The Very Beginning: Werner Forssmann

Although many anecdotal and sometimes purely historical reports bring to our knowledge the evidence that the human body and the vascular system were entered by our ancestors in an attempt to alleviate disease as early as 3000 years B.C., little doubt exists that the first documented vascular catheterization in a living human is the one performed by Werner Forssmann on himself in 1929 [1]. This young, quiet, introverted surgical resident at Eberswelde Hospital was prompted by the need to develop a safe and effective way to deliver life-saving drugs into the hearts of patients suffering from cardiac arrest. He was convinced that inserting a catheter into the right side of the heart through the venous system was by far safer than a direct intracardiac injection, and pursued the realization of this concept working alone, on himself, given the resistance of his medical colleagues. What happened exactly is not entirely clear, since several versions of this story exist [2, 3]; what holds true is that Forssmann obtained an X-ray to show that the urethral catheter he had inserted through his left basilic vein had advanced into his right atrium (Fig. 15.2). This is the first documented human cardiac catheterization.

## 15.3 From Nonselective to Selective Coronary Angiography

The idea of injecting radiopaque contrast medium into the coronary arteries during normal cardiac activity matured very slowly over almost 2 decades. In the 1940s, selective angiographic visualization of the coronary arteries was considered dangerous and possibly fatal. Therefore, if one aimed at studying the anatomy and pathology of the coronary arteries in patients, indirect methods of visualization had to be pursued.

The simplest of all was to perform aortography, using a catheter positioned just above the aortic valve. However, catheter injection performed under normal circulatory conditions had several drawbacks. Contrast medium is rapidly flushed away by blood ejected from the left ventricle. Consequently, a large amount of contrast medium is required, and this can be administered only using large-bore catheters, since the injection rate is maximally dependent on catheter diameter. Also, X-ray acquisition requires a fast sequence (5–6 films per second). Moreover, the quality of the image obtained was sometimes poor, especially in patients with a high heart rate or dilated aorta.

Thus, researchers devised several alternative methods to enhance the diagnostic performance of pan-aortography. The first was synchronized diastolic injection, but the results, due to the poor technology available, were unsatisfactory [4, 5]. Another possibility for overcoming these limitations was to reduce cardiac output for a limited, controlled period of time, through the induction of hypotension and bradycardia. This would allow the administration of a much lower amount of contrast medium through smaller catheters and to obtain adequate imaging of the coronary arteries with a single still frame. The protocols included the administration of drugs such as acetylcholine [6], proposed by Arnulf in Lyon, or trimethaphan [7], as suggested by Pinet and Gravier; alternatively, augmentation of intrabronchial pressure obtained during general anesthesia with intratracheal balloon inflation, as described by Nordenstrom [8], induced reflex hypotension/bradycardia of a similar nature.

Of all these methods, acetylcholine administration became the most popular because it was considered safe, fast-acting and reversible, although intravenous injection sometimes required very high doses [9].

An alternative approach used by Dotter and Frische consisted of positioning a double-lumen balloon catheter in the ascending aorta and inflating it until occlusion of the vessel occurred so that contrast medium injection would follow the path of least resistance through the coronary arteries [10].

Many nonselective coronary angiograms were obtained in different laboratories using these techniques, alone or in combination, and different laboratories often developed individual protocols.

These concepts were dramatically reconsidered after the casual experience of Mason Sones in 1959. A catheter positioned in the ascending aorta just above the aortic valve to obtain pan-aorto-coronary angiography dropped inadvertently into the right coronary artery while contrast medium was being injected. The subsequent injection of 30 ml of contrast agent induced transient ventricular standstill but no fibrillation. After a pause and cough resuscitation, the patient recovered with normal sinus rhythm [11]. The first selective coronary angiography had thus been performed, unintentionally. As the patient survived without damage, Sones realized that selective injection of an adequate amount of contrast medium into a coronary artery was not only feasible, but also extremely more informative than a nonselective injection (Fig. 15.3).

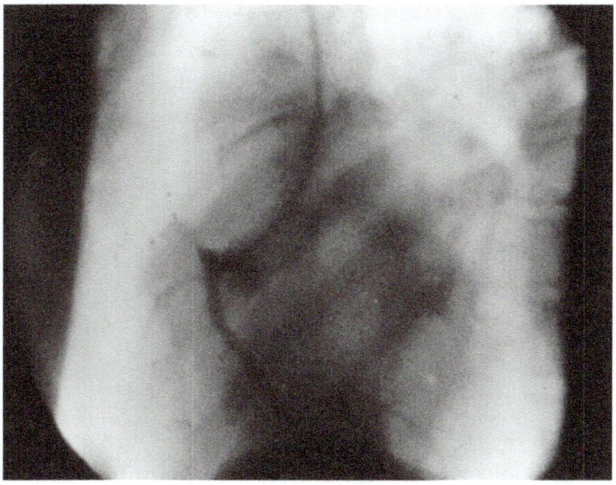

**Fig. 15.3** The first selective coronary angiogram performed accidentally by Mason F. Sones in 1958

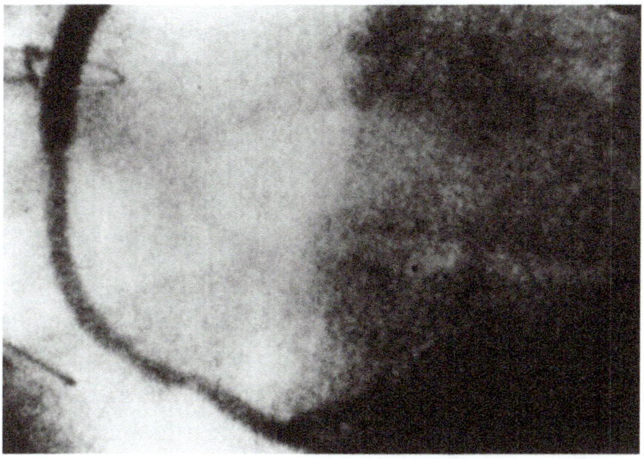

**Fig. 15.4** The first selective angiogram of a saphenous bypass graft performed by Mason F. Sones in 1967

Therefore, he rapidly dedicated himself to developing a specially designed catheter to electively engage the coronary ostia. The vascular approach consisted of a right brachial artery cut-down. Soon after, Sones could describe his experience of the first 1,500 consecutive coronary angiograms before the 8th Annual Meeting of the American College of Cardiology in 1959: three procedural deaths had occurred and the incidence of ventricular fibrillation was 2 % [12]. In 1967, the first saphenous vein graft was visualized angiographically (Fig. 15.4).

## 15.4 From Direct Puncture to Cut-Down to Percutaneous Approach

The aorta and left-sided cardiac chambers were initially entered for pressure measurement and angiography through direct needle puncture, either antegrade or retrograde. Percutaneous left ventricular puncture was performed initially by

**Table 15.1** Various approaches to the left heart through direct puncture

| | |
|---|---|
| *Left atrial puncture* | |
| Posterior transthoracic | Bjork et al. [41] |
| Transbronchial | Facquet et al. [42] |
| Suprasternal | Hansen et al. [43] |
| *Left ventricular puncture* | |
| Subxiphoid | Smith et al. [44] |
| Apical | Brock et al. [45] |

Reboul and Racine in 1933 [13]. Other direct approaches to cardiac chambers are summarized in Table 15.1. Of all these aggressive, cumbersome, and hazardous approaches, the only direct puncture technique that has survived from those times to obtain an established role in cardiac catheterization and intervention is the transseptal left atrial access, first developed by Ross in 1959 [14].

As shown in the previous paragraph, in the 1950s, coronary arteriography (either selective or nonselective) was mainly performed using brachial artery cutdown, according to the Sones technique.

The Sones technique was modified by Ricketts and Abrams with the introduction of two new catheters of modified design, aimed at selective engagement of coronary ostia from a percutaneous femoral approach in 1962 [15]. The catheters were exchanged using a spring guide. Aortography was first performed through a femoral artery cut-down by Farinas in 1941 [16].

All these experiences were carried out mainly by radiologists and surgeons and required some knowledge of surgical techniques and, most of all, a high dose of recklessness. Cardiologists were mainly interested in cardiac catheterization, pressure measurements, and hemodynamics [17], a fascinating field of invasive-based pathophysiology that for the sake of conciseness we will forcedly neglect.

In 1953, Dr. Sven Seldinger first described the technique of percutaneous arterial puncture by means of a specially designed steel needle containing an obturator [18]. A simplified method of arterial puncture consists of a single thin-walled needle to gain direct access to the artery with a single wall puncture only. An essential part of the technique was the insertion of a long, flexible guidewire advanced through the needle into the vessel. Seldinger designed himself such a wire consisting of a round cross-sectional wire tightly coiled on a central wire core. The advantages of direct puncture were immediately evident for both safety and the patient's comfort. This apparently simple technical development must be considered essential in enabling cardiologists to perform safely angiographic procedures, without the need for surgical experience. However, almost 10 years passed before the percutaneous approach to entering the vascular system for coronary angiography was applied [15].

## 15.5 From Femoral to Radial Artery

After the fundamental experience developed by Judkins [19], the percutaneous femoral approach became the standard for coronary angiography and left heart catheterization. When this access was technically not feasible, the brachial artery remained as an alternative, initially via surgical cut-down, then, thanks to the progressive reduction in sheath size, percutaneously as well [20]. Also, since 1965, the axillary route was demonstrated to be feasible by Wiedner et al., but never became popular [21], mainly because of the difficulties encountered in obtaining adequate hemostasis and the relatively high frequency of brachial plexus compression [22].

Although radial access for coronary angiography had already been obtained by Bertrand in 1974 [23], Lucien Campeau from the Montreal Heart Institute [24] was the first to propose the radial artery as a default access site for coronary angiography in 1989. Potential advantages of this approach originated from a series of observations. First, it was noted that patients with a long duration of invasive arterial monitoring through the radial artery often developed a total occlusion of the vessel, but this occurred without symptoms or clinical consequences. Second, the radial artery has no significant venous vessel or nerve branch adjacent to its course, thus making the occurrence of nervous/vascular complications highly unlikely. Finally, the downsizing of coronary catheters over time made radial artery access for diagnostic purposes less traumatic. The first series published by Campeau included 100 patients, with a 90 % success rate. From that time, the radial approach was extended to percutaneous intervention and is now routinely performed in many laboratories all over the world. Despite improved material technology and expanded experience, the initial success rate has improved by only 5 % in over 20 years [25].

Over a 50-year period, the contribution of coronary angiography to cardiovascular medicine has been of paramount importance (Table 15.2).

## 15.6 From Dotter to Gruentzig

The history of vascular intervention begins with the fortuitous experience of Charles Dotter, radiologist at Oregon University. He developed a technique for dilatation of peripheral arteries after the observation that a guidewire, inadvertently advanced past an arterial narrowing during diagnostic angiography, induced an improvement in the angiographic patency of the vessel. This inadvertent therapeutic maneuver marked the beginning of the era of vascular intervention, and for this achievement, Dotter was recognized as its father. The concept developed by Dotter consisted of gently advancing coaxial catheters of progressively larger size across a vascular narrowing so as to open up the vessel enough to restore flow and resolve ischemia (Fig. 15.5). After attempts performed on cadavers, the first patient undergoing peripheral treatment with the use of Dotter's

**Table 15.2** The contribution of coronary angiography over 5 decades

| Decade | Contribution |
|---|---|
| 1950s | Selective coronary arteriography introduced by Mason Sones |
| | The first human studies using an in vivo marker for severity and extent of CAD |
| 1960s | Earliest natural history studies of proven CAD |
| | Dynamic visualization of LV performance |
| | Demonstration of prompt and complete revascularization by CABG |
| 1970s | Refinement of natural history studies of unoperated CAD patients |
| | Discovery of the benefit of CABG vs medical treatment in subsets of patients |
| | Delineation of coronary vasospasm and Prinzmetal's angina |
| | Significance of coronary pathoanatomy (ulceration, thrombus, dissection, aneurysm, collaterals, bridging) |
| | Introduction of PTCA and delineation of restenosis |
| | First angiographic evidence of clot lysis in a coronary vessel |
| 1980s | Dawn of the thrombolytic era |
| | Demonstration of spontaneous fibrinolysis during 24 h of acute occlusion |
| | Plaque regression studies |
| | Delineation of the pathogenesis of myocardial infarction from studies outlining angiographic progression to myocardial infarction |
| | Estimates of coronary flow using TIMI flow rates and TIMI frame counts |
| | Comparison of PCI vs CABG for revascularization outcomes |
| 1990s | Establishment of the stent era |
| | Studies of the coronary microcirculation by myocardial blush |
| | Brachytherapy, late stent thrombosis and pharmacotherapy |
| | Newer imaging devices (intravascular ultrasound, MRI) |

Modified from: Ryan [46]. With permission

*CAD* coronary artery disease, *CABG* coronary artery bypass surgery, *PTCA* percutaneous transluminal coronary angioplasty, *TIMI* Thrombolysis in myocardial infarction, *LV* left ventricle

technique was an elderly diabetic lady with advanced leg ischemia who required a "salvage" procedure to avoid amputation. The vascular dilatation was performed on 16 January 1964, required the use of two catheters, and was successful, both angiographically and clinically [26].

Dotter's technique was considered a rather crude treatment for atherosclerotic obstructions. Damage to the vascular wall, distal embolization or thrombotic occlusion were considered potentially major drawbacks to this technology, which

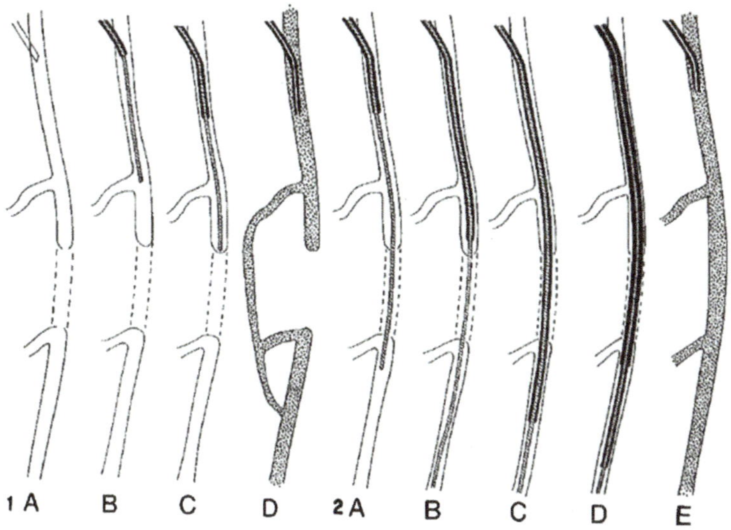


**Fig. 15.5** Schematic illustration of transluminal recanalization according to Dotter's technique. Panel 1, from *A* to *D*. The artery is punctured and a catheter is introduced over a guidewire; then, angiography is obtained. Panel 2, from *A* to *E*. The guide is advanced through the occluded segment and coaxial catheters of increasing size are advanced to the distal lumen, until vessel patency is completely restored

never gained much attention by colleagues, and overt opposition from vascular surgeons. However, in contrast to the American medical community, much interest developed in Europe concerning Dotter's technique. Many investigators, among which Portsmann and Wierny [27], Zeitler and Muller [28], van Andel [29], Dow and Hardwick [30], and many others performed peripheral angioplasties using Dotter's principles and published series of them. Clearly, however, these principles were not applicable to coronary arteries. No matter how much the profile of these coaxial catheters could be improved, the small size of the coronary arteries, combined with the tortuosity and the motion of the cardiac cycle, rendered this approach prohibitive in cardiology.

A different device had to be developed and the idea that it should be a balloon-based technology was growing among scientists. Incidentally, non-coronary applications of balloon therapy were established (Table 15.3). The critical step consisted of adding an inflatable balloon at the distal tip of the catheter, allowing for the system to be more flexible and of smaller size. Unfortunately, the balloons available for medical use were made of latex, because this was the only known material for catheterization in humans and was derived from urethral probes. When inflated against the resistance of a vascular plaque, latex undergoes remarkable deformation and inflates almost exclusively where least resistance is met: thus, the vessel is dilated in the healthy segments adjacent to the lesion while the plaque remains unchanged. This is exactly the opposite of what was required to treat atherosclerotic vessels.

**Table 15.3** Balloon technologies in medicine

| Author | Year | Use |
|---|---|---|
| Arnott | 1819 | Dilate urethral stenosis |
| Reybard | 1855 | Dilate urethral stenosis |
| Plummer | 1906 | Dilate esophageal stenosis |
| Foley | 1927 | Tamponade of bleeding after urethral surgery |
| Gianturco | 1950 | Vascular dilatation |
| Fogarty | 1963 | Removal of vascular emboli |

Initial developments were made by Gianturco (cited in [31]), who dilated a femoral artery in 1971 with a balloon made of polyolefin; by Portsmann [32], who built a prototype of a latex balloon that was caged on Teflon struts; and by Dotter himself [33], who modified Portsmann's catheter by inserting woven fiberglass between the balloon and the Teflon struts, but failed to solve the problem because these "caged" balloons induced plaque fragmentation and distal embolization.

The clinical scenario remained relatively stagnant until the advent of Andreas Gruentzig, a young German physician who was shifting his interests from internal medicine to vascular radiology and whose personality had been destined to make an unprecedented leap forward in the development of cardiovascular medicine ever since.

Gruentzig was convinced that the principle of balloon dilatation was correct but realized that its practical realization was far from being adequate for clinical use. After moving to Zurich from Engelskirchen, he began to study how he could add a balloon to the Dotter's catheter. The answer to this question came along with the help of professor Hopff, an engineer who worked in a nearby Institute of in Zurich University and was an expert in the field of plastic polymers. He explained to Gruentzig that polyvinylchloride (PVC) could represent the solution to the problem. This "new" material exhibited favorable characteristics of elastic memory after thermal treatment. This meant a reasonable correspondence between developed pressure and achieved balloon size, and, more importantly, these features were reproducible. Thus, the first prototype of the coronary balloon was developed. Gruentzig, whose kitchen table was transformed into an extemporary laboratory, used small PVC tubing originally designed as insulation for electric wires, and inflated them with air obtaining a localized dilatation of the tubing. An outer larger tube was advanced onto the previous one so as to confine the diameter of the segment, which assumed a sausage shape. The structure of this device consisted of a single lumen. Holes in correspondence of the balloon segment allowed liquid to enter for inflation and be aspirated for deflation.

This principle constitutes the structural basis for virtually all developed catheter-based technology for coronary dilatation from that time onward.

These concepts are clearly outlined by Abele [34]: "The objective of dilatation are numerous and not easy to achieve. They are: -to open the vessel lumen (….); -to perform the opening in such a manner that the vessel stays open; -to create a smooth inner surface without rough transition; -to produce no distal debris; -to create minimum interference or disruption of the arterial wall structure. The Gruentzig-style balloon (….) -once in the lesion applies radial force only; -there is no axial component; -has a smooth outer shape and surface; -has a controlled diameter (…); -can be introduced percutaneously and manipulated like an angiographic catheter; -can operate next to obstructions and around curves; -can be made in many different sizes and shapes".

Although the beginning of the coronary angioplasty era is traditionally set at 16 September 1977, when the first procedure was performed by Gruentzig on the proximal left anterior descending coronary artery of a 37-year-old salesman, as many as 15 procedures had already been performed since May that year in San Francisco by Gruentzig and Myler.

One year earlier, in November 1976, Gruentzig presented for the first time the results of his experiments at the American Heart Association meeting. There, he met Richard Myler, a cardiologist from San Francisco. From that encounter, a professional collaboration and personal friendship began. They studied the application of coronary balloon dilatation intraoperatively, in patients undergoing coronary artery bypass surgery, and demonstrated the safety and feasibility of the procedure in human patients, confirmed by post-operative angiography [35].

Contrary to Dotter's first angioplasty, Gruentzig chose an elective young patient with a single tight proximal lesion of the left anterior descending coronary artery. The choice was influenced by the available material, whose poor trackability and flexibility prevented the treatment of more distal lesions, but more so by a previous negative experience. In 1976, a severely ill middle-aged man with triple vessel disease and left main stenosis was proposed to Gruentzig for balloon dilatation since he had been rejected for bypass surgery. However, this patient had very poor peripheral circulation and the procedure was attempted from a left brachial approach, but was then abandoned due to the inability to selectively engage the left ostium. The patient subsequently died of recurrent infarction. In this regard, Gruentzig said: "the case taught me that if you start a method you should start with an ideal case and not with end-stage disease and this has been the truth for so many other colleagues being in a similar position later in time."

That first coronary angioplasty performed on 16 September 1977 was not just a technical and procedural success, but more so a clinically long-term effective treatment for coronary atherosclerosis (Fig. 15.6).

Two balloon inflations were performed and were well tolerated by the patient; the distal coronary pressure, measured through the catheter lumen, rose nicely after dilatation and the procedure was soon terminated without the need for further instrumentation. This result translated into a negative exercise test and had persisted until angiographic control 10 years later.

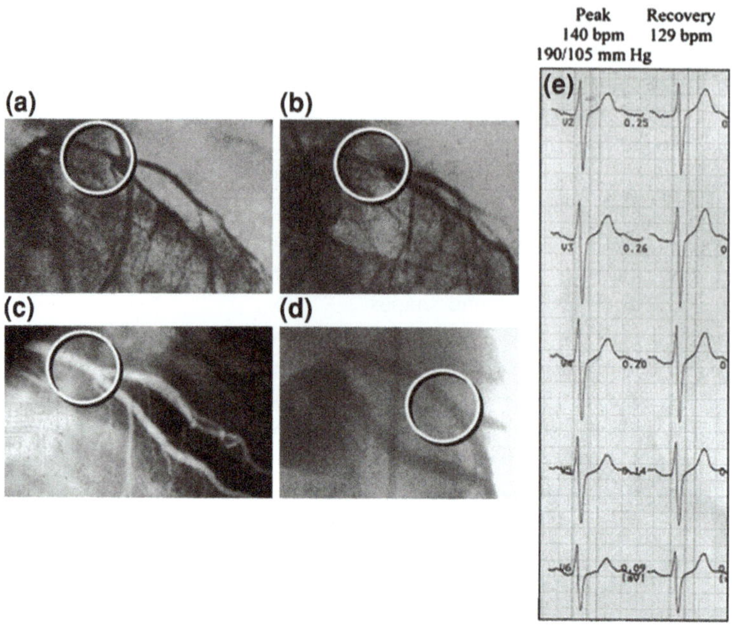


**Fig. 15.6** The first coronary angioplasty. Left panel **a** the lesion before dilatation, **b** after the procedure; **c** 10 years and **d** 23 years later. Right panel The long-term excellent functional result of the procedure

Starting from that first, durable success, Gruentzig soon expanded the applications of the technique, performing dilatations of left main coronary artery and multivessel disease in one session. Subsequent developments in angioplasty technology were "fast and furious." In 1984, in the USA, coronary angioplasty became the prevalent revascularization procedure surpassing bypass surgery [36].

## 15.7 From Over-the-Wire to the Monorail System

The original balloon catheter developed by Gruentzig was a double lumen catheter carrying the balloon at its distal tip; one lumen was connected to the balloon and used to inflate and deflate it with fluid; the second was filled with saline and used to measure the pressure gradient across the stenotic site, which was a physiological measure of success.

The first balloon specifically designed for coronary arteries was conceived by Simpson et al. and was advanced on a freely movable wire [37].

However, it became soon apparent that, given the available technology, more than one balloon was needed to dilate a tight lesion: a small one to open up the lesion and a second one of adequate size to fully dilate the vessel. Retrieving the first balloon and advancing the second one across the lesion after the first dilatation was, however, dangerous. Thus, the 3-m long steerable guidewire was developed by Kaltenbach to maintain a safe access to the lesion while exchanging the balloon [38].

Although feasible and effective, this method was clearly cumbersome, required assistance by a second operator and some skill by the first operator. In search for a solution, the monorail system was developed by Dr. Bonzel et al. with the help of the Schneider Company and obtained a patent in 1984. This technology was based on the principle that instead of elongating the guidewire, the balloon exchangeability could be obtained by shortening the catheter, or at least the coaxial part of the catheter, by developing a non-coaxial system in which the wire could exit the catheter lumen as distal as possible [39]. The system rapidly became popular and now covers >90% of all coronary interventional procedures performed worldwide.

## 15.8 Obstacles, Jealousy, Misunderstanding

*"So many of the procedures that have come since have been developed against conventional wisdom and, as with the first coronary angioplasty, have required courage and conviction of the pioneering physicians"*

Gary S. Roubin

Being a pioneer very often brings along problems, frustrations and conflicts. Interventional cardiology is no exception to this rule. Here are just a few examples:

1. Dr. Forssmann was dismissed for not mentioning the clinic in his publication.
2. Dr. Seldinger was not allowed to leave the hospital to present his paper describing the new technique at the annual congress of the Northern Association of Medical Radiology in Helsinki.
3. Dr. Dotter was thwarted by the medical community in Portland, Oregon, for his new technique, which was rejected in his own country.
4. Concerning Andreas Gruentzig, the words of Bernard Meier clearly depict the scenario [40]: "The term "mobbing" had not been invented yet, but who cares about the term? Andreas was clearly disprivileged when it came to promotions in Zurich. He had the smallest office among his colleagues, had to pay for secretarial help from private sources…and was rarely praised for success but regularly reprimanded for failures."

## 15.9 Conclusion

To conclude this concise overview of the scientific and technical developments in the field of coronary angiography and intervention, let us acknowledge the contributions provided by many more of the distinguished scientists that were essential to the progress of invasive cardiology over the past 150 years (Table 15.4).

**Table 15.4** Contributions made to the development of invasive cardiology over the past 150 years

| Year | Author | Catheterization/angiography | Imaging |
|---|---|---|---|
| 1855 | Reybard | Urethral dilatation with latex balloon | |
| 1895 | Roentgen | | X-rays |
| 1912 | Unger | First intra-arterial injection of drug | |
| 1924 | Brooks | First intra-arterial injection of contrast medium | |
| 1929 | Forssmann | First catheterization in a human patient | |
| 1929 | Lichtenberg and Swick | | Thorotrast—uroselectan |
| 1932 | De Carvalho | First angiography in a human patient (pulmonary) | |
| 1933 | Rausthoi | Coronary angiography in dogs | |
| 1941 | Farinas | First aortography via femoral cut-down | |
| 1953 | Seldinger | Catheter replacement of the needle | Fluoroscopic image amplifier |
| 1956 | Gidlund | | First modern high pressure contrast injector and biplane roll film changer |
| 1956 | Axen and Lind | | Biplane rapid filming |
| 1958 (October) | Sones | First selective coronary angiogram | |
| 1959 | Arnoulf | Nonselective coronary angiogram with cardiac arrest using acetylcholine | |
| 1959 | Dotter | Nonselective coronary angiogram with aortic occlusive balloon | |
| 1959 | Sones | First Sones catheter | |
| 1962 | Ricketts | Percutaneous femoral coronary angiography | |

(continued)

**Table 15.4** (continued)

| Year | Author | Catheterization/angiography | Imaging |
|---|---|---|---|
| 1963 | Hanafee | Axillary approach | |
| 1964 | Dotter | First peripheral angioplasty in a human patient | |
| 1967 | Sones | First selective angiogram of a saphenous bypass graft | Cineangiograms |
| 1973 | Portsmann | Balloon in cage | |
| 1974 | Bertrand | Radial approach by arteriotomy | |
| 1974 | Gruentzig and Hopff | First balloon | |
| 1977 (May) | Gruentzig and Myler | First coronary angioplasties in the operating room | |
| 1977 (September) | Gruentzig | First coronary balloon angioplasty in a human patient | |
| 1981 | Fergusson and Kamada | Percutaneous brachial approach | |
| | | | Cranial/caudal views |
| | | | Digital lab |
| 1989 | Campeau | First series of radial coronary angiography published | |

## References


1. Forssmann W (1929) Die Sonderung des rechten Herzens. Klin Wschr, 8
2. Splittgerber F, Harken DE (1991) Catheterization of the right heart by Werner Forssmann. Cardiac Chronicle 4:13–15
3. Warren JV (1980) Fifty years of invasive cardiology: Werner Forssmann (1904–1979) and his unusual success story. Am J Med 69:10–12
4. Richards LS, Thal AP (1958) Phasic dye injection control system for coronary arteriography in the human. Surg Ginec Obst 107:739
5. Urschel HC Jr, Roth EJ (1959) Electronically controlled coronary arteriography. Ann Surg 150(2):275–289
6. Arnulf G (1959) Methodical arteriography of the coronary vessels using acetylcholine. Arch Mal Coeur Vaiss 52:1121–1139
7. Pinet F, Gravier J, Pinet A (1959) Nouvelle méthode d'aortographie. Semin Hop 35:1855–1860
8. Nordenstrom B (1960) Contrast examination of the cardiovascular system during increased intrabronchial pressure. Acta Radiol (Stockholm) Suppl 200:1–110
9. Gensini G (1963) Coronary angiography. Prog Cardiovasc Dis 6(2):155–188

10. Dotter C, Frische L (1958) Visualization of the coronary circulation by occlusion aortography: a practical method. Radiology 71:502–524
11. Cheng TO (2004) The cough that resuscitated Dr. Mason Sones's first patient undergoing selective coronary angiography. Cathet Cardiovasc Interv 63(3):398
12. Sones FM (1959) Coronary arteriography. In: 8th Annual Convention of the ACC, Philadelphia
13. Reboul H, Racine M (1933) La ventriculographie cardiaque expérimentale. Presse Med 41:763–767
14. Ross J Jr (1959) Transseptal left heart catheterization. a new method of left atrial puncture. Ann Surg 149:395–401
15. Ricketts HJ, Abrams HL (1962) Percutaneous selective coronary cine arteriography. JAMA 181:620–624
16. Farinas PL (1941) A new technique for the arteriographic examination of the abdominal aorta and its branches. Am J Roentgenol 45:641–645
46. Cournand A (1975) Cardiac catheterization. Development of the technique, its contribution to experimental medicine and its initial application in man. Almqvist and Wiksell, Uppsala
18. Seldinger SJ (1953) Catheter replacement of the needle in percutaneous arteriography, a new technique. Acta Radiol 39:368–376
19. Judkins MP (1967) Selective coronary arteriography. I. Percutaneous transfemoral technique. Radiology 89:815–824
20. Ferguson DJG, Kamada RO (1981) Percutaneous entry of the brachial artery for left heart catheterization using a sheath. Cathet Cardiovasc Diagn 7:111–114
21. Wiedner W, MacAlpin R, Hanafee W, Kattus A (1965) Percutaneous transaxillary selective coronary arteriography. Radiology 85:652–657
22. Hessel SJ, Adams DF, Abrams HL (1981) Complications of angiography. Radiology 138:273–281
23. Bertrand ME, Ketelers JY, Carré A, Ginestet A, Lemaire P, Warembourg H (1974) Une nouvelle voie d'abord pour l'exploration hemodynamique des cavités cardiaque gauche utilisant l'artère radial au dessous du plì du coude. Coeur Med Interne 13:345–346
24. Campeau L (1989) Percutaneous radial artery approach for coronary angiography. Cathet Cardiovasc Diagn 16:3–7
25. Brueck M, Bandorski D, Kramer W, Wieczorek M, Höltgen R, Tillmanns H (2009) A randomized comparison of transradial versus transfemoral approach for coronary angiography and angioplasty. JACC Cardiovasc Interv 2(11):1047–1054
26. Dotter CT, Judkins MP (1964) Transluminal treatment of arteriosclerotic obstruction: description of a new technique and a preliminary report of its application. Circulation 30:654–670
27. Portsmann W, Wierny L (1967) Intravasale Rekanalisation inoperabiler arterieller Obliterationen. Zentralbl Chir 92:1586–1589
28. Zeitler E, Muller R (1969) Erste Ergebnisse mit der Katheter-Rekanalisation nach Dotter bei arterieller Verschlusskrankheit. Fortschr Roentgenstr III:345–352
29. Van Andel GJ (1976) Percutaneous transluminal angioplasty: the Dotter procedure. Excerpta Medica, Amsterdam
30. Dow J, Hardwick C (1966) Transluminal arterial recanalization. Lancet I:73–74
31. Geddes LA, Geddes LE (1993) The catheter introducers. Mobium Press, Chicago
32. Portsmann W (1973) Ein neuer Korsett-Ballonkatheter zur transluminalen Rekanalisation nach Dotter unter besonderer Berucksichtigung von Obliterationen an den Beckenarterien. Radiol Diagn 14:239–244
33. Dotter CT (1974) Transluminal iliac artery dilatation. Nonsurgical catheter treatment of atheromatous narrowing. JAMA 230:117–124
34. Abele JE (1980) Balloon catheters and transluminal dilatation: technical considerations. Am J Radiol 135:901–906

35. Gruentzig AR, Myler RK, Hanna ES, Turina ML (1977) Coronary transluminal angioplasty (Abstr). Circulation 55:56–84
36. Douglas JS Jr (1998) Approaches to the patient with prior bypass surgery. In: Topol EJ (ed) Textbook of cardiovascular medicine. Lippincott-Raven, Philadelphia, pp 2101–2118
37. Simpson JB, Baim DS, Robert EW, Harrison DC (1982) A new catheter system for coronary angioplasty. Am J Cardiol 49:1216–1222
38. Kaltenbach M (1984) The long wire technique—a new technique for steerable balloon catheter dilatation of coronary artery stenosis. Eur Heart J 5:1004–1009
39. Bonzel T, Wollschlager H, Kasper W, Meinertz T, Just H (1987) The sliding rail system (monorail): description of a new technique for intravascular instrumentation and its application to coronary angioplasty. Z Kardiol 76 [Suppl 6]:119–122
40. Meier B (2006) The first coronary angioplasties in Zurich. In: Bertrand ME (ed) the evolution of cardiac catheterization and interventional cardiology. Iatric press, St. Albany
41. Bjork VO, Malmstrom G, Uggla LG (1953) Left auricular pressure management in man. Ann Surg 138:718–725
42. Facquet J, Lemoine LM, Alhomme P, Lefebvre J (1952) La mesure de la pression auriculaire gauche par la voie transbronchique. Arch Mal Coeur Vaiss 45:741–745
43. Hansen AT, Fabricius J, Pedersen A, Sandoe E (1953) Suprasternal puncture of the left atrium and great vessels: experience from 500 punctures. Am Heart J 63:443–450
44. Smith PW, Wilson CW, Cregg HA, Klassen KP (1954) Cardioangiography. J Thorac Surg 28:273–280
45. Brock R, Milstein BB, Ross DN (1956) Percutaneous left ventricular puncture in the assessment of aortic stenosis. Thorax 11:163–171
46. Ryan TJ (2002) The coronary angiogram and its seminal contribution to cardiovascular medicine over five decades. Circulation 106:752–756

# Right Cardiac Catheterization After the Advent of CPB

16

Achille Gaspardone and Giuilo G. Stefanini

*Memento audere semper.*
Gabriele D'Annunzio

**Abstract**

In 1968 Harold Jeremy Swan and William (Vilem) Ganz invented the pulmonary arterial catheter, which represented one of the most practical devices in cardiology when it became commercially available in 1970. Observing the functioning of sailing boats in calm water of the coast of Santa Monica, Swan realized the effectiveness of a spinnaker in contrast to only a main and jib sailing rigging. This idea was the theoretical basis for the application of a balloon at the tip of a vascular catheter to navigate in the calm waters of the venous circulation.

In 1968 Harold Jeremy Swan and William (Vilem) Ganz invented the pulmonary arterial catheter, which represented one of the most practically used devices in cardiology when it became commercially available in 1970 (Fig. 16.1). Observing the functioning of sailing boats in calm water of the coast of Santa Monica, Swan observed the effectiveness of a spinnaker in contrast to only a main and jib sailing rigging. This observation was the theoretical basis for the application of a balloon at the tip of a vascular catheter to navigate in the calm waters of the venous circulation [1]. Later Ganz added the thermistor, a temperature probe located 3 cm behind the catheter tip, to measure cardiac output by the thermodilution technique. Within a few years a number of changes had been applied to the catheter, in order to allow calculation of oxygen consumption, shunt calculation in congenital heart diseases, right atrial, right ventricular, pulmonary artery and wedge pressures, right atrial and

A. Gaspardone (✉) · G. G. Stefanini
Department of Medicine, Division of Cardiology, Ospedale S Eugenio, Rome, Italy
e-mail: a_gaspardone@yahoo.com

M. Picichè (ed.), *Dawn and Evolution of Cardiac Procedures*,
DOI: 10.1007/978-88-470-2400-7_16, © Springer-Verlag Italia 2013

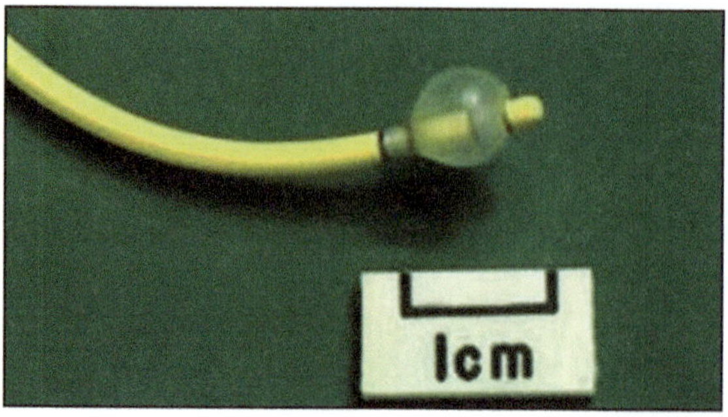


**Fig. 16.1** The pulmonary artery flow-directed balloon catheter: the Swan–Ganz catheter

ventricular pacing, and administration of drugs through the inner infusion lumen [2–18]. Initially introduced into clinical practice without substantial supporting evidence, recent retrospective studies and randomized controlled trials have not shown any positive benefit with the use of this catheter [2, 9–14]. Ramsey and co-authors investigated the role of the pulmonary artery catheter in a retrospective cohort study from 56 community-based hospitals in the USA [14]. A total of 13,907 patients undergoing non-urgent coronary surgical revascularization were reviewed in order to assess the impact of pulmonary artery catheters on in-hospital mortality, length of stay in the intensive care unit, total length of stay, and hospital costs. Around 58 % of the reviewed patients received a pulmonary artery catheter during the hospitalization. After adjustment for baseline clinical characteristics, hospital size and number of pulmonary artery catheters used in the year of interest, patients receiving a pulmonary artery catheter compared with patients who did not receive a pulmonary artery catheter were at higher risk of in-hospital mortality (RR 2.10; 95 % confidence interval, 1.40–3.14; $P < 0.001$). The authors concluded that the use of pulmonary artery catheterization for patients undergoing non-urgent myocardial surgical revascularization was associated with an increased risk of in-hospital mortality, a longer hospital stay, and higher total costs [14]. Notwithstanding, a prospective, randomized, controlled trial [11] showed no significant difference in mortality between patients managed with a pulmonary artery catheter compared with those patients managed without a pulmonary artery catheter. Moreover, further evidence from a randomized controlled trial supported these findings, showing no significant differences in mortality with or without the pulmonary artery catheter at day 14 [10]. In a pooled analysis of two large randomized clinical trials, pulmonary artery catheterization was associated with increased mortality, with the exception of patients in cardiogenic shock [18].

In 2005, Harvey and colleagues conducted a randomized controlled trial in 1,041 patients in intensive care, finding no difference in hospital mortality between critically ill patients managed with or without a pulmonary artery catheter [12]. Wheeler et al. [13] investigated the hemodynamic management guided by either pulmonary artery catheterization or central venous catheterization among patients with acute lung injury. The authors reported that treatment guided by the pulmonary artery catheter did not improve the outcomes of patients presenting with shock, suggesting that the pulmonary artery catheter should not be routinely used in the management of acute lung injury.

This evidence has called into question the role of the pulmonary artery catheter [15]. Recently, Leibowitz stated that cardiac filling pressures do not correlate with accepted standards of intravascular volume determination and left ventricular filling compared with echocardiographic findings, leaving the intensivist in "an intellectual bind" [16]. Benjamin and colleagues reported that pressure measurements performed by echocardiography and the pulmonary artery catheter disagreed in 55 % of comparative examinations among patients in the intensive care setting [17]. Indeed trans-esophageal echocardiography has been suggested as an alternative method; however, several authors pointed out that this latter technique is limited in its use owing to intermittent assessments and that it necessitates the use of skilled operators [15]. Inaccurate measurements and interpretation of the data continue to represent a major problem, leading to inappropriate and potentially harmful interventions. Moreover, central venous catheterization is certainly still required as it is necessary to facilitate administration of fluids, drugs, and parenteral nutrition [13]. Several authors have also suggested that still no conclusion can be drawn on the role of the pulmonary artery catheter in critically ill patients, since the findings of the available studies should be cautiously interpreted and eventually used for the development of more effective treatment strategies [1, 17].

Finally, pulmonary artery catheterization still maintains a crucial role for the differential diagnosis of pulmonary artery hypertension, as no other test can provide such an accurate diagnosis of precapillary, post-capillary, or mixed hemodynamic types of pulmonary arterial hypertension [12].

In conclusion, right heart catheterization continues to be the gold standard in diagnosing patients with elevated right heart pressures, although this technique has complications. The development of noninvasive techniques has progressed; however, prospective clinical trials are lacking. Right heart catheterization is indicated only in patients with complex medical problems or in those patients in whom important hemodynamic measures are only obtainable with its use. It is important to note that the use of the pulmonary artery catheter is a monitoring procedure and not a treatment. When viewed in this context, the pulmonary artery catheter provides the clinician with the advantage of continuous hemodynamic monitoring that could assist the trained health care professional in the application of therapeutic treatments before the development of symptomatic decompensation.

## References


1. Berry D (2011) William (Vilem) Ganz, 1919–2009, cardiologist and co-inventor of the Swan-Ganz catheter which revolutionized cardiovascular investigations. Eur Heart J 32(6): 655–664
2. Chatterjee K (2009) The Swan-Ganz catheters: past, present, and future. A viewpoint. Circulation 119:147–152

3. Savage AP, Picard M, Hopkins CC et al (1993) Complications and survival of multilumen central venous catheters used for total parenteral nutrition. Br J Surg 80:1287–1290
4. Marini JJ (1986) Acute lung injury. Hemodynamic monitoring with the pulmonary artery catheter. Crit Care Clin 2:551–572
5. Moser KM, Spragg RG (1983) Use of the balloon-tipped pulmonary artery catheter in pulmonary disease. Ann Intern Med 98:53–58
6. Aikawa N, Martyn JA, Burke JF (1978) Pulmonary artery catheterization and thermodilution cardiac output determination in the management of critically burned patients. Am J Surg 135:811–817
7. Gilbertson AA (1974) Pulmonary artery catheterization and wedge pressure measurement in the general intensive therapy unit. Br J Anaesth 46:97–104
8. Liggett SB, St John RE, Lefrak SS (1987) Determination of resting energy expenditure utilizing the thermodilution pulmonary artery catheter. Chest 91:562–566
9. Cohen MG, Kelly RV, Kong DF et al (2005) Pulmonary artery catheterization in acute coronary syndromes: insights from the GUSTO IIb and GUSTO III trials. Am J Med 118:482–488
10. Richard C, Warszawski J, Anguel N et al (2003) Early use of the pulmonary artery catheter and outcomes in patients with shock and acute respiratory distress syndrome: a randomized controlled trial. JAMA 290:2713–2720
11. Rhodes A, Cusack RJ, Newman PJ et al (2002) A randomised, controlled trial of the pulmonary artery catheter in critically ill patients. Intensive Care Med 28:256–264
12. Harvey S, Harrison DA, Singer M et al (2005) Assessment of the clinical effectiveness of pulmonary artery catheters in management of patients in intensive care (PAC-Man): a randomised controlled trial. Lancet 366:472–477
13. Wheeler AP, Bernard GR, Thompson BT et al (2006) Pulmonary-artery versus central venous catheter to guide treatment of acute lung injury. N Engl J Med 354:2213–2224
14. Ramsey SD, Saint S, Sullivan SD et al (2000) Clinical and economic effects of pulmonary artery catheterization in nonemergent coronary artery bypass graft surgery. J Cardiothorac Vasc Anesth 14:113–118
15. Rubenfeld GD, McNamara-Aslin E, Rubinson L (2007) The pulmonary artery catheter, 1967–2007: rest in peace? JAMA 298:458–461
16. Leibowitz AB (2003) Who benefits from pulmonary artery catheterization? Crit Care Med 31:2805–2806
17. Benjamin E, Griffin K, Leibowitz AB et al (1998) Goal-directed transesophageal echocardiography performed by intensivists to assess left ventricular function: comparison with pulmonary artery catheterization. J Cardiothorac Vasc Anesth 12:10–15
18. Vincent JL, Pinsky MR, Sprung CL et al (2008) The pulmonary artery catheter: in medio virtus. Crit Care Med 36:3093–3096

# The History of Research on Coronary Stenting

# 17

Fabrizio Tomai and Leonardo De Luca

*Any sufficiently advanced technology is indistinguishable from magic*

Arthur C. Clarke

**Abstract**

There are few technical developments that have changed the face of interventional cardiology as much and as rapidly as the practice of the placement of intracoronary stents. The first stents were implanted in the coronary arteries of humans more than 20 years ago; since then, there have been significant developments in their technology, the most notable of which has been the introduction of drug-eluting stents. Nowadays, newer stents have been developed that are currently undergoing pre-clinical and clinical trials with promising early results.

In May 1977 Gruentzig and Myler performed the first coronary angioplasty during coronary artery bypass graft (CABG) surgery in San Francisco, and a few months later performed the first coronary angioplasty in an awake patient in Zurich, Switzerland [1]. In 1978, Gruentzig described the first series of percutaneous transluminal coronary angioplasty (PTCA), performed successfully in five patients [2]. The technique involved advancement of a balloon-tipped catheter into a narrowed coronary artery, inflation of the balloon to cause plaque compression, and removal of the catheter after balloon deflation. However, in the first 50 patients who underwent PTCA, the primary success rate was only 64 % and emergency CABG was required in 14 % [3]. As experience with PTCA grew, its success rate increased to approximately 90 % and emergency CABG decreased to 1 % respectively (Fig. 17.1).

F. Tomai (✉) · L. De Luca
Department of Cardiovascular Sciences, Interventional Cardiology Unit, European Hospital, Rome, Italy
e-mail: f.tomai@tiscali.it

L. De Luca
e-mail: leo.deluca@libero.it

M. Picichè (ed.), *Dawn and Evolution of Cardiac Procedures*, DOI: 10.1007/978-88-470-2400-7_17, 

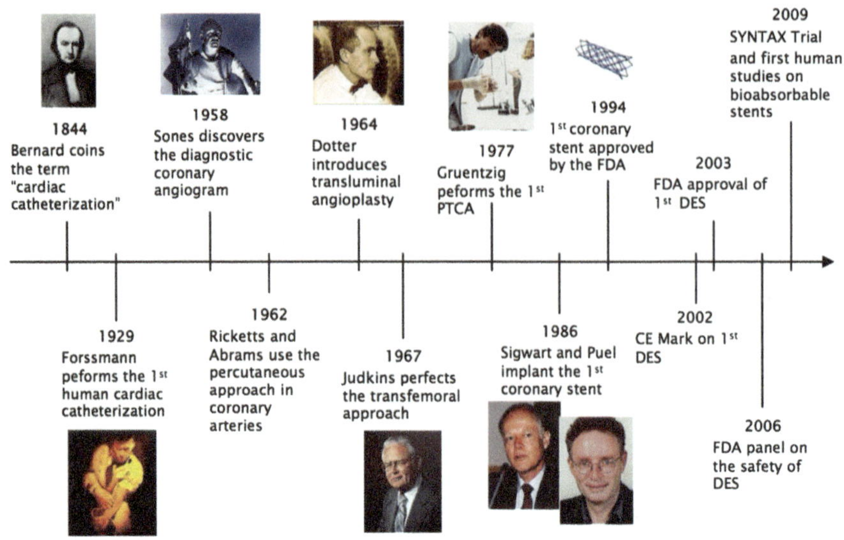


**Fig.17.1** Milestones in the history of percutaneous coronary intervention and development of coronary stents

## 17.1 The Development of Coronary Stents

The idea of using foreign bodies to maintain arterial luminal integrity was introduced by the Nobel laureate Alexis Carrel in 1912 when he described experiments in which paraffin-covered glass and metal tubes were implanted into canine thoracic aorta [4]. Dotter and Judkins reintroduced the concept of using an implantable prosthetic device to maintain the luminal diameter of diseased vessels in 1964 [5]. Years later, Rousseau et al. developed flexible, self-expanding, stainless-steel mesh tubes, which were implanted into canine coronary arteries [6]. In 1985, Palmaz et al. introduced the use of balloon-mounted stents in peripheral arteries [7]. Interest in stent implantation in human coronary arteries intensified after Schatz et al. reported the results of successful percutaneous implantation of stainless steel slotted tube coronary stents in canine coronary arteries [8]. With the hope that acute occlusion and restenosis could be alleviated, Jacques Puel in Toulouse, France, and Ulrich Sigwart in Lausanne, Switzerland, deployed the first human coronary stents after PTCA in 1986 [9]. Sigwart et al. also first described the use of this stent for arterial dissection. The stent, acting as a scaffold, optimized lumen integrity by tracking down dissection flaps against the vessel wall, and providing mechanical support to offset elastic recoil during PTCA [10]. In 1993, bare-metal stents (BMS) were approved in the United States to treat acute and threatened vessel closure after failed PTCA. Subsequent studies confirmed the efficacy of percutaneous coronary intervention (PCI), with stenting as an alternative to avoid emergency CABG surgery after failed PTCA [11].

In 1993, two landmark trials, the Belgium Netherlands Stent Arterial Revascularization Therapies Study (BENESTENT) [12] and the North American Stent Restenosis Study (STRESS) [13], confirmed that, compared with PTCA, coronary stenting significantly improved angiographic and clinical outcomes, thus establishing elective coronary stent implantation as an accepted standard of care. These studies also prompted the Food and Drug Administration (FDA) to approve BMS for elective use in the United States.

In 1997 a randomized, single-center study first demonstrated that in patients with symptomatic isolated stenosis of the proximal left anterior descending coronary artery, stenting had advantages over standard PTCA in that it was associated with both a lower rate of restenosis and a better clinical outcome [14]. By 1999, more than 80 % of all PCIs involved stent insertion.

Although BMS implantation effectively eliminated acute vessel closure, initial trials reported acute (<24 h) and subacute (24 h to 30 days) stent thrombosis (ST) rates of approximately 20 % [15]. Thrombosis had long been recognized as a serious complication of stent implantation in both animal and early clinical studies; aggressive anticoagulation attempts were implemented to prevent this. Two practices led to a dramatic reduction in the incidence of ST in BMS: first, the use of intravascular ultrasound and high balloon pressures to optimize apposition of the stent struts to the vessel wall, and second, the replacement of anticoagulation with dual-antiplatelet therapy. The combination of a thienopyridine with aspirin became the cornerstone of antithrombotic prophylaxis [16]. Their combined effects resulted in superior antithrombotic activity compared with conventional anticoagulation in initial studies and reduced the incidence of BMS thrombosis to the current rate of 1%.

## 17.2 Coronary Stents and Restenosis

Despite the advancements made with BMS implantation, they are still associated with a 20–25 % restenosis rate within 6 months of implantation [17]. Lesion complexities, comorbidities (diabetes, renal insufficiency) increase this incidence. Although initial stent placement prevents acute recoil, the stent struts traumatize the vascular wall provoking an inflammatory reaction followed by an exaggerated proliferative response within the media and adventitia, which produces greater neointimal formation compared with PTCA-induced restenosis [18]. In-stent restenosis incidence peaks at 3 months, reaches a plateau between 3 and 6 months, but can persist beyond 1 year after stent deployment [19]. Reintervention attempts to prevent in-stent restenosis have included PTCA, atherectomy, repeat stenting, drug-eluting balloons, laser, and brachytherapy (intracoronary delivery of a radioactive isotope). Brachytherapy increases stent margin restenosis and delays endothelialization, leading to a 15 % stent thrombotic occlusion rate, with an overall failure rate of 30 %. Adding pharmacological therapies, such as prednisone at immunosuppressive doses has also shown remarkable long-term efficacy in reducing ischemic recurrences in nondiabetic patients with a marked inflammatory response after stenting [20].

**Table 17.1** Summary of major randomized clinical trials of SES or PES versus BMS in different clinical settings

| Study | Publication | Number of patients | Clinical and procedural setting | Binary in-stent restenosis (DES vs BMS), % | MACE (DES vs BMS), % | TLR (DES vs BMS), % |
|---|---|---|---|---|---|---|
| RAVEL | N Engl J Med 2002;346:1773–80 | SES ($n$ = 120) vs BMS ($n$ = 118) | Elective simple lesions | 0.0 vs 26.6 | 5.8 vs 28.8 | 0.0 vs 23.7 |
| C-SIRIUS | J Am Coll Cardiol 2004;43:1110–5 | SES ($n$ = 50) vs BMS ($n$ = 50) | Elective lesions | 0.0 vs 45.5 | 4.0 vs 18.0 | 4.0 vs 18.0[a] |
| E-SIRIUS | Lancet 2003;362:1093–9 | SES ($n$ = 175) vs BMS ($n$ = 177) | Elective long lesions, small vessels, overlapped stents | 3.9 vs 41.7 | 8.0 vs 22.6 | 4.0 vs 20.9 |
| SIRIUS | N Engl J Med 2003;349:1315–23 | SES ($n$ = 163) vs BMS ($n$ = 159) | Elective lesions | 3.2 vs 35.4 | 8.3 vs 23.2 | 4.9 vs 20.2[a] |
| MISSION! | J Am Coll Cardiol 2008;51:618–26 | SES ($n$ = 158) vs BMS ($n$ = 152) | STEMI | 2.3 vs 22.6 | NA | 3.2 vs 11.2 |
| SESAMI | J Am Coll Cardiol 2007;49:1924–30 | SES ($n$ = 160) vs BMS ($n$ = 160) | STEMI | 9.3 vs 21.3 | 6.8 vs 16.8 | 4.3 vs 11.2[a] |
| STRATEGY | JAMA 2005;293:2109–17 | SES ($n$ = 87) vs BMS ($n$ = 88) | STEMI | 7.5 vs 28 | 18.4 vs 31.8 | 5.7 vs 20.5 |
| TYPHOON | N Engl J Med 2006;355:1093–104 | SES ($n$ = 355) vs BMS ($n$ = 357) | STEMI | 3.5 vs 20.3 | 5.9 vs 14.6 | 5.6 vs 13.4[a] |
| SCANDSTENT | J Am Coll Cardiol 2006;47:449–55 | SES ($n$ = 163) vs BMS ($v$ = 159) | Complex CAD | 2.0 vs 30.6 | 4.3 vs 29.9 | 2.5 vs 29.3[a] |

(continued)

**Table 17.1** (continued)

| Study | Publication | Number of patients | Clinical and procedural setting | Binary in-stent restenosis (DES vs BMS), % | MACE (DES vs BMS), % | TLR (DES vs BMS), % |
|---|---|---|---|---|---|---|
| TAXUS-I | Circulation 2003;107:38–42 | PES ($n = 31$) vs BMS ($n = 30$) | Simple lesions | 0.0 vs 10.4 | 3.3 vs 10.0 | 0.0 vs 10.0 |
| TAXUS-II Slow release | Circulation 2003;108:788–94 | PES ($n = 131$) vs BMS ($n = 136$) | Simple lesions | 2.3 vs 17.9 | 10.9 vs 22.0 | 4.7 vs 12.9 |
| TAXUS-II Moderate release | Circulation 2003;108:788–94 | PES ($n = 135$) vs BMS ($n = 134$) | Simple lesions | 4.7 vs 20.2 | 9.9 vs 21.4 | 3.8 vs 16.0 |
| TAXUS-IV | N Engl J Med 2004;350:221–31 | PES ($n = 662$) vs BMS ($n = 652$) | Simple lesions | 5.5 vs 24.4 | 8.5 vs 15.0 | 3.0 vs 11.3[a] |
| TAXUS-V | JAMA 2005;294:121–23 | PES ($n = 577$) vs BMS ($n = 579$) | Complex lesions | 13.7 vs 31.9 | 15.0 vs 21.2 | 8.6 vs 15.7[a] |
| TAXUS-VI | Circulation 2005;112:3306–13 | PES ($n = 219$) vs BMS ($n = 227$) | Long complex lesions | 9.1 vs 32.9 | 16.4 vs 22.5 | 6.8 vs 18.9 |
| HORIZONS-AMI | N Engl J Med 2009;360:1946–59 | PES ($n = 2{,}257$) vs BMS ($n = 749$) | STEMI | 8.2 vs 21.0 | 8.0 vs 7.9 | 4.3 vs 7.2[a] |

*BMS* bare-metal stent(s), *MACE* major adverse cardiovascular events (a composite of death, myocardial infarction, and target lesion revascularization), *NA* not available, *PES* paclitaxel-eluting stent(s), *SES* sirolimus-eluting stent(s), *STEMI* ST-segment elevation myocardial infarction, *TLR* target lesion revascularization

[a] Ischemia-driven

Several changes in design and structure of BMSs performed since their introduction significantly improved their trackability, flexibility and crossability so that technical success is at present around 99 %. For instance, an alternative to the stainless steel that constitutes initial coronary stents is cobalt chromium (CoCr), which exhibits superior radial strength and improved radio-opacity, allowing for thinner stent struts (less than 100 μm). CoCr stents have been shown to be associated with a favorable impact on restenosis rate, which, however, has been dramatically reduced only with the advent of drug-eluting stents (DES).

## 17.3 The Advent of DES

Drug-eluting stents were developed to prevent neointimal hyperplasia (medial hyperproliferation) and consequent restenosis, while preserving vessel architecture compromised by PTCA. By coating a BMS with a polymer containing antiproliferative material that inhibits neointimal hyperplasia, cardiologists hoped that these devices would eliminate restenosis and the need for reintervention. The first-generation DES locally release either sirolimus or paclitaxel from a nonresorbable polymer. Both agents effectively inhibit vascular smooth cell migration and proliferation, although by different intracellular mechanisms [21].

In the United States, the FDA granted expedited review of both DES, and approved sirolimus-eluting stents (Cypher®, Cordis Corporation) for use in April 2003, while paclitaxel-eluting stents (Taxus®, Boston Scientific) were approved in March 2004. Initial approval was based on the results of randomized controlled trials with carefully selected patient populations (Table 17.1). These trials demonstrated the superior ability of both sirolimus-DES and paclitaxel-DES to reduce neointimal hyperplasia, restenosis, and reintervention compared with BMS, reaching a binary restenosis rate of 8 % and target lesion revascularization of 6 % at 1 year [22–24]. Both types of DES have shown continued efficacy in preventing restenosis when studied 4 years after initial deployment [25, 26]. Although a meta-analysis of randomized trials comparing paclitaxel-DES with sirolimus-DES revealed significantly higher restenosis rates with the former ($P = 0.001$), clinical outcomes (death and MI) were similar in both groups [27].

In 2005, at the height of clinical enthusiasm, 85 % of all stents implanted in the United States and Europe were DES.

## 17.4 Risks and Complications with Des

In recent years, several patient-based meta-analyses were performed that reassuringly demonstrated the overall comparable outcomes between DES and BMS in terms of death and MI, at both short- and long-term follow-up [26, 28–30]. The largest of these studies, by Stettler et al. [30], reported a similar risk of death for patients treated with SES, PES, or BMS.

### 17.4.1 Off-Label Indications

The current on-label indications for DES use, as approved by the US FDA are limited to simple lesions: for SES, de novo lesions $\leq$30 mm in length in native coronary arteries with reference vessel diameters of 2.5–3.5 mm, and for PES de novo lesions $\leq$28 mm in native coronary arteries 2.5–3.75 mm in diameter. It follows that off-label indications represent a higher-risk population with more complex lesion morphologies and unstable clinical presentations.

Numerous observational studies demonstrated that the use DES for off-label indications was associated with poorer clinical outcomes in terms of death, MI, and repeat revascularization compared with DES use for on-label indications [31].

### 17.4.2 Stent Thrombosis

Interest from the scientific community as well as regulatory agencies and the public is now focused on ST because of the associated incidences of death ($\sim$20 to 40 %), myocardial infarction ($\sim$50 to 70 %) and repeat revascularization. The pathophysiology of ST includes stent-, procedure-, and patient-related factors and can occur with either BMS or DES [32]. Early events may be related to residual target lesion thrombus or dissection, stasis, stent underexpansion, or a combination of these. Following DES deployment, late incomplete stent apposition demonstrated by intravascular ultrasound, due to the gradual dissolution of thrombus or positive arterial remodeling, has not been convincingly linked to adverse outcomes [33]. Late ST may be more frequently related to incomplete healing and/or inadequate neointimal coverage [34]. Although a correlation has been observed between uncovered DES struts and ST, endoluminal mural thrombus may be present despite neointimal coverage and may reflect underlying inflammation related to the drug-delivery polymer.

At present ST after DES implantation amounts to around 0.5 % per year, an incidence similar to that observed with BMS [35].

### 17.4.3 Stent Fracture

Since the introduction of DES, stent fractures have also been reported in small studies and case reports. The reported rate of DES fracture in coronary arteries ranges from 1 to 8 %, although much of the available literature is derived from single-center studies that are heterogeneous in their study methods [36]. A higher risk of stent fracture may be associated with the right coronary artery location, excessive tortuosity or angulation of the vessel, overlapping stents, and longer stents. The closed-cell design of the Cypher stent has been associated with increased rigidity that may increase the risk of stent fracture. Stent fracture has been shown by most studies to be associated with a statistically increased incidence of focal in-stent restenosis, and some have shown an increased risk of target lesion revascularization. Other complications observed with stent fracture include stent thrombosis, coronary aneurysms, myocardial infarction, and sudden death.

### 17.4.4 Coronary Artery Aneurysms

Coronary artery aneurysms are a rare complication of stenting, whose true incidence, clinical course, and treatment are largely unknown. Nevertheless, studies report an incidence between 0.3 and 6.0 % after DES and BMS implantation respectively [37]. There are a number of postulated causes for these coronary artery aneurysms, some of which are specific for DES. In general, mechanical causes include the use of oversized balloons or stents, high-pressure balloon inflations, and atherectomy—all of which can cause residual dissection and deep arterial wall injury eventually leading to aneurysm formation. Of note for DES, the elution of antiproliferative drugs and/or the presence of a polymer can lead to delayed re-endothelialization, inflammatory changes in the medial wall, and hypersensitivity reactions, all of which can result in coronary artery aneurysm formation. Coronary artery aneurysms can be associated with restenosis, whereas turbulent and sluggish blood flow in the area of the aneurysm, coupled with a metallic stent, can predispose patients to the risk of ST and/or distal embolization [38].

## 17.5 New Stents and Future Directions

### 17.5.1 New Generation DES

The new generation DES utilize CoCr, and elute drugs with the aid of more biostatic and biocompatible polymers than are found on the first-generation DESs.

The new generation DES with the largest amount of scientific evidence are the zotarolimus-eluting stent (ZES) and the everolimus-eluting stent (EES).

The Endeavor stent (Medtronic Inc., Minnesota, USA) has a polymer that releases zotarolimus, a sirolimus analog, within 14 days of stent deployment, and causes less inflammation compared with the polymer on the Cypher SES stent. Indeed, compared with first-generation DES, data have indicated a relatively poorer performance of ZES at short-term follow-up, as indicated by significantly higher late loss and numerically greater TLR [39]. However, longer follow-up has shown significant reductions in the absolute difference in TLR between ZES and SES/PES [40].

The Xience V stent (Abbott Vascular, Santa Clara, CA, USA) consists of the Multilink Vision CoCr platform with a biocompatible polymer eluting everolimus, a synthetic derivative of sirolimus. Clinical data consist of both real-world registries, and randomized trials comparing EES with BMS and PES [41]. Results have consistently demonstrated the safety and efficacy of the EES, together with low rates of ST out to long-term follow-up [42]. The Xience PRIME EES, which represents the latest development of the Xience V stent, has a CoCr platform with a new enhanced stent delivery system that enables the stent to be more flexible and deliverable.

### 17.5.2 Bifurcation Stents

Dedicated bifurcation stents are an exciting technology as they are an attempt to find specific technological solutions to a specific subset of coronary lesions. However, the first-generation bifurcation stents, tested in clinical studies and multicenter registries only [43], did not achieve a high device success rate and resulted in restenosis rates ranging from 30 to 55 %. Second-generation drug-eluting devices have only recently been introduced [44]. In this regard, the Axxess Plus biolimus-eluting stent demonstrated a favorable rate of restenosis for the main branch and side branch, although most patients required at least one other stent implanted in the bifurcation [44]. A number of first-in-man studies and multicenter registries are ongoing and the results are eagerly awaited to establish if these new devices will become a good alternative to current bifurcation strategies in different bifurcation scenarios.

### 17.5.3 Stents with Novel Coatings

Innovative coronary stents with a modified coating with anti-inflammatory, bacteria-resistant, or anti-platelet aggregation and pro-healing qualities, are currently under evaluation in pre-clinical studies and small first-in-man clinical trials. However, their potential efficacy in reducing ST and restenosis needs to be confirmed in large clinical studies with longer periods of follow-up [45].

Other attractive solutions for reducing ST and restenosis are coronary stents with highly biocompatible coating and a drug release system based on the use of reservoirs on the stent's outer surface to ensure a targeted drug release toward the vessel wall.

### 17.5.4 DES Without Durable Polymer

In an effort to address concerns related to DES, such as long-term safety, with particular reference to stent thrombosis, newer stents have been developed that include: DES that are polymer-free and DES with biodegradable polymers. Interest has focused on these stents because initially after implantation, they may theoretically offer the antirestenotic benefits of a standard DES, whereas once the polymer has biodegraded, they speculatively may offer the safety profile of a BMS. The safety and efficacy of BioMatrix Flex (Biosensors Int., CA, USA), a biolimus-eluting stent system with abluminal biodegradable polymer has been demonstrated in the LEADERS (Limus Eluted from A Durable versus ERodible Stent coating), a multi-center randomized study in which 1,707 patients eligible for PCI received either the BioMatrix Flex or the Cypher Select stent [46]. At 3 years' follow-up there was a nonsignificant trend toward a lower rate of major adverse cardiac events in patients treated with the BioMatrix Flex stent compared with those treated with the Cypher Select stent, especially in patients with ST-elevation MI, complex coronary disease, and multivessel disease. Presently, the ISAR-TEST 3 (Intracoronary Stenting and Angiographic Restenosis Investigators–Test Efficacy of Rapamycin-Eluting Stents With Different Polymer Coating Strategies) represents the only comparison of three stents with different types of polymer and the same antiproliferative drug [47]. This noninferiority study randomized 605 patients to rapamycin-eluting stents with a durable polymer, a biodegradable polymer, or a stent that was polymer-free. At the 6- to 8-month angiographic follow-up, the biodegradable polymer stent met its pre-specified criterion for noninferiority in terms of in-stent late lumen loss, whereas the polymer-free stent failed to achieve noninferiority.

Fully biodegradable stents (BDS) offer several potential advantages over conventional bare or drug-coated metallic stents [48]. These include potential reductions in adverse events such as ST, because drug elution and vessel scaffolding are only provided by the stent until the vessel has healed, and as such, no triggers for ST, such as non-endothelialized stent struts, or drug polymers are present long term. The absence of these foreign materials may also reduce the requirements for long-term DAPT, reducing the risk of associated bleeding complications and making further stent implantation easier, avoiding stent-in-stent implantation or complex by-pass grafting. The safety and feasibility of the first-generation BDS implant was assessed in 30 low-risk patients with de novo coronary lesions who were enrolled in the prospective, open-label, multicenter ABSORB (a bioresorbable everolimus-eluting coronary stent system for Patients With Single De Novo Coronary Artery Lesion) study [49]. The study demonstrated the clinical safety of the BDS as there was only one ischemia-driven major adverse event (non-Q-wave MI) at 6 months, whereas no major adverse clinical events were reported in the following 30 months. Of note, no ST has been observed at up to 3 years' follow-up. Ongoing experimental studies will clarify whether BDS might be superior in terms of safety and efficacy to current new-generation DES.

## 17.6 Conclusions

Coronary stents, which were first developed in the mid-1980s, revolutionized the practice of interventional cardiology. The introduction of DES led to significant reductions in restenosis rates and improved outcomes, also expanding indications for PCI in patients with complex coronary artery disease. The persisting concerns over ST have led to improvements in stent design and technology. It is clear that no single stent design and polymer type will be suitable for all patients and lesion types. Therefore, a more individualized choice of stent, taking into account patient and lesion characteristics will be important factors influencing stent selection in the future.

## References


1. Mueller RL, Sanborn TA (1995) The history of interventional cardiology: cardiac catheterization, angioplasty, and related interventions. Am Heart J 129:146–172
2. Gruntzig A (1978) Transluminal dilatation of coronary-artery stenosis. Lancet 1:263
3. Gruntzig AR, Senning A, Siegenthaler WE (1979) Nonoperative dilatation of coronary-artery stenosis: percutaneous transluminal coronary angioplasty. N Engl J Med 301:61–68
4. Nobel's Lectures (1967) Physiology or Medicine 1901–1921. Elsevier Publishing Company, Amsterdam
5. Dotter CT, Judkins MP (1964) Transluminal treatment of arteriosclerotic obstruction. Description of a new technique and a preliminary report of its application. Circulation 30:654–670
6. Rousseau H, Puel J, Joffre F et al (1987) Self-expanding endovascular prosthesis: an experimental study. Radiology 164:709–714
7. Palmaz JC, Sibbitt RR, Reuter SR et al (1985) Expandable intraluminal graft: a preliminary study. Work in progress. Radiology 156:73–77
8. Schatz RA, Palmaz JC, Tio FO et al (1987) Balloon-expandable intracoronary stents in the adult dog. Circulation 76:450–457
9. Sigwart U, Puel J, Mirkovitch V et al (1987) Intravascular stents to prevent occlusion and restenosis after transluminal angioplasty. N Engl J Med 316:701–706
10. De Feyter PJ, de Jaegere PP, Serruys PW (1994) Incidence, predictors, and management of acute coronary occlusion after coronary angioplasty. Am Heart J 127:643–651
11. Roubin GS, Cannon AD, Agrawal SK et al (1992) Intracoronary stenting for acute and threatened closure complicating percutaneous transluminal coronary angioplasty. Circulation 85:916–927
12. Serruys PW, de Jaegere P, Kiemeneij F, The Benestent Study Group et al (1994) A comparison of balloon-expandable-stent implantation with balloon angioplasty in patients with coronary artery disease. Benestent Study Group. N Engl J Med 331:489–495
13. Fischman DL, Leon MB, Baim DS, The stent restenosis study investigators et al (1994) A randomized comparison of coronary-stent placement and balloon angioplasty in the treatment of coronary artery disease. Stent restenosis study investigators. N Engl J Med 331:496–501
14. Versaci F, Gaspardone A, Tomai F et al (1997) A comparison of coronary-artery stenting with angioplasty for isolated stenosis of the proximal left anterior descending coronary artery. N Engl J Med 336:817–822
15. Serruys PW, Strauss BH, Beatt KJ et al (1991) Angiographic follow-up after placement of a self-expanding coronary-artery stent. N Engl J Med 324:13–17
16. Schomig A, Neumann FJ, Kastrati A et al (1996) A randomized comparison of antiplatelet and anticoagulant therapy after the placement of coronary artery stents. N Engl J Med 334:1084–1089
17. Moliterno DJ (2005) Healing Achilles–sirolimus versus paclitaxel. N Engl J Med 353:724–727
18. Hoffmann R, Mintz GS (2000) Coronary in-stent restenosis—predictors, treatment and prevention. Eur Heart J 21:1739–1749
19. Hirshfeld JW Jr, Schwartz JS, Jugo R, The M-heart investigators et al (1991) Restenosis after coronary angioplasty: a multivariate statistical model to relate lesion and procedure variables to restenosis. The M-heart investigators. J Am Coll Cardiol 18:647–656
20. Ribichini F, Tomai F, De Luca G et al (2011) CEREA-DES investigators. Immunosuppressive therapy with oral prednisone to prevent restenosis after PCI. A multicenter randomized trial. Am J Med 124:434–43
21. Woods TC, Marks AR (2004) Drug-eluting stents. Annu Rev Med 55:169–178
22. Dangas GD, Claessen BE, Caixeta A et al (2010) In-stent restenosis in the drug-eluting stent era. J Am Coll Cardiol 56:1897–1907
23. Tomai F, Petrolini A, De Luca L et al (2010) Rationale and design of the randomized comparison of XiEnce V and Multilink VisioN coronary stents in the sAme muLtivessel patient with chronic kidney disease (RENAL-DES) study. J Cardiovasc Med 11:310–317

24. Tomai F, Reimers B, De Luca L et al (2008) Head-to-head comparison of sirolimus- and paclitaxel-eluting stent in the same diabetic patient with multiple coronary artery lesions: a prospective, randomized, multicenter study. Diabetes Care 31:15–19
25. Hill RA, Dundar Y, Bakhai A et al (2004) Drug eluting stents: an early systematic review to inform policy. Eur Heart J 25:902–919
26. Stone GW, Moses JW, Ellis SG et al (2007) Safety and efficacy of sirolimus- and paclitaxel eluting coronary stents. N Engl J Med 356:998–1008
27. Kastrati A, Dibra A, Eberle S et al (2005) Sirolimus-eluting stents vs paclitaxel eluting stents in patients with coronary artery disease: meta-analysis of randomized trials. JAMA 294:819–825
28. Kastrati A, Mehilli J, Pache J et al (2007) Analysis of 14 trials comparing sirolimus-eluting stents with bare-metal stents. N Engl J Med 356:1030–1039
29. Kirtane AJ, Gupta A, Iyengar S et al (2009) Safety and efficacy of drug-eluting and bare metal stents: comprehensive meta-analysis of randomized trials and observational studies. Circulation 119:3198–3206
30. Stettler C, Wandel S, Allemann S et al (2007) Outcomes associated with drug-eluting and bare-metal stents: a collaborative network meta-analysis. Lancet 370:937–948
31. Win HK, Caldera AE, Maresh K et al (2007) Clinical outcomes and stent thrombosis following off-label use of drug-eluting stents. JAMA 297:2001–2009
32. Iakovou I, Schmidt T, Bonizzoni E et al (2005) Incidence, predictors, and outcome of thrombosis after successful implantation of drug-eluting stents. JAMA 293:2126–2130
33. Serruys PW, Daemen J (2007) Are drug-eluting stents associated with a higher rate of late thrombosis than bare metal stents? Late stent thrombosis: a nuisance in both bare metal and drug-eluting stents. Circulation 115:1433–1439
34. Kuchulakanti PK, Chu WW, Torguson R et al (2006) Correlates and long-term outcomes of angiographically proven stent thrombosis with sirolimus- and paclitaxel-eluting stents. Circulation 113:1108–1113
35. Roukoz H, Bavry AA, Sarkees ML et al (2009) Comprehensive meta-analysis on drug-eluting stents versus bare-metal stents during extended follow-up. Am J Med 122(581):e1–e10
36. Nakazawa G, Finn AV, Vorpahl M et al (2009) Incidence and predictors of drug-eluting stent fracture in human coronary artery a pathologic analysis. J Am Coll Cardiol 54:1924–1931
37. Aoki J, Kirtane A, Leon MB et al (2008) Coronary artery aneurysms after drug-eluting stent implantation. J Am Coll Cardiol Intv 1:14–21
38. Alfonso F, Perez-Vizcayno MJ, Ruiz M et al (2009) Coronary aneurysms after drug-eluting stent implantation: clinical, angiographic, and intravascular ultrasound findings. J Am Coll Cardiol 53:2053–2060
39. Eisenstein EL, Leon MB, Kandzari DE et al (2009) Long-term clinical and economic analysis of the endeavor zotarolimus-eluting stent versus the cypher sirolimus-eluting stent 3 year results from the ENDEAVOR III trial (randomized controlled trial of the Medtronic Endeavor drug [ABT-578] eluting coronary stent system versus the cypher sirolimus-eluting coronary stent system in de novo native coronary artery lesions). J Am Coll Cardiol Intv 2:1199–1207
40. Leon MB, Mauri L, Popma JJ et al (2010) A randomised comparison of the endeavor zotarolimus-eluting stent versus the TAXUS paclitaxel eluting stent in de novo native coronary lesions: 12 month outcomes from the ENDEAVOR IV trial. J Am Coll Cardiol 55:543–554
41. Stone GW, Midei M, Newman W et al (2008) Comparison of an everolimus-eluting stent and a paclitaxel-eluting stent in patients with coronary artery disease: a randomized trial. JAMA 299:1903–1913
42. Kedhi E, Joesoef KS, McFadden E et al (2010) Second-generation everolimus-eluting and paclitaxel-eluting stents in real-life practice (COMPARE): a randomised trial. Lancet 375:201–209
43. Latib A, Colombo A, Sangiorgi SM (2009) Bifurcation stenting: current strategies and new devices. Heart 95:495–504
44. Verheye S, Agostoni P, Dubois CL et al (2009) 9 month clinical, angiographic, and intravascular ultrasound results of a prospective evaluation of the Axxess self-expanding

biolimus A9-eluting stent in coronary bifurcation lesions: the DIVERGE (Drug-eluting stent intervention for treating side branches effectively) study. J Am Coll Cardiol 53:1031–1039
45. Garg S, Serruys PW (2010) Coronary stents: looking forward. J Am Coll Cardiol 56:S43–S78
46. Windecker S, Serruys PW, Wandel S et al (2008) Biolimus-eluting stent with biodegradable polymer versus sirolimus-eluting stent with durable polymer for coronary revascularisation (LEADERS): a randomized non-inferiority trial. Lancet 372:1163–1173
47. Byrne RA, Kufner S, Tiroch K et al (2009) Randomised trial of three rapamycin-eluting stents with different coating strategies for the reduction of coronary restenosis: 2 year follow-up results. Heart 95:1489–1494
48. Ormiston JA, Serruys PWS (2009) Bioabsorbable coronary stents. Circ Cardiovasc Interv 2:255–260
49. Serruys PW, Ormiston JA, Onuma Y et al (2009) A bioabsorbable everolimus-eluting coronary stent system (ABSORB): 2 year outcomes and results from multiple imaging methods. Lancet 373:897–910

# The History of Percutaneous Valvuloplasty

# 18

Alessandro Fontanelli

*What is now proved was only once imagined.*
William Blake

**Abstract**

The cardiointerventional era began in 1953 with the first percutaneous interventional procedure consisting of a wire pulmonary valvuloplasty performed by Rubio-Alvarez. In 1964 Dotter and Judkins performed the dilatation of the peripheral arteries using a coaxial double catheter with an outer diameter of 8 and 12 French respectively, which allowed for a mechanical dilatation of leg arterial stenosis. Nine years later, Porstmann described the first catheter with a latex balloon, but the first modern balloon catheter was reported by Gruentzig in 1976: it was a sausage-shaped polyvinyl chloride balloon at the tip of a double lumen catheter. In one year the indications for percutaneous dilatation were expanded from the iliac to the renal and coronary arteries. For these reasons percutaneous coronary balloon angioplasty can be considered the evolution of the Dotter technique and the Rubio-Alvarez procedures, and the current balloon percutaneous valvuloplasty a further application.

The cardiointerventional era began in 1953 with the first percutaneous interventional procedure consisting of a wire pulmonary valvuloplasty performed by Rubio-Alvarez [1]. In 1964 Dotter and Judkins performed the dilatation of the peripheral arteries using a coaxial double catheter with an outer diameter of 8 and 12 French respectively, which allowed for a mechanical dilatation of leg arterial stenosis [2]. Nine years later, Porstmann described the first catheter with a latex balloon [3], but the first modern catheter-balloon was reported by Gruentzig in 1976: it was a sausage-shaped polyvinyl chloride balloon at the tip of a double lumen catheter [4]. In 1 year the indications for percutaneous dilatation were expanded from iliac to renal

A. Fontanelli (✉)
Cardiac Surgery Unit, Department of Cardiovascular Science,
San Bortolo Hospital, Vicenza, Italy
e-mail: fontanelli.cardiovi@ulssvicenza.it

M. Picichè (ed.), *Dawn and Evolution of Cardiac Procedures*,
DOI: 10.1007/978-88-470-2400-7_18, © Springer-Verlag Italia 2013

and coronary arteries [5]. For these reasons percutaneous coronary balloon angioplasty can be considered the evolution of the Dotter technique and the Rubio-Alvarez procedures, and the current balloon percutaneous valvuloplasty a further application.

## 18.1 The Percutaneous Pulmonary Balloon Valvuloplasty

The percutaneous pulmonary balloon valvuloplasty (PPBV) was described firstly by Semb and coworkers in 1979: the procedure was performed using a Rashkind-type catheter that was passed into the main pulmonary artery of a newborn affected by tight pulmonary stenosis and severe tricuspid incompetence. The inflation of the balloon and its withdrawal through the stenotic valve produced an important clinical benefit to the patient [6]. Subsequently, Kan and coworkers in 1982 described the first percutaneous dilatation of a pulmonary valve stenosis performed by a dedicated balloon [7, 8]. Several months later Pepine and coworkers used a polyethylene balloon with a size of 20 × 40 mm for the same purpose [9]. In April 1983 Mullins performed the first dilatation of a pulmonary valve in a 6-month-old baby at the St. Luke's hospital in Houston.

Pulmonary valve stenosis accounts for approximately 20 % of all cases of congenital cardiac disease. In the absence of dysplasia, the percutaneous pulmonary dilatation procedure is the easiest method, performed transvenously using a femoral approach [10]. The accepted indication is a valvular gradient that exceeds 40 mmHg at rest, and the dilatation is performed by means of an oversized balloon or by two balloons. The double balloon technique is preferred in order to avoid arterial pressure drop during the inflation [11]. The disappearance of the waist provoked by the stenotic valve on the balloon is the most reliable marker of the efficacy of the dilatation. There were technical improvements over time to prevent two different and severe hemodynamic consequences that can appear during or immediately after the procedure. The first concern involves the drastic fall in arterial pressure during single balloon inflation. This is brought about by total blockage of the arterial flow by the balloon, which is 30 % larger than the pulmonary annulus. The second issue involves the infundibular pressure gradient due to the basal hypertrophy and to the post-dilatation hyperdynamic status of the infundibulum. The double balloon technique has been developed in order to avoid these two complications, and it has been coupled with intravenous beta-blocker administration prior to valvuloplasty. The two balloons inflated simultaneously permit residual flow through the valve thereby avoiding the arterial pressure drop, similarly beta blockers prevent infundibular obstruction and the consequent flow reduction.

The long-term results of dilatations are excellent [12, 13] and they compare favorably with surgical procedures [14].

## 18.2 The Percutaneous Aortic Balloon Valvuloplasty

On 23 September 1985, in Rouen, Alain Cribier performed the first percutaneous dilatation of an aortic valve degenerative stenosis [15]. He later described the procedure in a documentary fashion: "The patient was symptomatic for dyspnea and angina, she has a tight aortic stenosis with a 90 mmHg gradient and normal coronary arteries. At this time the surgical risk is considered too high because of her age and because she is a diabetic and obese. The procedure was performed by cut-down of the humeral artery to approach easily the ascending aorta and to facilitate crossing of the stenotic valve. The dilatation was performed with extreme caution beginning with an 8 mm balloon later followed by a 10 mm and then by a 12 mm balloon. The gradient was decreased by 50 % in comparison to baseline. In the following days the clinical improvement was exciting".

Great enthusiasm was generated both by Cribier's study involving 92 patients [16] and by the opening of the first dedicated course for this technique offered in February 1987 at Rouen. Widespread interest was directed to PABV as a palliative treatment for elderly patients with calcified aortic stenosis [17, 18].

This technique has been used in symptomatic patients who were at high risk of aortic valve replacement including very elderly patients, others with severe comorbidities or a severe depression in left ventricular function [19, 20].

The final aortic valve area obtained by PABV is most likely related to the underlying valve pathology: in rheumatic stenosis the crack of the fused commissures is the most important mechanism, but in degenerative calcified valves the fracture of the calcium deposit on the aortic leaflets is predominant. In 1991, data about a multicenter trial conducted in the USA were published in *The Journal of the American College of Cardiology* and many concerns were raised about the mid-term restenosis rate, which clearly represented the main limitation of the PABV [21]. ACC/AHA guidelines recommended PABV as a class 2b indication for elderly patients with a surgical indication, but not amenable to valve replacement [22]. In the late 1990s the technique was progressively abandoned due to the increased number of patients accepted for surgical valve replacement and because of the high restenosis rate. For the latter reason a strategy based on multiple staged PABV was suggested for nonsurgical patients and repeated dilatations have shown to offer a higher survival rate of about three years compared with patients who undergo only a single PABV [23]. Concurrently clinical better improvement was usually maintained by the multiple dilatation strategy [24].

In 2002 PBAV started to play an ancillary role related to the new procedure of transcatheter aortic valvular implantation (TAVI) pioneered again by A. Cribier and his team [25]. In a few years TAVI, consisting of a stent-valve transcatheter implantation under rapid pacing, via either a transapical or a transfemoral access, represented the ideal strategy for elderly patients with decompensated isolated aortic stenosis with a high logistic surgical euroSCORE (above 20 %) [26, 27]. Concomitant severe co-morbidities, left ventricular dysfunction or a critical preoperative state due to acute low cardiac output, represent the more frequent reasons for a high-risk surgical operation. If unstable high-risk patients are suitable for biological heart valve implantation and technical skills are acquired by the team, primary TAVI is the logical step forward instead of performing PBAV as a "bridge" to open AVR.

Nowadays, in some rare cases (e.g., apical thrombus and severe peripheral vascular disease in patients with nonsurgical indications) a bailout PBAV performed through a subclavian or a humeral access prior to standard AVR can be taken into consideration. Similarly, for young AS patients in cardiogenic shock and multi-organ failure an urgent PBAV for restoration of the patient's hemodynamics, as a bridge to AVR, appears to be an option as long as no randomized trial is available. For these young patients, the use of cardiopulmonary bypass for urgent surgical AVR is at very high risk, so it is not encouraged, while TAVI, consisting of a biological valve implantation, is not considered because of the unknown long-term durability of the prosthesis.

## 18.3 The Percutaneous Mitral Balloon Valvuloplasty

Historically, surgical commissurotomy was the standard treatment for repair of mitral stenosis. The first single-balloon valvuloplasty of the mitral valve was described by Inoue et al. in 1984, but the first clinical application of a prototype balloon catheter was previously performed in a 33-year-old man on 3 June 1982 by the same operators [28]. PMBV has since become the treatment of choice for mitral stenosis.

First, Inoue, a cardiac surgeon, developed the concept that a thickened and deteriorated mitral valve could be widened by a synthetic balloon and subsequently the double-balloon technique was introduced in Saudi Arabia as an alternative method to the single-balloon valvuloplasty [29]. Initially, the double balloon catheter technique was not widely utilized until the low profile single catheter with the shaft connected to two balloons in parallel became available. The easier double balloon technique requires the use of a floating balloon catheter to cross the mitral valve and then the positioning of two guide wires in the apex of the left ventricle. The simplicity and ease of use of the Inoue latex-balloon has led to it almost replacing the cumbersome, time-consuming and technically demanding double balloon technique [30, 31]. The Inoue balloon catheter remains to date the most commonly used technique for PMBV [32].

Meier in 1986 proposed a trefoil balloon that was a combination of three parallel balloons with a single shaft [29]: the potential advantages of this device were the single interatrial septum perforation, the residual transvalvular flow during the dilatation, and the high pressure of inflation tolerated from the single smaller balloon. Taking into consideration the oval shape of the mitral valve, the bifoil balloon was proposed by Medina and associates and specifically designed for mitral valvuloplasty [33, 34].

An original technique, an alternative to transvenous anterograde valvuloplasty, was suggested in 1987 by Babic [35], in order to avoid damage to the chordae tendinae and large perforations in the interatrial septum. According to this retrograde technique, the balloon dilating catheters were advanced percutaneously through the femoral arteries over two guide wires connecting the venous and the arterial circulations. Previously a Swan–Ganz floating catheter was advanced through a trans-septal sheath from the right femoral vein into the left atrium and then it was inflated with carbon dioxide and advanced through the left ventricle into the aortic root. A long guide wire was advanced via the Swan–Ganz floating catheter from the right femoral vein into the aortic root where it was snared by the retrieval catheter and brought out of the body through the left femoral artery [36].

The wire became the rail for the balloon catheter introduced into the femoral artery and advanced over the loop into the left ventricle up to 2–3 cm from the apex after which it was placed across the mitral valve. The results obtained by this technique were good, but it was in reality too complex for most of the operators.

It has been 30 years since the introduction of PMBV and the publication of the first results concerning patients submitted to this procedure: in this period, small technique variations were incorporated but the method remains essentially unmodified. However, the cost of this easier procedure is high which represents a real limitation for countries with restricted financial resources. Moreover, it is well known that the option of an imperfect sterilization procedure introduces potential hazards and decreases performance. For these reasons in 1999, Cribier [37] proposed a new metallic device, similar to the Tubb's dilator used during closed surgical commissurotomy, which could replace the latex balloon for the percutaneous commissurotomy/dilatation of the mitral valve. The advantage of this device, because it is a metallic material, is that it enables appropriate sterilization, thus making it possible for the device to be reused several times without any loss of performance, and significantly reducing costs.

In clinical decision-making, anatomical assessment is important in determining contraindications to the PMBV and assists in defining prognostic considerations [38]. Echographic assessment allows for the classification of patients into anatomical groups with similar predictive outcomes. Most authors use the Wilkins score [39] others, like Cormier [40] use a more general assessment of valve anatomy. In performing PMBV the American Heart Association (AHA)/American College of Cardiology (ACC) guideline recommendations are well established [41].

Currently, the Inoue technique is confirmed to be the most widely used method for PMBV. In comparison to the double-balloon technique, it has similar efficacy with the additional benefit of presenting lower intra- and peri-procedural risks. Recently, PMBV has been demonstrated to reduce the incidence of ischemic cerebral stroke in patients with symptomatic rheumatic mitral stenosis [42].

If compared with surgical mitral commissurotomy, mitral valvuloplasty with the balloon technique shows similar or greater success rates and better long-term outcome [43, 44].

## 18.4 The Percutaneous Balloon Tricuspid Valvuloplasty

Tricuspid valve stenosis is an uncommon disease and mostly represents a rheumatic fever sequela. A clinically significant stenosis is diagnosed when the diastolic gradient is >5 mmHg. Rheumatic tricuspid stenosis is generally associated with mitral valve disease and, in some cases, the aortic valve is involved as well. Percuaneous balloon tricuspid valvuloplasty (PTBV) has been described since 1987 [45] and the double balloon technique was suggested most often [46, 47]. Sometimes PTBV and mitral or aortic dilatation has been combined [48, 49].

Other causes of flow obstruction include tricuspid congenital atresia or stenosis, right atrial or metastatic tumors, the carcinoid syndrome [50], bacterial endocarditis, particularly in association with a pacemaker lead [51], and degenerated biological prosthetic valve for which PTBV can be a reasonable therapeutic alternative [52, 53]. The long-term outcome of such a procedure remains unclear. Tricuspid regurgitation greater than mild is considered a contraindication to valvotomy, in spite of the fact that a few patients with moderate regurgitation have been successfully treated. Tumor masses, vegetations, and thrombi are contraindications to valvotomy.

Most published data available so far deal with single case reports and there is far less experience with tricuspid valvotomy than with mitral valvotomy [45–50]. Valve areas generally increase from less than 1 to almost 2 $cm^2$. While some stenosis persists, this change in area is sufficient to produce a significant reduction in the transvalvular pressure gradient and a decrease in right atrial pressure. Experience with the Inoue balloon indicates that single balloon techniques may be as effective as the previous double balloon techniques [54].

Recognizing that there are no published studies that compare percutaneous balloon valvotomy with surgical valvuloplasty, and that only limited long-term results have been published, few conclusions are appropriate, even though the history of PTBV started in 1987. The data that are available indicate that PTBV is effective and is associated with a low morbidity.

## 18.5 Conclusions

Interventional cardiologists have pioneered the procedures of percutaneous valvuloplasty, overcoming general skepticism and demonstrating the technique's validity and efficacy when correct indications are respected. The procedure's success rate has also been enhanced by improvement in the field of imaging. Percutaneous valvuloplasty represents not only a valid therapeutic option, but it also lays the foundation for more sophisticated and definitive techniques such as TAVI.

## References


1. Rubio-Alvarez V, Limon-Larson R (1954) Treatment of pulmonary valvular stenosis and tricuspid stenosis with a modified cardiac catheter. Program Abstract II Second World Congress on Cardiology, Washington, DC, p 205
2. Dotter CT, Judkins MP (1964) Transluminal treatment of arteriosclerotic obstruction: description of a new technique and a preliminary report of its application. Circulation 30:654–670
3. Wierny L, Plass R, Porstmann W (1974) Long-term results in 100 consecutive patients treated by transluminal angioplasty. Radiology 112(3):543–548
4. Gruentzig AR, Turina MI, Schneider JA (1976) Experimental percutaneous dilatation of coronary artery stenosis (abstract). Circulation 53:11–I81
5. Gruentzig A, Senning A, Siegenthaler W (1979) Nonoperative dilatation of coronary artery stenosis: percutaneous transluminal coronary angioplasty (PTCA). N Engl J Med 301:61–68
6. Semb BKH, Tijonneland S, Stake G (1979) Balloon valvulotomy of congenital pulmonary valve stenosis with tricuspid valve insufficiency. Cardiovasc Intervent Radiol 2:239–241
7. Kan JS, White RI, Mitchell SE et al (1982) Percutaneous balloon valvuloplasty: a method for treating congenital pulmonary valve stenosis. N Engl J Med 307(9):540–542

8. Kan JS, White RI Jr, Mitchell SE et al (1984) Percutaneous transluminal balloon valvuloplasty for pulmonary valve stenosis. Circulation 69(3):554–560
9. Pepine CJ, Gessner IH, Feldman RL (1982) Percutaneous balloon valvuloplasty for pulmonary valve stenosis in the adults. Am J Cardiol 50:1442–1445
10. McCrindle BW (1994) Independent predictors of long-term results after balloon pulmonary valvuloplasty. Circulation 89:1751–1759
11. Park JH, Yoon YS, Yeon KM et al (1987) Percutaneous pulmonary valvuloplasty with a double-balloon technique. Radiology 164:715–718
12. Al-Kasab S, Ribeiro PA, Al-Zaibag M et al (1988) Percutaneous double balloon pulmonary valvotomy in adults: One-to-two year follow-up. Am J Cardiol 62:822–824
13. Stanger P, Cassidy SC, Girod DA, Kan JS, Lababidi Z, Shapiro SR (1990) Balloon pulmonary valvuloplasty: results of the valvuloplasty and angioplasty of congenital anomalies registry. Am J Cardiol 65:775–783
14. O'Connor BK, Beekman RH, Lindauer A, Rocchini A (1992) Intermediate-term outcome after pulmonary balloon valvuloplasty: comparison with a matched surgical control group. J Am Coll Cardiol 20:169–173
15. Cribier A, Souudi N, Berland J et al (1986) Percutaneous transluminal valvuloplasty of acquired aortic stenosis in elderly patients: an alternative to valve replacement? Lancet 1:63
16. Cribier A, Savin T, Berland J (1987) Percutaneous transluminal balloon valvuloplasty of adult aortic stenosis: report of 92 cases. J Am Coll Cardiol 9(2):381–386
17. O'Keefe JH Jr, Vlietstra RE, Bailey KR (1987) Natural history of candidates for balloon aortic valvuloplasty. Mayo Clin Proc 62(11):986–991
18. Safian RD, Berman AD, Diver DJ et al (1988) Balloon aortic valvuloplasty in 170 consecutive patients. N Engl J Med 319(3):125–130
19. Sprigings DC, Jackson G, Chambers JB (1988) Balloon dilatation of the aortic valve for inoperable aortic stenosis. BMJ 297(6655):1007–1011
20. Serruys PW, Luijten HE, Beatt KJ (1988) Percutaneous balloon valvuloplasty for calcific aortic stenosis. A treatment 'sine cure'? Eur Heart J 9(7):782–794
21. Percutaneous balloon aortic valvuloplasty (1991) Acute and 30-day follow-up results in 674 patients from the NHLBI balloon valvuloplasty registry. Circulation 84(6):2383–2397
22. Bonow RO et al (2006) ACC/AHA Guidelines for the management of patients with valvular heart disease a report of the American College of Cardiology/American Heart Association task force on practice guidelines. J Am Coll Cardiol 48(3):1–148
23. Ferguson JJ, Garza RA (1991) Efficacy of multiple balloon valvuloplasty procedures. J Am Coll Cardiol 17:1430–1435
24. Agarwal A, Kini AS, Attanti S (2005) Results of repeat balloon valvuloplasty for treatment of aortic stenosis in patients aged 59–104 years. Am J Cardiol 95(1):43–47
25. Cribier A, Eltchaninoff H, Bash A et al (2002) Percutaneous transcatheter implantation of an aortic valve prosthesis for calcific aortic stenosis: first human case description. Circulation 106:3006–3008
26. Zajarias A, Cribier AG (2009) Outcomes and safety of percutaneous aortic valve replacement. J Am Coll Cardiol 53(20):1829–1836
27. Walter T, Simon P, Dewey T et al (2007) Transapical minimally invasive aortic valve implantation. Multicenter experience. Circulation 116:1240–1245
28. Inoue K, Owaki T, Nakamura T, Kitamura F, Miyamoto N (1984) Clinical application of transvenous mitral commissurotomy by a new balloon catheter. J Thorac Cardiovasc Surg 87:394–402
29. Chen CR, Cheng TO (1995) Percutaneous balloon mitral valvuloplasty by the Inoue technique: a multicenter study of 4832 patients in China. Am Heart J 129:1197–1203
30. Rihal CS, Jr Holmes (1994) Percutaneous balloon mitral valvuloplasty: issues involved in comparing techniques. Cathet Cardiovasc Diagn Suppl 2:35–41
31. Inoue K, Feldman T (1993) Percutaneous transvenous mitral commissurotomy using the Inoue balloon catheter. Cathet Cardiovasc Diagn 28:119–125

32. Al Zaibag M, Ribeiro PA, Al Kasab S (1986) Percutaneous double-balloon mitral valvotomy for rheumatic mitral-valve stenosis. Lancet 1:757–761
33. Medina A, Bethencourt A, Coello I et al (1988) Utilizacion de un Nuevo cateter bibalon para la valvuloplastia mitral percutanea transatrial. Rev Esp Cardiol 41:477–480
34. Patel J, Vythilingum S, Mitha AS (1990) Balloon dilatation of the mitral valve by a single bifoil (2 × 19 mm) or trefoil (3 × 15 mm) catheter. Br Heart J 64(5):342–346
35. Babic UU, Grujicic S, Popovic Z et al (1992) Percutaneous transarterial balloon dilatation of the mitral valve: five years experience. Br Heart J 67:185–189
36. Babic UU, Pejcic P, Djurisic Z et al (1986) Percutaneous transarterial balloon valvuloplasty for mitral valve stenosis. Am J Cardiol 57:1101–1104
37. Cribier A, Eltchaninoff H, Koning R et al (1999) Percutaneous mechanical mitral commissurotomy with a newly designed metallic valvulotome. Circulation 99:793–799
38. Fatkin D, Roy P, Morgan JJ (1993) Percutaneous balloon mitral valvotomy with the Inoue single-balloon catheter commissural morphology as a determinant of outcome. J Am Coll Cardiol 21:390–397
39. Wilkins GT, Weyman AE, Abascal VM (1988) Percutaneous balloon dilatation of the mitral valve: an analysis of echocardiographic variables related to outcome and the mechanism of dilatation. Br Heart J 60:299–308
40. Iung B, Cormier B, Ducimetiere P et al (1996) Immediate results of percutaneous mitral commissurotomy. Circulation 94:2124–2130
41. Bonow RO, Carabello BA, Kanu C et al (2006) ACC/AHA 2006 guidelines for the management of patients with valvular heart disease: a report of the American College of Cardiology/ American Heart Association task force on practice guidelines (writing committee to revise the 1998 guidelines for the management of patients with valvular heart disease): developed in collaboration with the Society of Cardiovascular Anesthesiologists. Circulation 114: e84–e231
42. Liu TJ, Lai HC, Lee WL et al (2008) Percutaneous balloon commissurotomy reduces incidence of ischemic cerebral stroke in patients with symptomatic rheumatic mitral stenosis. Int J Cardiol 123:189–190
43. Turi ZG, Reyes VP, Raju BS et al (1991) Percutaneous balloon versus surgical closed commissurotomy for mitral stenosis: a prospective, randomized trial. Circulation 83:1179–1185
44. Arora R, Nair M, Kalra GS et al (1993) Immediate and long-term results of balloon and surgical closed mitral valvotomy: a randomized comparative study. Am Heart J 125:1091–1094
45. Al-Zaibag M, Ribeiro P, Al-Kasab S (1987) Percutaneous balloon valvotomy in tricuspid stenosis. Br Heart J 57(1):51–53
46. Khalilullah M, Tyagi S, Yadav BS et al (1987) Double-balloon valvuloplasty of tricuspid stenosis. Am Heart J 114:1232–1233
47. Ribeiro P, Al-Zaibag M, Al-Kasab S et al (1988) Percutaneous double balloon valvotomy for rheumatic tricuspid stenosis. Am J Cardiol 61:660–662
48. Bethencourt A, Medina A, Hermandez E et al (1990) Combined percutaneous balloon valvuloplasty of mitral and tricuspid valves. Am Heart J 119:416–418
49. Berland J, Rocha P, Mechmerche R et al (1990) Percutaneous valvuloplasty for combined mitral and tricuspid stenosis: results in 3 cases. Arch Mal Coeur 83:1585–1589
50. Mullins PA, Hall JA, Shapiro LM (1990) Balloon dilatation of tricuspid stenosis caused by carcinoid heart disease. Br Heart J 63(4):249–250
51. Unger P, Clevenbergh P, Crasset V et al (1997) Pacemaker-related endocarditis inducing tricuspid stenosis. Am Heart J 133:605
52. Wren C, Hunter S (1989) Balloon dilatation of a stenosed bioprosthesis in the tricuspid valve position. Br Heart J 61:65–67
53. Chow W-H, Cheung K-L, Tai Y-T et al (1990) Successful percutaneous balloon valvuloplasty of a stenotic tricuspid bioprosthesis. Am Heart J 119:666–668
54. Shaw TRD (1992) The Inoue balloon for dilatation of the tricuspid valve: a modified over-the-wire approach. Br Heart J 67:263–265

# Percutaneous Closure of Atrial and Ventricular Septal Defects

# 19

Achille Gaspardone and Giulio G. Stefanini

*Multa non quia difficilia sunt non audemus, sed quia non audemus sunt difficilia*

Lucius Annaeus Seneca

**Abstract**

Catheter occlusion of atrial septal defects has its roots in the 1950s, with early devices being implanted during closed-heart surgery without cardiopulmonary bypass. In 1974 King and Mills performed the first percutaneous atrial septal defects (ASD) closure in six dogs, by the use of a device introduced through a 23 F catheter. Two years later, the same device was successfully used in a 17-year-old girl. Since the mid-1980s an impressive development of materials and technique has prompted wide use of invasive procedures for the percutaneous closure of atrial and ventricular septal defects. The development of interventional techniques for closure of atrial and ventricular septal defects has completely changed the therapeutic approach to these diseases and has provided a new important tool for the treatment of these potentially dreadful clinical conditions, with a remarkable improvement in patients' quality of life and prognosis. At present more than 80 % of patients with ASD can be treated percutaneously and an increasing number of patients with ventricular septal defects (VSD) are recommended to undergo percutaneous closure. Financial estimates indicate that the economic impact of this new treatment technology is to the order of $30 billion per year and it appears to be constantly increasing, as shown by the 58-fold increase in the use of this new therapeutic approach in the last 10 years.

A. Gaspardone (✉) · G. G. Stefanini
Department of Medicine, Division of Cardiology,
Ospedale S. Eugenio, Rome, Italy
e-mail: a_gaspardone@yahoo.com

M. Picichè (ed.), *Dawn and Evolution of Cardiac Procedures*,
DOI: 10.1007/978-88-470-2400-7_19, 

Atrial septal defects (ASD) represent almost 10 % of congenital heart defects [1–3]. ASD is observed three-fold more frequently among women than men, and almost 70 % of ASD are positioned in the superior portion of the inter-atrial septa (ostium secundum). ASD are usually well tolerated by patients; indeed, subjects with an ASD have few symptoms and the diagnosis is usually made by chance. ASD closure remains controversial, particularly among patients older than 40 years [4–7]; nevertheless, the indication is commonly accepted whenever the ASD determines a right ventricle overload with $Qp/Qs \geq 1.5$ [7–10]. Since 1960, surgical closure of ASD has been considered a safe and effective intervention [11]. Patients undergoing this procedure have an excellent long-term prognosis with a similar life expectancy and only a small increase in the risk of supraventricular arrhythmias compared with normal subjects [12, 13]. Ventricular septal defects (VSDs) are the most common congenital heart defects in both children and adults [14]. Their documented incidence has increased significantly with the development of echocardiography. VSD are diagnosed in up to 5 % of live births, with an estimated prevalence of simple VSDs in the adult population of 0.3 per 1,000. VSD hemodynamics is influenced by the size of the defect, the pressure gradient between left and right ventricles, and pulmonary vascular resistance. Surgical repair of congenital VSDs is safely performed with a low risk of mortality (1–5 %); however, complications include complete atrioventricular block, as well as other conduction disturbances, chylothorax, phrenic nerve injury, postpericardiotomy syndrome, and neurological sequelae of cardiopulmonary bypass. While in the early era 80 % closure failure and 3 % complete atrioventricular block rates were reported among patients undergoing control catheterization at long-term follow-up, eight more recent studies report residual shunting in 30 % and complete atrioventricular block in up to 3 % of patients, with pacemaker implantation occurring in 10 per 10,000 patient-years and endocarditis in 16 per 10,000 [15]. It is noteworthy that most residual shunts after surgical closure are insignificant, and a reintervention is rarely required [15].

## 19.1 Atrial Septal Defects

Catheter occlusion of atrial septal defects has its roots in the 1950s, with early devices being implanted during closed-heart surgery without cardiopulmonary bypass (Fig. 19.1). In 1974 King and Mills performed the first percutaneous ASD closure in six dogs, by the use of a device introduced through a 23 F catheter [16]. Two years later, the same device was successfully used in a 17-year-old girl [17].

In 1987 and 1989, Lock and Rashkind developed a smaller device (15 F guiding catheter, "USCI-Bard clamshell umbrella") and performed a series of closures in lambs [18]. However, due to frequent fractures of the metal components, this device was dropped very early. During the 1990s several new models were proposed and studied, such as the "CardioSEAL atrial septal occluder" and the "Starflex" (both based on the structure of the "clamshell device") [19], the

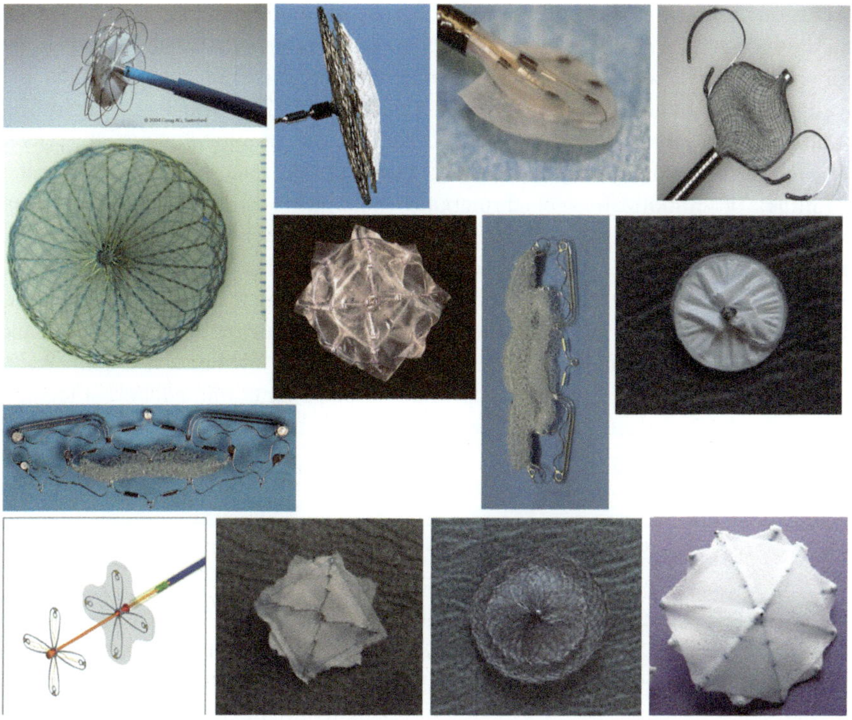

Fig. 19.1 Devices developed for atrial septal defect and patent foramen ovale percutaneous closure

"Sideris buttoned occluding device" [20], the "atrial septal defect occlusion system—ASDOS" [21], and the "Angel-wing self-centering device" [22]. In 1996, Sharafuddin and colleagues described the use of a new double-disk device made of nitinol developed by Amplatz, the "Amplatzer Septal Occluder" [23, 24]. The main advantage of this device is the possibility of retrieving it even after a complete delivery. In 2000 a new double helix device ("Helex") was proposed; however, the experimental studies limited the use of this device to the closure of patent foramen ovale [25]. In June 2007, a new bioabsorbable closure device was introduced onto the European market, (BioSTAR—NMT Medical, Boston, MA, USA), with the aim of reducing the synthetic metallic structure and hence avoiding potential complications such as erosion, thrombus formation, and intra-atrial mechanical encumbrance.

Accurate patient selection and operator's experience represent two cornerstones of ASD percutaneous closure. Several reports showed rates of successful closure without residual shunt and procedural complication ranging from 85 to 100 % [26]. Percutaneous closure is feasible in up to 80 % of patients with ostium secundum ASD, after an adequate angiographic and echocardiographic evaluation. Mainly ASD size and rim characteristics play a role in determining patient exclusion from a percutaneous strategy. Procedural complication rate has significantly decreased with the increasing operators' experience; nevertheless, they are still observed in a considerable amount of cases and therefore have to be taken into account when planning a percutaneous ASD closure [26]. The following procedural complications have been associated with the use of all the available devices: air embolization (1 %) mainly due to air entrapment into the delivery catheter (Mullins) or embolization of thrombotic material (1–2 %); pulmonary artery perforation due to the stiffness of the guidewire used for sizing balloon and device delivery (<1 %); functional alterations of atrioventricular valves (1 %); systemic or pulmonary venous thromboembolism (1 %); atrial perforation leading to cardiac tamponade (1–2 %); transient supraventricular arrhythmias (1–3 %); and device malapposition and/or acute embolization (2–10 %). Finally, a non-significant residual shunt is observed in up to 10 % of patients immediately after percutaneous ASD closure. As it relates to long-term follow-up, the few published series did not raise any safety issues.

## 19.2 Ventricular Septal Defects

As for ASD closure, the potential benefits of percutaneous VSD closure, without open heart surgery and cardiopulmonary bypass, appear intuitive. In 1987, Lock and co-authors attempted percutaneous closure of seven postinfarction or congenital VSDs in six patients, by the use of Rashkind double umbrella devices [27]. In all cases the authors managed to successfully cross the VSDs; nevertheless, one device embolized immediately into the pulmonary artery and all four patients with postinfarction VSD died from increasing VSD shunting within several days. In the following years, the Rashkind double umbrella as well as other devices originally designed for the closure of different intracardiac defects were used with variable success. Besides the very high residual shunt rates (35–100 %), the major drawbacks were the large delivery sheaths required (11 F), a complex implantation technique, the inability to reposition the device, and the interference with aortic and tricuspid valves. In 1998 a dedicated device—the Amplatzer VSD occluder—became available and Thanopoulos et al. [28] and Hijazi et al. [29] reported initial applications in children. The main advantages of the Amplatzer membranous and muscular VSD occluders are the possibility of redeploying or removing the device after initial positioning (until it remains screwed on the delivery wire), the smaller delivery sheaths (7–9 F), the higher closure rates attributable to its mechanism of closure (stenting of the defect with the waist of the device), and its round shape minimizing the potential for valvular or tissue injury. In 50 patients undergoing percutaneous closure of muscular VSDs [30], by the use of Sideris ($n = 2$) and Amplatzer muscular VSD occluder ($n = 48$), device success was 100 %, without residual shunt by transthoracic echocardiography at 24 h, and no late complications. In a phase I multicentre clinical trial including 35 patients treated with the Amplatzer membranous VSD occluder [31]—the only device specifically designed for perimembranous VSD closure—the authors reported a 9 % device success, with a complete closure rate of 96 % at 6 months by transthoracic echocardiography. All patients survived, but 9 % of patients had serious complications (one permanent complete atrioventricular block requiring pacemaker implantation after 3 months, one peri-hepatic bleeding requiring transfusions, and one failed transcatheter device retrieval with rupture of the tricuspid valve chordae tendinae requiring surgical device removal, tricuspid valve repair, and VSD closure), and various other adverse events occurred in 15 other patients (43 %). One additional patient (2 %) developed complete atrioventricular block requiring pacemaker implantation 16 months after device implantation. In a European multicenter trial [32], 54 pediatric patients underwent transcatheter VSD closure with the Amplatzer membranous VSD occluder, showing a 91 % device success and a 94 % complete occlusion rate at 1 year—as assessed by transthoracic echocardiography. Principal procedural complications—precluding device implantation—included severe bradycardia with hemodynamic compromise in 2 patients (4 %), and transient Mobitz II (2:1) atrioventricular block in 1 patient (2 %). Moreover, 2 patients (4 %) suffered device embolization into the descending aorta with percutaneous removal and successful closure with a second device, and 1 patient (2 %) developed late complete atrioventricular block requiring pacemaker implantation. Finally, data from a partially incomplete international registry including 100 patients [33] showed 93 % device success and 84 % complete closure rate at 6 months' follow-up. Complications were observed in 29 patients (29 %), including complete atrioventricular block requiring pacemaker implantation in 2 patients.

## 19.3 Conclusions

The development of interventional techniques for closure of atrial and ventricular septal defects has completely changed the therapeutic approach to these diseases and has provided a new important tool for the treatment of these potentially dreadful clinical conditions, with a remarkable improvement of patients' quality of life and prognosis. At present more than 80 % of patients with ASD can be treated percutaneously and an increasing number of patients with VSD are proposed for percutaneous closure. Financial estimates indicate that the economic impact of this new treatment technology is to the order of $30 billion per year and it appears to be constantly increasing, as shown by the 58-fold increase in the use of this new therapeutic approach in the last 10 years.

## References

1. Bedford DE, Papp C, Parkinson J (1941) Atrial septal defect. Br Heart J 3:37–38
2. Dave KS, Pakrashi BC, Woolder GH et al (1973) Atrial septal defect in adults: clinical and hemodynamic results of surgery. Am J Cardiol 31:7–14

3. Campbell M (1970) Natural history of atrial septal defects. Br Heart J 32:820–826
4. Webb G (2001) Do patients over 40 years of age benefit from closure of an atrial septal defect? Heart 85:249–250
5. Jemielity M, Dyszkiewicz W, Paluszkiewicz L, Perek B, Buczkowski P, Ponizynski A (2001) Do patients over 40 years of age benefit from surgical closure of an atrial septal defect? Heart 85:300–303
6. Ward C (1994) Secundum atrial septal defect: routine surgical treatment is not of proven benefit. Br Heart J 71:219–223
7. Connelly MS, Webb GD, Sommerville J et al (1998) Canadian consensus conference on adult congenital heart defects. Can J Cardiol 14:395–452
8. Murphy GJ, Gersh BJ, McGoon MD et al (1990) Long-term outcome after surgical repair of isolated atrial septal defect: follow-up at 27–32 years. N Engl J Med 323:1644–1650
9. Shah D, Azar M, Oakley CM et al (1994) Natural history of secundum atrial septal defect in adults after medical or surgical treatment: a historical prospective study. Br Heart J 71: 224–228
10. Konstantinides S, Geibel A, Olschewski M et al (1995) A comparison of surgical and medical therapy for atrial septal defect in adults. N Engl J Med 333:469–473
11. Meijboom F, Hess J, Szatmari A et al (1993) Long-term follow-up (9–20 years) after surgical closure of atrial septal defect at a young age. Am J Cardiol 72:1431–1434
12. Gatzoulis MA, Freeman MA, Siu SC et al (1999) Atrial arrhythmias and surgical closure of atrial septal defect in adults. N Engl J Med 340:839–846
13. Berger F, Vogel M, Kramer A et al (1999) Incidence of atrial flutter/fibrillation in adults with atrial septal defect before and after surgery. Ann Thorac Surg 68:75–78
14. Minette MS, Sahn DJ (2006) Ventricular septal defects. Circulation 114:2190–2197
15. Kidd L, Driscoll DJ, Gersony WM et al (1993) Second natural history study of congenital heart defects. Results of treatment of patients with ventricular septal defects. Circulation 87:138–151
16. King TD, Mills NL (1974) Nonoperative closure of atrial septal defects. Surgery 75:383
17. King TD, Mills NL (1976) Secundum atrial septal defect: nonoperative closure during cardiac catheterization. JAMA 235:2506–2509
18. Lock JE, Rome JJ, Davis R, Van Praagh S, Perry SB, Van Praagh R, Keane JF (1989) Transcatheter closure of atrial septal defects. Exp stud Circ 79:1091–1099
19. Carminati M, Giusti S, Hausdorf G et al (2000) A European multicentric experience using the cardio seal and starflex double umbrella devices to close interatrial communications holes within oval fossa. Cardiol Young 10:519–526
20. Zamora R, Sideris EB (2000) Results of transvenous occlusion of secundum atrial septal defects with the fourth generation buttoned device: comparison with first, second and third generation devices. International buttoned device trial group. J Am Coll Cardiol 36(2): 583–592
21. Sievert H, Babic UU, Hausdorf G, Schneider M, Hopp HW, Pfeiffer D, Pfisterer M, Friedli B, Urban P (1998) Transcatheter closure of atrial septal defect and patent foramen ovale with ASDOS device (a multi-institutional European trial). Am J Cardiol 82(11):1405–1413
22. Rickers C, Hamm C, Stern H, Hofmann T, Franzen O, Schrader R, Sievert H, Schranz D, Michel-Behnke I, Vogt J, Kececioglu D, Sebening W, Eicken A, Meyer H, Matthies W, Kleber F, Hug J, Weil J (1998) Percutaneous closure of secundum atrial septal defect with a new self centering device ("angel wings"). Heart 80(5):517–521
23. Sharafuddin MJA, Gu X, Titus J et al (1997) Transvenous closure of secundum atrial septal defects: preliminary results with a new self-expanding nitilol prosthesis in swine model. Circulation 95:2162–2168
24. Berger F, Ewert P, Bjornstad PG, Dahnert I, Krings G, Brilla-Austenat I, Vogel M, Lange PE (1999) Transcatheter closure as standard treatment for most interatrial defects: experience in 200 patients treated with the Amplatzer septal occluder. Cardiol Young 9(5):468–473

25. Sievert H, Wilson N, Trepels T et al (2001) Catheter closure of patent foramen ovale: experience with the new Helex occluder. Eur Heart J 22:42 (Abstract Supplement)
26. Wilkinson JL (1999) Can transcatheter closure of atrial septal defect be regarded as a "standard" procedure? Cardiol Young 9:458–461
27. Lock JE, Block PC, McKay RG et al (1988) Transcatheter closure of ventricular septal defects. Circulation 78:361–368
28. Thanopoulos BD, Tsaousis GS, Konstadopoulou GN et al (1999) Transcatheter closure of muscular ventricular septal defects with the Amplatzer ventricular septal defect occluder: initial clinical applications in children. J Am Coll Cardiol 33:1395–1399
29. Hijazi ZM, Hakim F, Al-Fadley F et al (2000) Transcatheter closure of single muscular ventricular septal defects using the Amplatzer muscular VSD occluder: initial results and technical considerations. Cathet Cardiovasc Interv 49:167–172
30. Arora R, Trehan V, Thakur AK et al (2004) Transcatheter closure of congenital muscular ventricular septal defect. J Interv Cardiol 17:109–115
31. Fu YC, Bass J, Amin Z et al (2006) Transcatheter closure of perimembranous ventricular septal defects using the new Amplatzer membranous VSD occluder: results of the U.S. phase I trial. J Am Coll Cardiol 47:319–325
32. Thanopoulos BV, Rigby ML, Karanasios E et al (2007) Transcatheter closure of perimembranous ventricular septal defects in infants and children using the Amplatzer perimembranous ventricular septal defect occluder. Am J Cardiol 99:984–989
33. Holzer R, de Giovanni J, Walsh KP et al (2006) Transcatheter closure of perimembranous ventricular septal defects using the Amplatzer membranous VSD occluder: immediate and midterm results of an international registry. Cathet Cardiovasc Interv 68:620–628

# Evolution of Homografts and Prosthetic Heart Valves

# 20

Marco Picichè

> *La science est due à des accidents heureux, à des hommes déraisonnables, à des désirs absurdes, à des questions saugrenues, à des amateurs de difficultés.*
>
> Paul Valery


**Abstract**

The history of heart valve replacement research comprises three rubrics: homografts, bioprostheses, and mechanical heart valves. The first prosthesis implanted was a mechanical valve in 1952. In rapid and overlapping succession, and despite numerous difficulties and failures, all three replacement types were in use by the early 1960s. Shape, design, size, volume, strength, durability, biocompatibility, ease of implantation, noise—every aspect was investigated in a swirl of industry competition to describe the optimal valve profile. Initially, mechanical valves attracted the most attention—witness the hundreds of models created at that time vs today where stented, stentless, transcatheter, and sutureless biological prostheses claim the spotlight.


The history of heart valve replacement research comprises three rubrics: homografts, bioprostheses, and mechanical heart valves. The first prosthesis implanted was a mechanical valve in 1952. In rapid and overlapping succession, and despite numerous difficulties and failures, all three replacement types were in use by the early 1960s.


M. Picichè (✉)
Cardiac Surgery Unit, San Filippo Neri Hospital,
Via Martinotti 20, 00135 Rome, Italy
e-mail: m.piciche@sanfilipponeri.roma.it; marcopiciche.history@libero.it



M. Picichè (ed.), *Dawn and Evolution of Cardiac Procedures*,
DOI: 10.1007/978-88-470-2400-7_20,

## 20.1 Homografts

At the time Bailey, Brock, and Lillehei were using closed or direct vision commissurotomy of the aortic valve to relief stenosis, Gordon Murray in Toronto was experimenting with homografts to treat aortic insufficiency. He performed a thoracotomy in dogs and placed a homograft in the descending thoracic aorta. Murray observed that if the native aortic valve functioned adequately then the implanted homograft stayed open and inactive. But when he made the native aortic valve incompetent, the homograft functioned with normal opening and closing—some of the dogs lived up to 9 months [1]. In 1955 Murray put to use a clinical application by operating on a 22-year-old patient. The successful operation consisted of a left thoracotomy, descending aortic cross clamping (7 min), and a homograft implant—the patient was symptom-free at the 6-year follow-up [2, 3]. Three more patients were managed similarly, with encouraging results. In Houston, Beall, Cooley, and DeBakey successfully reproduced this technique[4]. In 1961 Heimbecker in Toronto tried the first orthotopic aortic homograft implantation, but the patient died a few hours later. He attempted replacement of the mitral valve with aortic homografts in two patients, who both died [1, 5]. Meanwhile Alfred Gunning and Carlos Duran in Oxford were studying a method to achieve correct homograft orthotopic positioning [6]. They had not yet used their technique in humans when Donald Ross was forced by events to employ their application clinically [1]. While Ross was decalcifying an aortic valve, it was partially aspirated into the sucker catheter; he had no choice but to use Gunning and Duran's homograft implantation technique—and credited them for their work. That valve was not rejected and for 4 years it functioned adequately. Barratt-Boyes in New Zealand, and Kirklin, Angell, and Shumway in the United States adopted homografts in their practice [7]. In 1965 Weldon at the Johns Hopkins Hospital introduced homografts mounted on a frame (stent mounted) to simplify the implantation technique, and by the end of the 1960s these were used in the aortic, mitral, and tricuspid positions [8]. The hemodynamic performance was encouraging but the stents caused tissue failure within a few years and so were less durable than free hand-sewn homografts. Senning in Switzerland [9] and Ionescu [10] in Britain fashioned autogenous fascia lata into a trileaflet valve with unsatisfying results. Further attempts were made using dura mater and pericardium. In the early 1960s at Stanford University, Lower and Shumway first conceived the idea that an autogenous pulmonary valve could be used as an aortic valve substitute [11]. However, the first clinical operation based on this concept was not performed until 1967, by Ross [12]. Initially, the aortic valve was replaced by a pulmonary autograft as a subcoronary implant, and then later as an aortic root replacement. The pulmonary outflow tract was replaced first by an aortic homograft, or later by a pulmonary homograft. The Ross procedure is a complex operation requiring the removal and transplantation of a healthy valve with the risk of damaging the first septal branch of the left anterior descending artery. One problem with cadaveric homografts is their lack of cellular regeneration when used

in children as opposed to the live pulmonary autografts. These days, the Ross procedure's early outcomes are still excellent. However, beyond the 10-year follow-up, problems lurk—
frequent reoperations are required. Progress in prosthetic heart valve surgery calls into question the choice of the Ross procedure in adults.

## 20.2 Bioprosthetic Heart Valves

As a result of limited access to human cadaveric material, difficulty in finding adequately sized homograft sources, the risk of degeneration, the time-consuming and skill-intensive implantation techniques—in an era where cardiopulmonary bypass (CPB) and myocardial protection were not as safe as nowadays—research turned to heterograft valves. Porcine valves were first used due to their similarity to human valves. Duran and Gunning, in Oxford performed heterologous aortic valve transplantation in dogs [13] and attempted a porcine valve implant in a single human patient on 23 September 1964 [1]. The following year Binet, Carpentier, Duran, and Langlois published the first successful results on the porcine aortic valve operation in five patients [14]. The problem of heterologous graft preservation and the risk of host rejection spurred further research into chemical treatments. The search was to obviate the immunological response and avoid tissue degradation. At first Binet and associates placed heterologous valves into mercurial solution—O'Brien used formaldehyde [1, 14, 15]. The hypothesis was that these substances denature proteins and thereby minimize the rejection phenomenon. Despite its usefulness to histologists in arresting autolysis and fixing tissues, formaldehyde causes shrinkage and stiffness. Research efforts shifted to the use of glutaraldehyde. In his doctorate work in chemistry in Paris, Carpentier [1] went on to elucidate the advantages of tissue cross-linking factors—they arrest autolysis, cause neither stiffness nor shrinkage, increase collagen cross-linking and strength, and trigger no significant immunological response [16]. Regarding homografts, Carpentier said that there is "the practical problem of getting enough specimens of different sizes" and that if "the durability of the homograft depends upon the viability of the tissue, the durability of the heterograft depends on the stability of the tissue" [1]. He also mounted valves on a stent, and working with Charles Dubost in 1967, performed the first stented xenograft implant in the mitral position [17]. This represented a major step forward in mitral valve surgery because stented xenograft implants were technically easier to accomplish than aortic homograft implants. Kaiser and Hancock described a heterograft porcine valve treated with glutaraldehyde and mounted on a rigid support frame in 1969 [18]. Two years later Reis and Hancock reported a modification of this valve consisting of a rigid base ring with flexible posts that became commercially available as the Hancock porcine xenograft valve [19]. Edwards Laboratories and Carpentier developed the Carpentier–Edwards bioprosthesis—commercially available from 1976. The current term "bioprosthesis" was coined by Carpentier in 1970 because of its hybrid mechanical and biological nature [1, 20]. Aside from the advantage of being readily available in different sizes, stented tissue valves have a disadvantage in comparison to homografts—they have a smaller orifice and are intrinsically obstructive because of the space occupied by the stent and sewing ring. The next step in biological valve research focused on creating a valve that combined the advantages of stentless homografts and stented bioprostheses. The stentless aortic porcine xenograft, a fully scalloped valve for subcoronary implantation or as a porcine aortic root, met these criteria. Immediate results showed good hemodynamic performance and a low failure, endocarditis, and reoperation rate [21]. Research then shifted to bovine and equine pericardial valves. Industry advances significantly narrowed the hemodynamic differences between stented and stentless valves. Indeed, recent randomized trials show equivalent left ventricular mass regression for both valve types at the 1-year mark, and in the long term. In addition, stentless valves do not afford a superior clinical outcome after 12 years [22].

## 20.3 Mechanical Heart Valves

At the dawn of the prosthetic valve era, prostheses were almost always designed by surgeons. With the passage of time innovative bio-prosthetic and mechanical valve designs arose from research collaborations between surgeons and non-medical scientists. To test valves in the laboratory, sophisticated pulse duplicators were designed to reproduce the physiology and hemodynamics of the cardiac cycle. Detailed investigations into anticoagulation measures and the interaction of blood with prosthetic materials were required. Shape, design, size, volume, strength, durability, biocompatibility, ease of implantation, noise—every aspect was investigated in a swirl of industry competition to describe the optimal valve profile. Initially, mechanical valves attracted the most attention—witness the hundreds of models created at that time vs. today where stented, stentless, trans-catheter, and sutureless biological prostheses claim the spotlight.

Charles Hufnagel created the first mechanical prosthetic heart valve (Fig. 20.1A) in 1952 [23]. Initially, it consisted of a rigid methacrylate tube containing a methacrylate ball and was conceived to treat only aortic insufficiency. The rigid tube was implanted via a left thoracotomy following aortic cross-clamping with a non-suture technique based on fixation rings. The noisy methacrylate was later replaced with a quieter hollow nylon material coated with silicone rubber. Astonishingly these pioneering valves could function for up to three decades with a low thrombogenicity rate despite the absence of anticoagulant therapy. Hufnagel implanted more than 200 valves, demonstrating that foreign material could be permanently implanted in the circulatory system. This concept, nowadays obvious, was altogether novel 60 years ago.

In the second half of the 1950s, flexible fabric valves and single fabric leaflets were created by several researchers. Bahnson used jersey knit Teflon aortic cusps. One to three cusps could be used, but this method, published in 1960, was quickly abandoned because stiffening and degeneration appeared within 24 months [24].

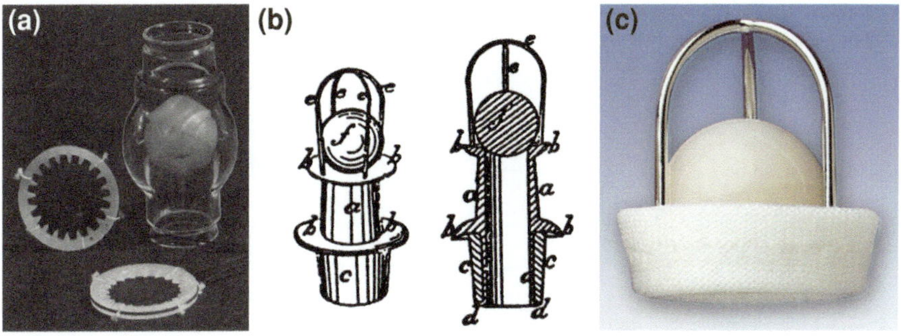


**Fig. 20.1** **a** Hufnagel's prosthesis, the first substitute for the function of a heart valve in the history of medicine. Courtesy of *Annals of Surgery* [40]. **b** William's bottle stopper design of 1858 (US patent No. 19323), which uses the ball and cage principle. **c** A model of caged-ball valve (aortic Starr–Edwards 1260, courtesy of Edwards Lifesciences)

In the CPB era, mechanical heart valves evolved into four different designs: caged ball, non-tilting disk, tilting disk valve, and the bileaflet. In 1958 Albert Starr was an instructor of surgery at the University of Oregon and Lowell Edwards was semi-retired from a brilliant engineering career. Many US military airplanes during World War II were equipped with Edwards's innovations. After retirement, Edwards turned his interest to medical projects—maybe his interest in heart valves arose from his experience with childhood rheumatic fever. A hard worker even as a biomedical engineer, he built a small laboratory next to his summer home—at night his wife often saw the forest trees illuminated by the light from his workshop [25]. A century earlier in 1858, a bottle stopper made from a cage containing a ball (Fig. 20.1B) was patented (US patent No. 19323) and this probably inspired Edwards's ball-and-cage valve design (Fig. 20.1C) [25]. Although his design differed in shape from human valves, Edwards believed that an engineer's goal is to replicate physiological function rather than human morphology. This concept was also embraced by Alain Carpentier in his work on mitral valve repair. Another source of inspiration was a paper published in 1958 by Ellis and Bulbulian, who described a caged ball valve implanted in dogs at the Mayo Clinic [26]. After Chesterman's first attempt at mitral valve replacement (Sheffield, 1955) using a Perspex valve in the patient who survived for 14 h [27], Nina Braunwald [28], Dwight Harken [29], George Magovern [30], and others attempted to implant mechanical mitral valves in humans. At the Chicago conference on prosthetic heart valves in September 1960 [25], many valve designs were on display, some strange and complicated—reminiscent of "man's early attempts to design a flying machine" [31]. By August, Starr had implanted the first Starr–Edwards (SE) valve (a methyl methacrylate cage holding a silicone rubber ball), but the patient died 10 h later [32]. Their second patient, Philip Admunson, received a Teflon and silicone valve on 21 September 1960 [33]. This was the first successful mitral valve replacement in a human patient, and he survived 15 years until a fatal fall from a ladder while painting his house [25]. Since the time of the first mitral valve

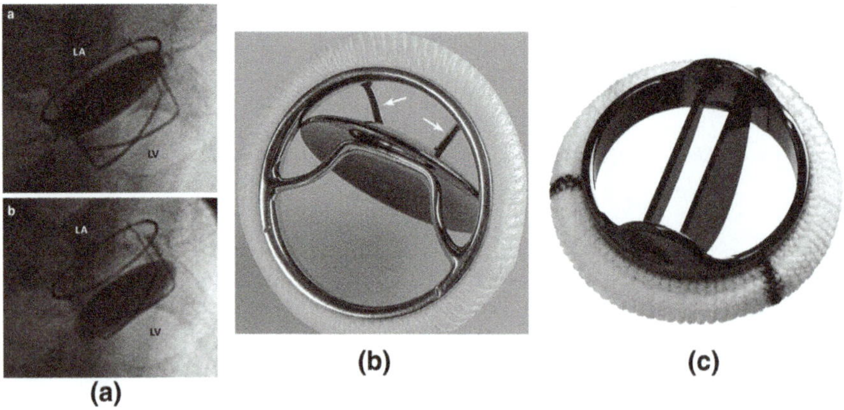


**Fig. 20.2** **a** A model of a non-tilting disk valve during *a* systole and *b* diastole (Harken's mitral valve). From: Hsi et al. [36] (Copyright 2003 by the Texas Heart® Institute, Houston). **b** A model of tilting disk valve (Bjork–Shiley, with convexo-concave disk. *Arrows* indicate sites of fractures (Courtesy of Sorin Group). **c** A model of a bileaflet valve (St. Jude prosthesis. Courtesy of St. Jude Medical)

SE models 6000/6120 and aortic valve SE models 1260/2400, nearly 300,000 valve implants have been done worldwide (although in recent decades only in undeveloped countries). By 2007 production had ceased [34].

The second wave of valve designs arose in the mid- to late 1960s and consisted of a satellite housing a non-tilting flat disk (Fig. 20.2A), i.e., the Kay–ShileyBeall–Surgitol, Cooley–Cutter, and Harken valves [35, 36]. The third design wave, the tilting flat disk valves, appeared in the late 1960s, emanating from the partnership of Swedish surgeon Viking Bjork and American engineer Donald Shiley [37]. Initially, the disk was constructed of Delrin polymer, but Delrin absorbed water and underwent configuration changes—it was replaced by pyrolytic carbon, a material that entered the medical field from the atomic energy industry. Vincent Gott, the co-inventor of the bileaflet Gott–Dagget valve, described a new test for the blood biocompatibility of materials. While casually reading Gott's paper, Jack Bokros, who worked for the General Atomic Company in San Diego, was inspired to test pyrolytic carbon and found that it was very blood biocompatible [35]. Between 1969 and 1986 297,000 Bjork–Shiley pyrolytic carbon flat disk prostheses were implanted in the mitral and aortic positions [38].

To improve the hemodynamics, a convexo-concave pyrolytic carbon disk was created, and the inlet and outlet struts were modified. The disk slid forward and down about 2 mm to enlarge the lesser valve orifice. This model was used from 1975 to 1986, during which time 86,000 valves were implanted [38]. Unfortunately, patients with the 29, 31, and 33 mm sizes suffered a 12% failure incidence, mainly because of strut fractures, in the 7-year post-operative interval and so valve production was eventually discontinued (Fig. 20.2B). Patients with the larger valves and the convexo-concave disks became candidates for prophylactic replacement [38].

The bileaflet valves were the fourth and final group of mechanical prostheses (Fig. 20.2C). Bhagabant Kalke, an Indian researcher working in Lillehei's laboratory, was inspired by the design of Indian tidal floodgates, which open with the outgoing tide and close with the incoming tide [38]. He conceived a valve with peripheral hinging leaflets and a central opening. This Kalke–Lillehei valve appeared in 1968 and was one of the first bileaflet designs [39]. The St. Jude was the first bileaflet prosthesis used on a large scale. Created by engineer Xinon Posis, surgeon Demetre Nicholoff, and Manuel Villafana, the founder of Cardiac Pacemaker Inc., it was named in honor of St. Jude Thaddeus, the patron of difficult cases—Villafana's son was recovering from a serious illness at the time [35].

From bottle stoppers to highly innovative designs, the evolution of prosthetic heart valves is a story of benefits for humanity emerging from intensive research—original ideas triggered chain reactions of thought and inquiry that, despite initial obstacles, led to safer devices and new therapeutic options.

## References

1. Westaby S, Bosher C (1997) Development of surgery for valvular heart disease. In: Landmarks in cardiac surgery. Isis medical media, Oxford, pp 139–174
2. Murray G, Roschlau W, Lougheed W (1956) Homologous aortic-valve-segment transplants as surgical treatment for aortic and mitral insufficiency. Angiology 7:466
3. Murray G (1960) Aortic valve transplants. Angiology 11:99
4. Beall ACJ, Morris GJ, Cooley D, De Bakey M (1961) Homotransplantation of the aortic valve. J Thorac Cardiovasc Surg 42:497
5. Heimbecker Ro, Baird RJ, Lajos TZ, Varga AT, Greenwood WF (1962) Homograft replacement of the human mitral valve. A preliminary report. Can Med Assoc J 5(86):805–809
6. Duran CG, Gunning AJ (1962) A method for placing a total homologous aortic valve in the subcoronary position. Lancet 2(7254):488–489
7. Shumacker HBJ (1992) The evolution of cardiac surgery. Indiana University Press, Bloomington
8. Weldon CS, Ameli MM, Morovati SS, Shaker IJ (1966) A prosthetic stented aortic homograft for mitral valve replacement. J Surg Res 6(12):548–552
9. Senning A (1967) Fascia lata replacement of aortic valves. J Thorac Cardiovasc Surg 54(4):465–470
10. Ionescu MI, Ross DN (1969) Heart-valve replacement with autologous fascia lata. Lancet 2(7616):335–338
11. Ross DN (1962) Homograft replacement of the aortic valve. Lancet 2:487
12. Lower RR, Stofer RC, Shumway NE (1961) Total excision of the mitral valve and replacement with the autologous pulmonic valve. J Thorac Cardiovasc Surg 42:696–702
13. Duran CG, Gunning AJ (1965) Heterologous aortic-valve transplantation in the dog. Lancet 1(7403):114–115
14. Binet JP, Carpentier A, Langlois J, Duran C, Colvez P (1965) Implantation of heterogenic valves in the treatment of aortic cardiopathies. C R Acad Sci Hebd Seances Acad Sci D 261(25):5733–5734 (in French)
15. Binet JP, Carpentier A, Langlois J (1966) Heterologous transplantation of the aortic valve. Langenbecks Arch Chir 316:800–802
16. Carpentier A, Lemaigre G, Robert L, Carpentier S, Dubost C (1969) Biological factors affecting long-term results of valvular heterografts. J Thorac Cardiovasc Surg 58(4):467–483

17. Carpentier A, Chanard JC, Laurens P, Guéry J, Harada H, Laurent D, Dubost C (1967) Use of aortic heterografts in treatment of mitral valvulopathy experimental basis and 1st clinical case. Mem Acad Chir 93(19):617–622
18. Kaiser GA, Hancock WD, Lukban SB, Litwak RS (1969) Clinical use of a new design stented xenograft heart valve prosthesis. Surg Forum. 20:137–138
19. Reis RL, Hancock WD, Yarbrough JW, Glancy DL, Morrow AG (1971) The flexible stent. A new concept in the fabrication of tissue heart valve prostheses. J Thorac Cardiovasc Surg 62(5):683–689
20. Black MM, Drury PJ, Tindale WBJ (1983) Twenty-five years of heart valve substitutes: a review. R Soc Med. 76(8):667–680
21. Stelzer PI (2008) Stentless aortic valve replacement: porcine and pericardial. In: Cohn LH (ed) Cardiac surgery in the adult. McGraw-Hill, New York, pp 915–934
22. Cohen G, Zagorski B, Christakis GT, Joyner CD, Vincent J, Sever J, Harbi S, Feder-Elituv R, Moussa F, Goldman BS, Fremes SE (2010) Are stentless valves hemodynamically superior to stented valves? Long-term follow-up of a randomized trial comparing Carpentier-Edwards pericardial valve with the Toronto stentless porcine valve. J Thorac Cardiovasc Surg 139(4):848–859
23. Hufnagel CA, Harvey WP, Rabil PJ, McDermott TF (1954) Surgical correction of aortic insufficiency. Surgery. 35(5):673–683
24. Bahnson HT, Spencer FC, Busse EF, Davis FW (1960) Cusp replacement and coronary artery perfusion in open operations on the aortic valve. Ann Surg 152(3):494–503
25. Matthews AM (1998) The development of the Starr-Edwards heart valve. Tex Heart Inst J 25(4):282–293
26. Ellis FH Jr, Bulbulian AH (1958) Prosthetic replacement of the mitral valve. I. Preliminary experimental observations. Proc Staff Meet Mayo Clin 33(21):532–534a
27. Norman AF (1991) The first mitral valve replacement. Ann Thorac Surg 51(3):525–526
28. Braunwald E (2001) Nina Starr Braunwald: some reflections on the first woman heart surgeon. Ann Thorac Surg 71 [2 Suppl]:S6–S7
29. Harken DE (1965) I A new caged-ball aortic and mitral valve. II. Monitoring and controlled respiration in critically ill patients. J Mt Sinai Hosp N Y 32:93–106
30. Magovern GJ, Cromie HW (1963) Sutureless prosthetic heart valves. J Thorac Cardiovasc Surg 46:726–736
31. Anonymous (1980) 20th Anniversary: The Starr-Edwards heart valve prosthesis. Ed-words 10(6):4–6
32. Pluth JR (1991) The Starr valve revisited. Ann Thorac Surg 51(2):333–334
33. Starr A, Edwards ML (1961) Mitral replacement: clinical experience with a ball-valve prosthesis. Ann Surg 154:726–740
34. Artificial heart valve. http://en.wikipedia.org/wiki/Artificial_heart_valve
35. DeWall RA, Qasim N, Carr L (2000) Evolution of mechanical heart valves. Ann Thorac Surg 69(5):1612–1621
36. Hsi DH, Ryan GF, Taft J, Arnone TJ (2003) A 29-year-old Harken disk mitral valve: long-term follow-up by echocardiographic and cineradiographic imaging. Tex Heart Inst J 30(4):319–321
37. Björk VO (1970) The central flow tilting disc valve prosthesis (Björk-Shiley) for mitral valve replacement. Scand J Thorac Cardiovasc Surg 4(1):15–23
38. Gott VL, Alejo DE, Cameron DE (2003) Mechanical heart valves: 50 years of evolution. Ann Thorac Surg 76(6):S2230–S2239
39. Lillehei CW, Nakib A, Kaster RL, Kalke BR, Rees JR (1989) The origin and development of three new mechanical valvemechanical valve designs: toroidal disc, pivoting disc, and rigid bileaflet cardiac prostheses. Ann Thorac Surg 48 [3 Suppl]:S35–S37
40. Hufnagel CA, Villegas PD, Nahas H (1958) Experiences with new types of aortic valvular prostheses. Ann Surg 147(5):636–644

# 21 The History of Research on Mitral, Tricuspid, and Aortic Valve Repair After the Advent of Cardiopulmonary Bypass

Ruggero De Paulis, Andrea Salica, Raffaele Scaffa and Luca Weltert

*When you're finished changing you're finished.*
Benjamin Franklin

**Abstract**
This chapter focuses on the history of research on mitral, aortic and tricuspid valve repair after the advent of cardiopulmonary bypass. Starting from the first findings in the early Fifties, the authors describe the most important steps in surgical research made during the decades, and the improvement of techniques.

## 21.1 The Mitral Valve

Gibbon in 1953 closed an inter-atrial septal defect with a total cardiopulmonary support using a pump screen oxygenator and thus began the era of open-heart surgery [1]and the birth of modern cardiac surgery. Clear vision allowed a direct approach to the mitral valve and laid the basis for developing valve replacement and valve repair techniques. Since the beginning of mitral valve surgery, the annulus had played a pivotal role in mitral valve repair and was the target of the first procedures. In 1957 Wooler et al. [2] repaired mitral valve regurgitation, reducing the length of the mural annulus with an asymmetric mattress suture through the commissural portion of the mitral valve annulus. In the same period Kay and Reed [3] proposed a similar procedure. These techniques were based on mattress sutures placed on the commissural area of the annulus and tied to obtain a reduction of the mitral orifice. Gerbode et al. in 1962 developed the first posterior

R. De Paulis (✉) · A. Salica · R. Scaffa · L. Weltert
Cardiac Surgery Department, European Hospital, Rome, Italy
e-mail: depauli@tin.it

M. Picichè (ed.), *Dawn and Evolution of Cardiac Procedures*,
DOI: 10.1007/978-88-470-2400-7_21, 

annular reduction performing a segmental plication of a single portion of the mural annulus at the level of a quadrangular excision of the posterior leaflet [4]. Paneth and Burr proposed a semi-circular reduction of the posterior annulus performing a running suture all along the mural annulus tied between the commissures [5]. These techniques were the first steps in mitral repair surgery, but produced inconsistent results. After valve prostheses were developed, the problem of valve disease appeared to be solved and for a while the repair techniques were somehow forgotten. Later on, Alain Carpentier introduced the "French correction" (1983), a fundamental step into the future of valve repair [6]. He described a new approach to the mitral valve based on a systematic approach to mitral lesions and suggested the principles of mitral repair. The main contribution was the classification of mitral valve lesions based on a "functional approach". This functional approach led to a simplification of mitral diseases where the lesions, based on leaflet motion, were divided into three types: Type 1, normal leaflet motion (leaflet perforation, annulus dilatation); type 2, excessive leaflet motion (mitral valve prolapse, Barlow's syndrome, fibro-elastic deficiency); type 3, restricted leaflet motion (mitral apparatus fusion, rheumatic disease, functional ischemic mitral dysfunction). In 1971, Carpentier also introduced the use of a rigid ring as a fundamental tool to restrict and reshape the mitral annulus, reduce tension on leaflets, and guarantee long-term results. Ring implantation was performed with a series of sutures placed through the entire mitral annulus circumference and then through the sewing in such a way as to proportionally reduce the valve area. An important aspect was the choice of the ring size, based on the area of the anterior leaflet of the mitral valve. These concepts have stood the test of time and ring annuloplasty remains a gold standard in mitral valve repair independently from the etiology of the disease. Apart from the use of a ring, Carpentier's contribution is also related to repair techniques. Quadrangular resection of the posterior leaflet (associated when necessary to a sliding plasty) is still the most widely accepted mitral repair procedure for posterior leaflet prolapse with excellent long-term follow-up; other more complex techniques like chordal transposition, chordal shortening and triangular resection have demonstrated inconsistent results. As an example, while chordal shortening showed unsatisfactory results at follow-up, chordal transposition demonstrated superior results, but it was considered a less reproducible technique. Parallel to Carpentier's proposal other reliable options were developed. In 1976, Duran introduced a flexible prosthetic ring to maintain annular motion during systolic contraction and to improve hemodynamic performance of the mitral valve during the cardiac cycle [7]. Flexible rings are still used in degenerative mitral diseases and the choice depends on the surgeon's preference. With time mitral repair has been shown to be superior to valve replacement in terms of survival and quality of life. The number of valve repairs has significantly increased and newer techniques have been developed. The use of Goretex to replace mitral chordae is certainly one of the major advances in the "second era" of mitral repair. Although efforts to find a substitute for elongated or ruptured chordae date back to the 1960s by January et al. [8] and Frater et al. [9] with the use of a "00" suture and autologous pericardium respectively, not until 1985 were ePTFE neo-chordae introduced into clinical practice [10]. Usually, an ePTFE suture is placed through the papillary muscle and then through the free margin of the prolapsed leaflet at the level of an elongated or ruptured chorda. After almost 20 years of use, neochordae implantation has shown good results for both posterior and anterior leaflet prolapse or flail [11]. Quite recently, in 1998, Alfieri and colleagues described a simple and reliable technique for treating anterior leaflet and bileaflet prolapse, creating a double-mitral orifice by anchoring with a suture the free edge of the prolapsing leaflet to the corresponding free edge of the opposite leaflet [12]. This technique, originally proposed for degenerative and functional regurgitation, has shown satisfactory results and is still a widely accepted option especially where other techniques have failed or appear difficult to apply. During the last decade several different ring designs have been introduced into the armamentarium of the cardiac surgeon. The original "classic" Carpentier ring was flat and rigid. Better knowledge of the mitral motion during the cardiac cycle has suggested the use of a ring with selective flexibility and a slight three-dimensional shape to better conform to the normal mitral annulus [13]. Open bands are also used with the consideration that the anterior portion of the mitral annulus is not, in fact, a true annulus, and that it does not dilate with time. Despite a more "normal" valve physiology, superior long-term clinical results with these rings or bands still need to be demonstrated. The most recent annuloplasty rings are somehow disease-specific and are shaped according to the underlying mitral pathology. A newer attitude based on respecting more than resecting the prolapsed segment of the valve is challenging the classic, basic concepts of mitral repair. New surgical approaches are appearing aiming at respecting the leaflet's tissue [14].

## 21.2 The Tricuspid Valve

The tricuspid valve (TV) has not received as much attention as the aortic or mitral valve, and lately has been referred to as the "forgotten valve". Almost 50 years have elapsed since the paper *The TV: A surgical challenge* pointed out the difficulty in the decision-making process and treatment of this right-sided valve [15]. Recently, it appeared evident that this valve was poorly understood at the time and had probably been left undertreated more than necessary. Tricuspid regurgitation (TR) is not a rare entity. Mostly, it is secondary to left-sided heart pathology, especially in mitral valve disease with the consequent pulmonary hypertension, right ventricular dilatation, and then tricuspid annular dilatation, in addition to tethering of the leaflets. In most cases of functional TR, the orifice dilatation is practically limited to the part of the annulus corresponding to the free wall of the right ventricle. In 15–30 % of the cases it may be organic and related to direct involvement of the TV by the rheumatic disease, infective endocarditis, trauma, and diffuse collagen disease. Whichever the type, TR has a significant impact on the clinical condition and the medium and long-term prognosis of the patients. Hence, it requires special consideration and a more aggressive treatment when associated with mitral and/or aortic valve surgery [16]. Despite a growing body of literature, controversy remains regarding the choice of repair versus valve replacement, the efficacy of different methods of annuloplasty, and the type of prosthesis to implant. Replacement of the TV is currently reserved for those rare occasions where the valve is no longer amenable to repair. Despite advances in surgery and peri-operative care, morbidity and mortality of TV replacement remain high, indicating that patients requiring TV replacement represent a high-risk group [17]. The choice of the prosthesis remains a subject of debate [18]. Several surgical approaches have been described for the repair of TV from the very simple economical "magic stitch" to various types and forms of rings. The goal of tricuspid repair is to reduce annular dilatation and lessen TV leaflet tethering, thereby stabilizing the annulus and increasing leaflet coaptation. Actually, in 1965, Kay was the first author to apply a reconstructive surgical technique for TR [19]. The operation consisted of creating a bicuspid valve by excluding the posterior leaflet with a consequent annular reduction. However, such a technique does not act on the anterior portion of the annulus, failing to prevent a possible subsequent dilatation of the anterior annulus. The De Vega [20] technique was introduced in 1972 in Madrid. It consists of two semi-circular sutures along the anterior and lateral portions of the TV, tied on both sides on pledgets over a 28- or 30-mm dilatator to avoid the purse string effect. It does not require prosthetic material, maintains annular flexibility and reduces the potential for conduction system injury. It is one of the most effective methods used in surgical correction of functional TR and has since been modified by others. In 1972 Cabrol described a similar technique ("over and over" suture) [21]. However, excessive tension on a continuous and single suture can cause recurrent TR owing to the bowstring or "guitar-string" phenomenon. Antunes and Girdwood [22] in 1983 incorporated Teflon pledgets into each stitch of the double suture to protect the outside surface of the endocardium. Revuelta and Garcia-Rinaldi's [23] technique was described in 1989, and consisted of the use of interrupted sutures bolstered in Teflon pledgets and placed around the posterior and anterior segments of the tricuspid annulus. This segmental tricuspid annuloplasty avoids tearing of the suture from the tricuspid annulus, "guitar-string valve incompetence," which leads to failure of De Vega annuloplasty early after surgery. Other techniques for TV repair include the use of customized semicircular annuloplasty using bovine pericardium [24] or autologous fixed pericardial C-shaped strip [25]. Basing his technique on pathological anatomical studies, Carpentier presented a remodeling semi-rigid prosthetic tricuspid ring annuloplasty to reconstruct the native valve geometry and selectively reduce the pathological dilatation of the posterior and anterior parts of the tricuspid annulus in 1974 [26]. Duran introduced a flexible prosthetic ring in 1975 to allow physiological motion of the tricuspid annulus during the cardiac cycle [7]. Nonetheless, most TV repairs are still either suture-based or done with rings originally conceived for mitral valve repair (e.g., the Cosgrove–Edwards flexible band) [27]. Newer three-dimensional rings mimicking the shape of the tricuspid annulus are now available [28]. Indeed, the work of several authors has shown that prosthetic annuloplasty guarantees less recurrent TR and is more durable than annular plication and suture annuloplasty. In recent years other techniques have been proposed: the edge-to-edge "Clover" technique, performed by suturing the free margins of the tricuspid leaflets in conjunction with ring annuloplasty [29]; anterior tricuspid leaflet augmentation, to increase leaflet coaptation and relief of tethered leaflets [30]; and a right ventricular reduction technique to plicate the wall by placement of two strips of felt on the epicardial surface. This method reduces the right ventricular cavity and approximates the papillary muscles [31]. Despite a half-century of experience in heart valve reconstruction, the TV has been considered a "second class structure" in cardiac surgery. Modern cardiac reconstructive surgery is paying more attention to this valve pathology with the surgical indication based more on the annular enlargement than on the degree of valve regurgitation.

## 21.3 The Aortic Valve

The concept of aortic valve repair has been present since the beginning of cardiac surgery. In the early 1950s aortic insufficiency presented sometimes as a complication of atrial defect repair, thus facing surgeons with unprecedented challenge. Some pioneers reported successful repair of aortic regurgitation owing to valvular fenestration and relief of aortic stenosis by means of commissural cuts and leaflet sculpturing. However, during the following years, while valve repair technique were continuously pursued in pediatric surgery, further refinements of repair techniques in the adult were somehow dampened by the development of artificial heart valve prostheses. As a consequence, aortic valve plasty was only considered for minimal organic lesions associated with other pathologies like infra-valvular stenosis. In the early 1980s, as trials of percutaneous aortic valve dilatation failed to consistently treat the aortic stenosis, it was also evident that valve prostheses were far from being perfect, leading to a long series of studies on structure–stress relations [32]. The concept of conservative treatment was therefore fueled again. Duran was one of the few constant believers of the efficacy of aortic valve conservative treatment, and the review of his work since 1974 established the basis for a systematic approach to aortic valve plasty. In his review [33], published in 1988, he identifies four possible procedures: commissurotomy, annuloplasty, cusp free edge unfolding, and supra-aortic crest enhancement. Even though at that time Duran was not alone in the realm of reconstructive aortic surgery, his vision was by far the more advanced, while other's experience was substantially limited to commissurotomy and decalcification, which were already well established long before [34]. His encouraging preliminary results led to a steep increase in the numbers of treated patients: if between 1974 and 1984 only 50 patients underwent conservative treatment, between 1988 and 1990 nearly half of his aortic valve operations were made conservatively. During the same period Cosgrove started a program of aortic valve conservative treatment for aortic regurgitation. His approach was directed at isolated valvular defects and he illustrated widely the technique of triangular resection of the free margin and the concept of lunula and interleaflet triangles and their role in a proper leaflet coaptation [35]. The 1990s brought to the attention the possibility of treating aortic insufficiency whenever it was due to aneurysmatic aortic pathology. In a short period of time two types of valve sparing were described: the remodeling technique proposed by Sarsam and Yacoub [36] and the reimplantation technique as introduced by David [37]. Both techniques used a Dacron graft to replace the whole aorta while sparing a normally functioning aortic valve. This new surgical approach raised interest in a better understanding of the aortic valve–aortic root relationship, both structurally and dynamically. Nonetheless, although it took almost a decade for these techniques to become standard practice, they also had the merit to fuel again interest in aortic valve repair. However, despite the interest, the vast majority of cardiac surgeons did not routinely perform aortic valve repair, as brilliantly depicted by Antunes in his late 1990s review *Aortic valve repair: still a dream?* [38]. Pericardium, either bovine or autologous, was found to be a good option for semilunar valves at the dawn of the new millennium. In 2002 both the French school of Carpentier [39] and the German school of Schäfers [40] suggested aortic cusp extension as a viable, standardized technique to treat either rheumatic aortic valve regurgitation or leaflet prolapse. Increased use of valve-sparing procedures continued to enlarge the experience of leaflet evaluation and of initial leaflet repair. By 2004 the first review of aortic valve repair was published in a major journal [41] and, most importantly, valve repair was compared with aortic valve replacement to evaluate whether it could be considered as a surgical option. A few months later another review of 160 patients operated on at the Mayo Clinic concluded that the repair of aortic valve regurgitation was a safe alternative to replacement. At the same time other emerging sites revealed their systematic approach and results: the Belgian School, under the guide of El Khoury [42] and the German school, under the guide of Schäfers [43]. The approach was becoming more technical and less artistic, trying to systematically analyze the organic valve lesion and tailoring the surgical treatment to each individual lesion. Both groups came to the same overall conclusions, that aortic valve repair was feasible even for complex mechanisms of aortic regurgitation with a systematic and individually tailored approach. With a low incidence of mortality and morbidity, for the first time aortic valve repair gained competitive status against valve replacement. At the same time, in 2005, Kumar and colleagues published the long-term follow-up studies of repairs of aortic stenosis with rheumatic causes, which also showed satisfactory results [44], thus demonstrating that this sort of repair had finally found success beyond Duran's single-center experience. In the following years the first reports on repairing a bicuspid valve were published [45]. The increasing diffusion of valve-sparing aortic root procedures led to a valuable knowledge increase, helping the approach to valve repair in cases of valve regurgitation without root dilatation; in both situations efficacy and durability showed comparable results [46]. Unlike the experience in a pediatric population, the pericardial patch extension for leaflet repair appeared to be a viable alternative in adults [47] where a similar rate of calcification was found in native valve tissue and in the pericardium used for the repair. Once the feasibility of the technique was established, the Belgian School followed the path of reproducibility, questioning some key points to make the procedure available to the average surgeon: accuracy and prediction of surgical repair ability via evaluation of functional anatomy by transesophageal echocardiography. Similar to Carpentier's theory at the time of the "French Correction" they distinguished three kind of mechanisms: type 1, normal leaflet motion, where the cause is the dilatation of the root at various levels; type 2, enhanced leaflet motion where the cause is mainly a cusp prolapse; and type 3, restrictive cusp motion, which is present often due to rheumatic or post-infective disease. A similar but more complex classification was also proposed by Lansac and colleagues along with a systematic approach to the various lesions of leaflet and root [48]. In late 2008 the efficacy of Goretex suspension for the treatment of cusp prolapse [49] was established and, compared with the now standard plication technique, it was found to be equally satisfactory in terms of duration. Recently, a series of articles re-proposed the old-fashioned techniques, like basal cusp enlargement, or cusp shaving for rheumatic insufficiency, or approached more complex anatomical situations like the extensive fenestration in myxomatous degeneration. Treatment of aortic regurgitation has now reached maturity, and only more experience will tell us whether the overwhelming success of conservative mitral surgery will be repeated.

## References


1. Gibbon JH Jr (1953) Application of a mechanical heart and lung apparatus to cardiac surgery, recent advance in cardiovascular physiology and surgery. University of Minnesota, Minneapolis, pp 107–113
2. Wooler GH, Nixon PGF, Grimshow VA, Watson DA (1962) Experiences with the repair of mitral valve in mitral incompetence. Thorax 17:49–57
3. Reed GE, Tice DA, Clauss RH (1965) Asymmetric exaggerated mitral annuloplasty: repair of mitral insufficiency with hemodynamic predictability. J Thorac Cardiovasc Surg 49:752–761
4. Gerbode F, Kerth WJ, Osborn JJ, Selzer A (1962) Correction of mitral insufficiency by open operation. Ann Surg 155:846–854
5. Burr LH, Krayenbuhl C, Sutton MS (1977) The mitral plication suture: a new technique of mitral valve repair. J Thorac Cardiovasc Surg 73:589–595
6. Carpentier A (1983) Cardiac valve surgery—the French correction. J Thorac Cardiovasc Surg 86:323–337
7. Duran CG, Ubago JLM (1976) Clinical and hemodynamics performance of a totally flexible prosthetic ring for atrioventricular valve reconstruction. Ann Thorac Surg 22:458–463
8. January LE, Fisher JM, Ehrenhaft JL (1962) Mitral insufficiency resulting from rupture of normal chordae tendineae. Report of a surgically corrected case. Circulation 26:1329–1333
9. Frater RW, Berghuis J, Brown AL Jr, Ellis FH Jr (1965) The experimental and clinical use of autogenous pericardium for the replacement and extension of mitral and tricuspid valve cusps and chordae. J Cardiovasc Surg (Torino) 6:215–228
10. David TE, Bos J, Rakowski H (1991) Mitral valve repair by replacement of chordate tendinae with polytetrafluoroethylene sutures. J Thorac Cardiovasc Surg 101:495–501

11. Salvador L, Mirone S, Bianchini R, Regesta T, Patelli F, Minniti G, Masat M, Cavarretta E, Valfrè C (2008) A 20-year experience with mitral valve repair with artificial chordae in 608 patients. J Thorac Cardiovasc Surg 135:1280–1287
12. Maisano F, Torracca L, Oppizzi M, Stefano PL, D'Addario G, La Canna G, Zogno M, Alfieri O (1998) The double orifice technique, a simplified method to correct mitral insufficiency. Eur J Cardiothorac Surg 13:240–246
13. Fedak PW, McCarthy PM, Bonow RO (2008) Evolving concepts and technologies in mitral valve repair. Circulation 117:963–974
14. Perier P, Hohenberger W, Lakew F, Batz G, Urbanski P, Zacher M, Diegeler A (2008) Toward a new paradigm for the reconstruction of posterior leaflet prolapse: midterm results of the "respect rather than resect" approach. Ann Thorac Surg 86:718–725
15. Grodin D, Lepage G, Castonguay Y, Meere C (1967) The tricuspid valve: a surgical challenge. J Thorac Cardiovasc Surg 53:7–20
16. Dreyfus GD, Corbi PJ, Chan KMJ et al (2005) Secondary tricuspid regurgitation or dilatation: which should be the criteria for surgical repair? Ann Thorac Surg 79:127–132
17. Topilsky Y, Khanna AD, Oh JK, Nishimura RA, Enriquez-Sarano M, Jeon YB, Sundt TM, Schaff HV, Park SJ (2011) Preoperative factors associated with adverse outcome after tricuspid valve replacement. Circulation 123(18):1929–1939
18. Rizzoli G, Vendramin I, Nesseris G, Bottio T, Guglielmi C, Schiavon L (2004) Biological or mechanical prostheses in tricuspid position? A meta-analysis of intra-institutional results. Ann Thorac Surg 77:1607–1614
19. Kay JH, Maselli-Campagna G, Tsuji HK (1965) Surgical treatment of tricuspid insufficiency. Ann Surg 162:53–58
20. De Vega NG (1972) La anuloplastia selective, regulable y permanente. Rev Esp Cardiol 25:555–556
21. Cabrol C (1972) Annuloplastie valvulaire: un nouveau procede. Nouv Press Med 1:1366
22. Antunes MJ, Girdwood RW (1983) Tricuspid annuloplasty: a modified technique. Ann Thorac Surg 35:676–678
23. Revuelta JM, Garcia-Rinaldi R (1989) Segmental tricuspid annuloplasty: a new technique. J Thorac Cardiovasc Surg 97:799–801
24. McCarthy PM, Bhudia SK, Rajeswaran J, Hoercher KJ, Lytle BW, Cosgrove DM, Blackstone EH (2004) Tricuspid valve repair: durability and risk factors for failure. J Thorac Cardiovasc Surg 127:674–685
25. Mohsen MO, Aziz Eglal Abd El, Salam Mustafa Abd El, Ramadan M (2002) Tricuspid annuloplasty with autologous fixed pericardial C-shaped strip: early and late results. J Egypt Soc Cardiothorac Surg 10(2):2001–2013
26. Carpentier A, Deloche A, Hanania G, Forman J, Sellier P, Piwnica A et al (1974) Surgical management of acquired tricuspid valve disease. J Thorac Cardiovasc Surg 67:53–65
27. Cosgrove DM 3rd, Arcidi JM, Rodriguez L, Stewart WJ, Powell K, Thomas JD (1995) Initial experience with the Cosgrove-Edwards annuloplasty system. Ann Thorac Surg 60:499–503; discussion 504
28. Filsoufi F, Salzberg SP, Coutu M, Adams DH (2006) A three-dimensional ring annuloplasty for the treatment of tricuspid regurgitation. Ann Thorac Surg 81:2273–2277
29. Lapenna E, De Bonis M, Verzini A et al (2010) The Clover technique for the treatment of complex tricuspid valve insufficiency: midterm clinical and echocardiographic results in 66 patients. Eur J Cardiothorac Surg 37:1297–1303
30. Dreyfus GD, Raja SG, John Chan KM (2008) Tricuspid leaflet augmentation to address severe tethering in functional tricuspid regurgitation. Eur J Cardiothorac Surg 34:908–910
31. Kappert U, Tugtekin SM, Ouda A et al (2008) Right ventricular reduction as an adjunct procedure in tricuspid valve repair. Ann Thorac Surg 85:e27–e29
32. Deck JD, Thubrikar MJ, Schneider PJ, Nolan SP (1988) Structure, stress, and tissue repair in aortic valve leaflets. Cardiovasc Res 22(1):7–16

33. Duran CG (1988) Reconstructive techniques for rheumatic aortic valve disease. J Card Surg 3(1):23–28
34. Shapira N, Lemole GM, Fernandez J, Daily PO, Dembitsky WP, O'Yek V, Haghighi P, Stewart J, Marsh DG, Bloor CM (1990) Aortic valve repair for aortic stenosis in adults. Ann Thorac Surg 50(1):110–120
35. Cosgrove DM, Rosenkranz ER, Hendren WG, Bartlett JC, Stewart WJ (1991) Valvuloplasty for aortic insufficiency. J Thorac Cardiovasc Surg 102(4):571–576; discussion 576–577
36. Sarsam MA, Yacoub M (1993) Remodeling of the aortic valve anulus. J Thorac Cardiovasc Surg 105(3):435–438
37. David TE (1994) Aortic valve repair in patients with Marfan syndrome and ascending aorta aneurysms due to degenerative disease. J Card Surg 9 [Suppl 2]:182–187
38. Antunes MJ (1997) Aortic valve repair: still a dream? Eur J Cardiothorac Surg 11(2):266–267
39. Grinda JM, Latremouille C, Berrebi AJ, Zegdi R, Chauvaud S, Carpentier AF, Fabiani JN, Deloche A (2002) Aortic cusp extension valvuloplasty for rheumatic aortic valve disease: midterm results. Ann Thorac Surg 74(2):438–443
40. discussion S1792–S1799
41. Carr JA, Savage EB (2004) Aortic valve repair for aortic insufficiency in adults: a contemporary review and comparison with replacement techniques. Eur J Cardiothorac Surg 25(1):6–15
42. El Khoury G, Vanoverschelde JL, Glineur D, Poncelet A, Verhelst R, Astarci P, Underwood MJ, Noirhomme P (2004) Repair of aortic valve prolapse: experience with 44 patients. Eur J Cardiothorac Surg 26(3):628–633
43. Langer F, Aicher D, Kissinger A, Wendler O, Lausberg H, Fries R, Schäfers HJ (2004) Aortic valve repair using a differentiated surgical strategy. Circulation 110 [11 Suppl 1]:267–273
44. Talwar S, Saikrishna C, Saxena A, Kumar AS (2005) Aortic valve repair for rheumatic aortic valve disease. Ann Thorac Surg 79(6):1921–1925
45. El Khoury G, Vanoverschelde JL, Glineur D, Pierard F, Verhelst RR, Rubay J, Funken JC, Watremez C, Astarci P, Lacroix V, Poncelet A, Noirhomme P (2006) Repair of bicuspid aortic valves in patients with aortic regurgitation. Circulation 114 [Suppl 1]:1610–1616
46. Lausberg HF, Aicher D, Kissinger A, Langer F, Fries R, Schäfers HJ (2006) Valve repair in aortic regurgitation without root dilatation—aortic valve repair. Thorac Cardiovasc Surg 54(1):15–20
47. De La Zerda DJ, Cohen O, Fishbein MC, Odim J, A Calderon C, Hekmat D, Dinov I, Laks H (2007) Aortic valve-sparing repair with autologous pericardial leaflet extension has a greater early re-operation rate in congenital versus acquired valve disease. Eur J Cardiothorac Surg 31(2):256–260
48. Lansac E, Di Centa I, Raoux F, Al Attar N, Acar C, Joudinaud T, Raffoul RA (2008) Lesional classification to standardize surgical management of aortic insufficiency towards valve repair. Eur J Cardiothorac Surg 33(5):872–878; discussion 878–880
49. de Kerchove L, Glineur D, Poncelet A, Boodhwani M, Rubay J, Dhoore W, Noirhomme P, El Khoury G (2008) Repair of aortic leaflet prolapse: a ten-year experience. Eur J Cardiothorac Surg 34(4):785–791

# History of Research on Myocardial Protection

# 22

Victor S. Costache, Cristian Martu, Nicolas Chavanis, Jean Philippe Frieh and Serban Stoica

*I only admire those who create as if a thousand years of peace wait ahead of our world.*

Mircea Eliade

**Abstract**

Since the early beginnings of cardiac surgery defining the ideal strategy for optimal myocardial protection became the new quest for the Holy Grail for cardiac surgeons worldwide. It was a quest rich in promising hypotheses that often became obsolete and criticised in order only to be readopted a few years later, not only by surgeons, but also by various researchers involved in cardiac physiology and pharmacology. The history of myocardial protection evolved in parallel with the development of new surgical techniques and with the advances in cardiopulmonary bypass that allowed increasingly safe cardiac surgery to be performed. The term myocardial protection includes an entire universe of pharmacological protocols, cardioplegic solutions with their various ways of administration, proper systemic and myocardial temperature control, backed by various devices (intra-aortic balloon pumps, ECLS), and optimal haemodynamic management. However, despite millions of patients operated on worldwide and hundreds of papers published on the subject, there is no universally accepted strategy for myocardial protection. In this chapter we intend to present the birth and the evolution of cardioplegic solutions with their various ways of administration, the existing alternative strategies and how to integrate all these concepts into the era of minimally invasive surgery.

V. S. Costache (✉) · C. Martu · N. Chavanis · J. P. Frieh
Cardiac Surgery, Centre Hospitalier de la Region d'Annecy, Metz Tessy, France
e-mail: victorscostache@gmail.com

S. Stoica
Cardiac Surgery, University Hospitals Bristol, Bristol, UK

M. Picichè (ed.), *Dawn and Evolution of Cardiac Procedures*,
DOI: 10.1007/978-88-470-2400-7_22, © Springer-Verlag Italia 2013

## 22.1 Advances in Physiology

Understanding cardiac physiology was one of the main points of interest, together with simultaneous research into pharmacology and cell biology. Despite significant advances in this field at the end of the 19th and the beginning of the 20th century, the step from laboratory research to the operating room was longer than in other surgical specialties, probably because the entire scientific and medical community was still under the shock after Theodore Billroth's statement that "any surgeon who wishes to preserve the respect of his colleagues, would never attempt to suture the heart."

However, in parallel with important discoveries in microbiology by Pasteur and Koch, the 19th century physiologist Otto Frank achieves a good understanding of cardiac muscle mechanisms while Starling publishes his theories on homeostasis [1] and on the regulation of cardiac energy output [2].

In the same period, Carl Friedrich Wilhelm Ludwig, a German physician, developed groundbreaking techniques for the study of isolated organs. His legacy, dating back to as early as the 1860s, inspired his collaborators from Leipzig and later on Sydney Ringer in London to continue the research into the actions of inorganic salts on isolated hearts and showed the effects of various ions on heart rhythm [3]. Ringer solutions are used even today in current clinical practice and serve as base for St Thomas-like cardioplegic solutions. Ringer was the first to publish in 1883 the antagonistic properties of potassium on cardiac contraction [4].

The beginning of the 20th century found the scientific community divided between myogenic versus neurogenic control of cardiac activity [5]. The Nobel Prize laureate in physiology, Alexis Carrel, was one of the first to state the importance of pharmacologically induced cardiac arrest, while trying to develop valve surgery. Defying Billroth's early statement, in the 1914 he said [6]: "The arresting of the circulation of the heart has already been performed in many ways by various experimenters. We ourselves have used all known methods of stopping the circulation through the heart". It is important to remember that neither Ringer's nor Carrel's work was greatly appreciated by the academic societies in Europe and while Carrel was forced to emigrate to North America, Ringer's work was continued later by American researchers, providing the basis for the ionic theory of cardiac activity.

While it had been acknowledged for many years that sodium, potassium and calcium ions are essential for cardiac activity, the second and third decades of the 20th century found several researchers trying to establish the precise role of each of these elements. Between 1929 and 1939 the pioneering works of D.R. Hooker, A.M. Baetjer and G.H. Zwikster showed that the heart could be reversibly arrested using potassium, while calcium was determined to be essential for the production of strong, mechanical contractions. Of course, all these breakthroughs in basic sciences had little application in the clinical practice of their time, as pharmacologically induced cardiac arrest needed haemodynamic support for a patient to survive, which came only after two decades when Gibbon started using the first heart–lung machine.

## 22.2 Hypothermia

In the late 1950s the heart–lung pump was successfully adopted at Toronto's Hospital for Sick Children by W.G. Bigelow, allowing him to introduce into clinical practice the technique of general body hypothermia. Described initially as a method for brain preservation during circulatory arrest, the use of hypothermia in heart surgery was presented at that time as the single most important element of myocardial protection [7]. At that time the main concern was avoiding air embolism, reducing foaming associated with the use of cardiopulmonary machines and operating on a quiet bloodless operative field; the mechanisms of ischaemia–reperfusion injury was not yet described yet, as most operations were performed on congenital cases and not on severely altered, ischaemic hearts.

Lewis and Taufic reported in 1953 on 26 dogs that were operated on using a hypothermic technique; at the end of their study, they added a case report of a 5-year-old girl who had undergone closure of her atrial septal defect in 1952 using hypothermia [8]. The patient recovered well after surgery and her postoperative convalescence was uneventful. Hypothermia alone was abandoned after the introduction of the bypass pump in 1955, as it was associated with myocardial injury due to alterations in cell fluidity and membrane integrity with production of myocardial oedema and a resulting decrease in ventricular output. In 1957 Sealy used moderate hypothermia (30 °C) produced by a more efficient heat exchanger as an adjunct to the heart–lung machine, initially to improve tolerance to low flows [9]. Two years later the concept of deep hypothermic arrest evolved and Drew published his first case reports [10]. Associated with cardiopulmonary bypass, hypothermia decreases myocardial oxygen consumption by 50 % for every 10 °C decrease in heart muscle temperature (Q10 effect) with the most important decrease in energy consumption taking place at 25 °C [11]. This technique remained at the stage of case report for a while before being reintroduced by Barratt-Boyes in the mid-1960s for infant cases and by Griepp from New York for extensive aortic arch surgery [12].

## 22.3 Cardioplegic Techniques

### 22.3.1 The Melrose Era

The concept of cardioplegia could not have been developed without the advances in cardiac physiology and related basic medical sciences that flourished at the end of the 19th century. Claude Bernard's early works on homeostasis defined the principle of a stable "internal milieu". Cardioplegic solutions contain a variety of components that are expected to arrest the heart rapidly in diastole, providing a quiet, bloodless operative field and offering reliable protection against ischaemia.

Gibbon's bypass machine gave birth to open heart surgery, but also to a new breed of researchers, mainly cardiac and vascular surgeons who were trying to find ways to perform heart surgery in a less lethal manner by trying to improve exposure and operative comfort. After reviewing Dr. Bernard's work and retrieving all the data published by Ringer, Hooker and Zwikster, Melrose and his colleagues at the Royal Postgraduate Medical School in London began experimentation with elective cardiac arrest. After successfully inducing a reversible pharmacological cardiac arrest by injecting more than 5 mg/mL of potassium citrate in dogs, Melrose and his associates demonstrated the possibility of achieving a 30-min reversible cardiac arrest and was the first to suggest that blood could be used as a reliable substrate for cardioplegia [13].

The first clinical study, on 34 patients, was performed in 1958, Melrose relying upon a solution of 25 % potassium citrate diluted 1 part in 9 in oxygenated blood [14]. In parallel, Sealy's group from Duke University published similar results after adding neostigmine to Melrose solution and was the first to use the term cardioplegia in the medical literature [15].

Gradually, as the technique evolved and was increasingly used by various surgical teams the first short-term terrible side-effects came out. Allen and Lillehei were the first to publish a word of caution regarding the Melrose technique, especially in patients presenting myocardial damage [16]. As some disappointing early clinical results started to come in, researchers tried to explain the mechanism of the failure of this technique. In 1959 Helmsworth reported the occurrence of unusual left ventricle tension, focal necrosis and irreversible ventricular fibrillation [17]. Similar results were soon published by various independent researchers, like Waldhausen and Björk, who finally stated that Melrose's technique seemed to be rather dangerous and doubtful [18]. High potassium citrate solutions were further discredited in 1960 when McFarland demonstrated histopathological evidence of focal myocardial necrosis and vascular injury in the left ventricles of patients deceased after undergoing heart surgery with the Melrose technique [19]. Melrose's critics suggested various alternatives or safer procedures for open heart surgery, Waldhausen advocated intermittent aortic occlusion, while Björk felt that hypothermic arrest was preferable.

## 22.3.2 Non-cardioplegic Techniques

When cardioplegic techniques fell into disgrace at the end of the 1960s, several methods were soon adopted in order to continue to perform open heart surgery: intermittent aortic occlusion/direct coronary perfusion, topical hypothermia or normothermic ischaemia.

*Direct coronary perfusion* became the preferred method for myocardial preservation in the 1960s and the beginning of the 1970s, after Kay and co-workers demonstrated that effective myocardial preservation can be achieved while performing direct cannulation of the coronary ostia and irrigating the coronary arteries with oxygenated blood. In order to improve operative comfort, the beating heart was soon replaced by electrically induced ventricular fibrillation. However, the disadvantages of this operative technique were soon noticed: reports of cannula-induced ostial stenosis or embolism, operative field flooding by coronary artery perfusion, deficient myocardial protection in the case of anatomical variations and finally evidence of possible subendocardial necrosis even when the coronary arteries were widely patent [20].

A variant of this technique is still used by a few surgical teams while performing coronary artery bypass using intermittent aortic cross-clamping with fibrillation and moderate hypothermic perfusion. The distal graft anastomosis is performed in a relative motionless field (during ventricular fibrillation) avoiding at the same time the consequences of profound metabolic changes that occur with more prolonged periods of ischaemia. Large series with good clinical results were published even recently [21, 22], suggesting that it is a safe technique in both elective and non-elective patients when performed by an experienced surgeon.

*Topical hypothermia* was introduced by Shumway and co-workers [23], who simply irrigated the suspended pericardial sac with cold saline at 4 °C. Shumway reported excellent results after using his technique for more than 10 years, with both coronary and valve surgery [7], but it never gained wide acceptance because of concerns regarding a limited safe arrest time, non-uniform cooling and phrenic nerve cold-induced palsy.

*Normothermic ischaemia* was popularised by Cooley starting from 1964, but its short ischaemic time and evidence of subendocardial necrosis made this method obsolete by the beginning of the 1970s [24]. A dreadful complication associated with this technique, the stone heart-which led operated myocardium in a state of irreversible ischaemic contraction, was described by Cooley himself.

### 22.3.3 Cardioplegia Reloaded: Intracellular, Extracellular or Blood

Although chemical cardioplegia was abandoned in North America, several European centres maintained their research programmes, trying to identify the problem related to the Melrose solution, suggesting that toxicity was probably due to high ionic concentrations rather than the chemical-induced electromechanical arrest itself.

It was in Berlin in the early 1960s that Hoelscher demonstrated, using recent advances in electron microscopy, the toxic effects of Melrose's solution to be caused by the chelating action of citrate ion that depletes intra- and extracellular stores of $Ca^{+2}$ and $Mg^{+2}$ [25]. Hoelscher used the membrane stabilizing effects of procaine amide and magnesium chloride in order to create a cardioplegic solution that allowed a rapid cardiac arrest and an uneventful recovery. His work was continued by Bretschneider, who was the first to coin the concept of "intracellular cardioplegia and elegantly described the logic behind each element of his solution. Low sodium concentrations mimic the same intracellular concentration of this ion, a calcium-free environment would prevent contraction while mannitol will maintain ideal osmolarity under the membrane-stabilising effects of procaine amide [26].

While the majority of cardiac surgeons of his time were struggling to perform open heart surgery with non-cardioplegic myocardial protection, Sondergaard courageously readopted chemical cardioplegia, using modified Bretschneider cardioplegic solutions. Interestingly, the first part of Sondergaard's protocol consisted of injecting a solution of blood and glucose while cooling the pericardial sac at 4 °C and secondly to infuse a No. 3 Bretschneider solution inducing cardiac arrest with excellent results in a clinical series of 100 patients [27].

Intracellular cardioplegia was not adopted on a large scale despite these encouraging results as most of Bretschneider's and Hoelscher's work was initially published in German and was in fact very much ahead of its time and contemporary surgical habits. However, a modified Bretschneider form of cardioplegia (the HTK solution) is gaining popularity in organ transplantation and in routine cardiac surgery.

Inspired by their German colleagues, Hearse and Braimbridge in the UK and Gay in the USA started to reinvent crystalloid cardioplegia by developing a solution with *extracellular* properties [28, 29]. Being convinced that the problems related to the use of the Melrose technique were high osmolarity and citrate, Hearse used an extracellular formula based on Krebs Henseleit bicarbonate buffer at 7.4 pH, 12 mM $K^+$, 1 mM procaine, 16 mM magnesium, 10 mM ATP and 10 mM creatine phosphate, demonstrating an improvement in aortic flow from 0 to 82 % after 30 min of normothermic ischaemia [28]. However, it was Tyers who elegantly demonstrated hyperosmolarity greater than 400 mOsm/l and excess citrate to be the main causes of the failures reported with the use of Melrose's crystalloid cardioplegia [30]. Braimbridge at St Thomas's Hospital in London then took Hearse's theories and put them into clinical practice in 1975, popularising the use of St Thomas cardioplegic solution No. 1, and demonstrating a similar degree of myocardial protection to that of non-cardioplegic techniques of his time (coronary perfusion) [31]. After further preclinical and clinical assessments Braimbridge and his co-workers improved their recipe, introducing the St Thomas solution No.2 (Plegisol), which essentially has a much lower calcium content and is still used in many cardiac surgical programmes [32].

Encouraged by the clinical results achieved by crystalloid cardioplegia, Buckberg's team working at the UCLA started to develop *blood cardioplegia* in the late 1970s [11]. Interestingly, the hypothesis that blood could be the ideal delivery vehicle for cardioplegia, was initially emitted by Melrose more than 20 years earlier [13, 33, 34]. Buckberg's group believed that blood has numerous advantages as it is readily available in the bypass pump limiting haemodilution in fragile patients, it offers a natural powerful buffering capacity because of its components (especially histidine imidazole groups), while erythrocytes contain endogenous oxygen free radical scavengers which may reduce oxygen-mediated injury during reperfusion [35, 36]. Several cardioplegic solutions were specifically developed to be mixed in a 4:1 ratio with blood, as classic cardioplegic solutions (Plegisol or HTK) were designed to work best on their own and would not provide the same level of protection when diluted with blood [37]. The renewed interest in blood as a vehicle gave birth to a variety of strategies of delivering cardioplegia; Salerno examined the effects of continuous warm-blood cardioplegia, initially experimentally and then clinically [38]. With this technique visualisation started to be a problem, especially in coronary surgery, despite the use of blowers, and several studies demonstrated no significant advantage over standard intermittent hypothermic cardioplegia [39, 40]. Currently, adepts of blood cardioplegia use a warm solution at the induction phase followed by a maintenance phase with cold cardioplegic replenishments at 20-min intervals to counteract non-coronary collateral washout, while a final "hot-shot" of warm blood solution irrigates the heart during recovery.

## 22.4 Techniques of Administration

As one may expect, the various strategies for myocardial protection gave birth to several routes of administration of the cardioplegic solutions: intermittent antegrade, continuous antegrade, antegrade via the graft, intermittent retrograde, continuous retrograde, alternate antegrade and retrograde, simultaneous antegrade and retrograde infusions.

When Melrose described his technique for chemical cardiac arrest, the cardioplegic solution was injected via a cannula into the aortic root, but soon, technical difficulties like porcelain aorta and diffuse coronary disease imposed the finding of alternative delivery methods. The importance of the coronary sinus and the possibility of irrigating the coronary arteries through the coronary veins had been described since the end of the 19th century by Pratt [41], but it was Lillehei, back in the 1950s, who first introduced into clinical practice coronary sinus cardioplegia for aortic surgery [42]. Retrograde delivery ensures a more homogeneous distribution of cardioplegia to regions of the heart that are poorly collateralised, allows delivery into a continuous manner—important in aortic surgery—and minimizes the risk of embolisation from saphenous vein grafts in redo patients. However, both experimental and clinical studies have revealed that the right ventricle is not adequately protected by retrograde cardioplegia on its own as the anterior region of the right ventricle is not drained by the coronary sinus and because of the various possible variations of coronary sinus anatomy [35]. Further studies proved that antegrade and retrograde routes are complementary as each supply different vascular beds; thus, Ihnken and Buckberg reported a technique of simultaneous cardioplegia delivery [43], which has been currently adopted by a large number of cardiac surgeons.

## 22.5 Minimally Invasive Surgery

The appearance of port-access surgery raised new challenges for optimal myocardial protection as surgeons realised that limited exposure and longer procedures require finding alternative methods of cardioplegia administration, ventricular venting and aortic occlusion. Delivering retrograde cardioplegia requires the use of a transjugular coronary sinus catheter that is placed by the anaesthetist under both fluoroscopic and TOE control. This procedure is tedious, may cause coronary sinus rupture and has a high rate of dislodgment during surgery [44]. All the above disadvantages, not to mention concerns regarding cost and time led several experienced teams to readopt single-dose intracellular cardioplegia, which has been proven in the past to ensure a safe cardiac arrest up to 180 min in duration, as their preferred technique of myocardial preservation, with excellent results [45, 46].

## 22.6 Conclusions

The concept of myocardial protection emerged 50 years ago and its development and progress were directly related to other advances in cardiac surgery. Several reliable methods of protection and delivery are available and they should be known by all those involved in patient management. Myocardial protection starts at the bedside on the very first day when the patient is assessed by the members of the "heart team" as long-term results after heart surgery are due, in part, to adequate myocardial protection. For example, the mechanism of action of beta blockers involves a key principle of myocardial protection: optimisation of energy supply/demand in the myocardium.

The history of myocardial protection proves that one should not rely on recent trends or fashion, but on the results of clinical studies. Despite several clinical trials, nobody could prove the superiority of blood cardioplegia over crystalloid cardioplegia, in terms of mortality and patient outcome. The advantages seen in animal research were never confirmed by solid clinical data. The development of minimally invasive surgery dealt another blow to "blood advocates", as problems related to exposure and cardioplegia delivery made the majority of experienced teams choose a more "user friendly" and reliable form of myocardial protection, the forgotten intracellular cardioplegia. Instead of searching for the absolute truth, further studies should be conducted to define which group of patients could benefit from a different but reliable strategy of myocardial protection. Criteria like the presence or absence of pathological findings (porcelain aorta, left main stenosis, diffuse coronary disease), surgical exposure (minimally invasive procedures), patient risk factors (poor left ventricular function, renal failure) or type of surgery (redo), and last but not least, each heart team's training capabilities, should be the defining end-points for the strategy to adopt during surgery.

However, the concept of myocardial protection is not a closed chapter as the continuous development of novel techniques imposes an obvious need to improve the current strategies of myocardial protection during heart surgery.

## References

1. Starling EH (1896) On the absorption of fluids from the connective tissue spaces. J Physiol 19(4):312–326
2. Starling EH, Visscher MB (1927) The regulation of the energy output of the heart. J Physiol 62(3):243–261

3. Miller DJ (2004) Sydney Ringer; physiological saline, calcium and the contraction of the heart. J Physiol 555(Pt 3):585–587
4. Ringer S (1883) A third contribution regarding the influence of the inorganic constituents of the blood on the ventricular contraction. J Physiol 4(2–3):222–225
5. Lee JA (1981) Sydney Ringer (1834–1910) and Alexis Hartmann (1898–1964). Anaesthesia 36(12):1115–1121
6. Carrel A (1914) Experimental operations on the orifices of the heart. Ann Surg 60(1):1–6
7. Griepp RB, Stinson EB, Shumway NE (1973) Profound local hypothermia for myocardial protection during open-heart surgery. J Thorac Cardiovasc Surg 66(5):731–741
8. Lewis FJ, Taufic M (1953) Closure of atrial septal defects with the aid of hypothermia; experimental accomplishments and the report of one successful case. Surgery 33(1):52–59
9. Sealy WC et al (1957) Hypothermia, low flow extracorporeal circulation and controlled cardiac arrest for open heart surgery. Surg Gynecol Obstet 104(4):441–450
10. Drew CE, Anderson IM (1959) Profound hypothermia in cardiac surgery: report of three cases. Lancet 1(7076):748–750
11. Buckberg GD et al (1977) Studies of the effects of hypothermia on regional myocardial blood flow and metabolism during cardiopulmonary bypass. I. The adequately perfused beating, fibrillating, and arrested heart. J Thorac Cardiovasc Surg 73(1):87–94
12. Hikasa Y et al (1967) Open heart surgery in infants with an aid of hypothermic anesthesia. Nihon Geka Hokan 36(4):495–508
13. Baker JB et al (1957) Arrest of isolated heart with potassium citrate. Lancet 273(6995):555–559
14. Gerbode F, Melrose D (1958) The use of potassium arrest in open cardiac surgery. Am J Surg 96(2):221–227
15. Sealy WC et al (1958) Potassium, magnesium, and neostigmine for controlled cardioplegia; studies on the deg using extracorporeal circulation and hypothermia. AMA Arch Surg 77(1):33–38
16. Allen P, Lillehei CW (1957) Use of induced cardiac arrest in open heart surgery; results in seventy patients. Minn Med 40(10):672–676
17. Helmsworth JA et al (1959) Myocardial injury associated with asystole induced with potassium citrate. Ann Surg 149(2):200–206
18. Bjork VO (1961) Methods for open heart surgery. Acta Chir Scand Suppl Suppl 283:75–83
19. Shiroishi MS (1999) Myocardial protection: The rebirth of potassium-based cardioplegia. Tex Heart Inst J 26(1):71–86
20. Najafi H et al (1971) Left ventricular hemorrhagic necrosis. Experimental production and pathogenesis. Ann Thorac Surg 12(4):400–410
21. Bonchek LI et al (1992) Applicability of noncardioplegic coronary bypass to high-risk patients. Selection of patients, technique, and clinical experience in 3000 patients. J Thorac Cardiovasc Surg 103(2):230–237
22. Raco L, Mills E, Millner RJ (2002) Isolated myocardial revascularization with intermittent aortic cross-clamping: experience with 800 cases. Ann Thorac Surg 73(5):1436–1439 discussion 1439–40
23. Shumway NE, Lower RR, Stofer RC (1959) Selective hypothermia of the heart in anoxic cardiac arrest. Surg Gynecol Obstet 109:750–754
24. Colapinto ND, Silver MD (1971) Prosthetic heart valve replacement. Causes of early postoperative death. J Thorac Cardiovasc Surg 61(6):938–944
25. Hoelscher B (1967) Studies by electron microscopy on the effects of magnesium chloride-procaine amide or potassium citrate on the myocardium in induced cardiac arrest. J Cardiovasc Surg (Torino) 8(2):163–166
26. Bretschneider HJ et al (1975) Myocardial resistance and tolerance to ischemia: physiological and biochemical basis. J Cardiovasc Surg (Torino) 16(3):241–260
27. Sondergaard T et al (1975) Cardioplegic cardiac arrest in aortic surgery. J Cardiovasc Surg (Torino) 16(3):288–290

28. Hearse DJ, Stewart DA, Braimbridge MV (1976) Cellular protection during myocardial ischemia: the development and characterization of a procedure for the induction of reversible ischemic arrest. Circulation 54(2):193–202
29. Gay WA Jr, Ebert PA (1973) Functional, metabolic, and morphologic effects of potassium-induced cardioplegia. Surgery 74(2):284–290
30. Tyers GF et al (1975) The mechanism of myocardial damage following potassium citrate (Melrose) cardioplegia. Surgery 78(1):45–53
31. Braimbridge MV et al (1977) Cold cardioplegia or continuous coronary perfusion? report on preliminary clinical experience as assessed cytochemically. J Thorac Cardiovasc Surg 74(6):900–906
32. Ledingham SJ, Braimbridge MV, Hearse DJ (1987) The St. Thomas' hospital cardioplegic solution. A comparison of the efficacy of two formulations. J Thorac Cardiovasc Surg 93(2): 240–246
33. Bentall HH, Melrose DG (1957) Elective cardiac arrest: lactic acid production in the arrested heart. J Physiol 135(2):38–39
34. Melrose DG et al (1955) Elective cardiac arrest. Lancet 269(6879):21–22
35. Buckberg GD (2002) Myocardial protection: entering the new millennium. J Card Surg 17(5):447–450
36. Buckberg GD (1995) Update on current techniques of myocardial protection. Ann Thorac Surg 60(3):805–814
37. Buckberg GD (1993) Myocardial protection: an overview. Semin Thorac Cardiovasc Surg 5(2):98–106
38. Salerno TA et al (1991) Retrograde continuous warm blood cardioplegia: a new concept in myocardial protection. Ann Thorac Surg 51(2):245–247
39. Lajos TZ et al (1993) Comparison of cold versus warm cardioplegia. crystalloid antegrade or retrograderetrograde blood? Circulation 88(5 Pt 2):II344–II3449
40. Jones EL et al (1995) Should the freehand allograft be abandoned as a reliable alternative for aortic valve replacement? Ann Thorac Surg 59(6):1397–1403 discussion 1403–1404
41. Pratt FH (1897) The circulation through the veins of thebesius. J Boston Soc Med Sci 1(15):29–34
42. Lillehei CW et al (1956) The direct vision correction of calcific aortic stenosis by means of a pump-oxygenator and retrograde coronary sinus perfusion. Dis Chest 30(2):123–132
43. Ihnken K et al (1994) The safety of simultaneous arterial and coronary sinus perfusion: experimental background and initial clinical results. J Card Surg 9(1):15–25
44. Lebon JS et al (2010) The endovascular coronary sinus catheter in minimally invasive mitral and tricuspid valve surgery: a case series. J Cardiothorac Vasc Anesth 24(5):746–751
45. Perier P et al (2008) Toward a new paradigm for the reconstruction of posterior leaflet prolapse: midterm results of the "respect rather than resect" approach. Ann Thorac Surg 86(3):718–725; discussion 718–725
46. Nloga J et al (2011) Mitral valve surgery in octogenarians: should we fight for repair? A survival and quality-of-life assessment. Eur J Cardiothorac Surg. 39(6):875–880

# Supra-Diaphragmatic Aortic Surgery: Evolution of Material, Techniques and Brain Protection

# 23

François Dagenais

> *There is no disease more conducive to clinical humility than aneurysm of the aorta.*
>
> William Osler

**Abstract**

The surgery of the thoracic aorta has evolved tremendously during the past 60 years. In the pre-CPB era pioneers have progressively perfected anastomotic techniques. The introduction of cardiopulmonary bypass facilitated the replacement procedures of the thoracic aorta. Experimental and clinical evaluations have led to better grafts, safer duration of brain and spinal cord ischemia, better perfusion techniques and operative techniques. More recently, thoracic stent–grafts dramatically reduced the mortality of high-risk patients requiring resection of the descending aorta albeit the presence of a favourable endovascular anatomy. Nowadays, dedicated multidisciplinary teams evaluate and treat patients with thoracic diseases with excellent outcomes owing to the skills and knowledge transmitted from their predecessors.

**Keywords**

Thoracic aorta · History · Brain protection

F. Dagenais (✉)
Department of Cardiac Surgery, Institut universitaire de cardiologie et pneumologie de Québec
Quebec Heart and Lung Institute, Québec, Canada
e-mail: francois.dagenais@chg.ulaval.ca

M. Picichè (ed.), *Dawn and Evolution of Cardiac Procedures*,
DOI: 10.1007/978-88-470-2400-7_23, 

## 23.1 Pre-Cardiopulmonary Era

Aneurysms were known since ancient Egypt. Antyllus, a Greek physician, suggested, even then, the ligation of arterial dilatation of the extremities with opening of the aneurysm [1]. This technique, however, did not gain widespread use. Ambroise Paré, a famous French surgeon of the 16th century, regarded ligation and opening of the aneurysm as a highly risky procedure, with an unacceptable rate of fatal bleeding. He further stated, referring to aneurysms of abdominal or thorax cavities, that "the aneurysms which happen in the internal parts are incurable" [2]. In 1785, John Hunter, an English surgeon, performed with success the treatment of a popliteal aneurysm by ligating proximally the superficial femoral artery [3]. Applying the technique of Hunter, other surgeons performed ligation of the aorta with the rationale to decrease the blood flowing through the aneurysm. However, this technique proved to be unsuccessful. To completely abolish the flow in the aneurysm, proximal and distal ligations were proposed. Surgeons were then faced with distal ischemia following these procedures. As an alternative approach, other physicians proposed the introduction of foreign material within the aneurysm to promote coagulation and thrombosis. Wrapping of aneurysms with agents such as cellophane was also suggested to promote fibrotic reaction and increase tensile time around the aneurysm wall [4]. These methods were championed until the fourth decade of the 20th century.

The first attempt to excise an aneurysm and preserve aortic continuity was done by Theodore Tuffier in 1902 [5], unsuccessfully. During the first decade of the 20th century, the experimental work on homografts and vascular anastomosis by Alexis Carrel and Charles Guthrie [6] led the pathway to a new era in vascular reconstruction. Another important breakthrough in vascular reconstruction was the discovery of heparin in 1918 by Jay McLean. However, heparin became clinically available only two decades later.

In 1944, Crafoord first performed a coarctation resection with an end-to-end aortic anastomosis using the technique described by Carrell [7]. The first successful treatment of a thoracic aneurysm was reported by Alton Ochsner in 1944 [8]. A 45-year-old man was operated on for a suspected mediastinal tumour on chest X-ray, which was found to be a saccular aneurysm of the descending aorta. The aneurysm was successfully excised and sutured following clamping of the base of the aneurysm. While an intern at the Johns Hopkins Hospital in 1945, Denton Cooley performed a resection of a pseudo-aneurysm of the ascending aorta with a similar technique to Ochsner's. Working on coarctation repair of the aorta, Robert Gross realised the importance of developing an aortic substitute when an end-to-end anastomosis was impossible [9]. In 1948, following extensive experimental work, Gross reported the use of a preserved arterial homograft for the treatment of coarctation of the aorta. Cooley and Michael DeBakey reported the first resection of a fusiform aneurysm in January 1953 with the aortic continuity restored with an aortic homograft [1]. The Houston team gained extensive experience and by 1955, DeBakey and Cooley teamed up to perform more than 245 repairs of aneurysms. Although aortic homografts proved to be initially acceptable, complications such as graft thrombosis, aneurysm formation, and infection led surgeons to explore new concepts of arterial substitutes. The efforts of William Blakemore and colleagues in the early 1950s led to the development of the first synthetic vascular graft known as Vinyon-N-Graft [10]. Subsequently, plastic fibres such nylon and polytetrafluoroethylene (also known as Teflon) were used with limited success. The graft technology used nowadays was stimulated by the discovery of Dacron by DeBakey. Early knitted Dacron grafts were flawed by excessive bleeding. Later, the development of a low porosity collagen impregnated graft proved to be much superior.

## 23.2 Post-Cardiopulmonary Bypass Era

The discovery of the heart–lung machine championed by John Gibbon in 1953 opened a new era in the management of the diseases of the thoracic aorta. The first resection of an ascending aortic aneurysm, under cardiopulmonary bypass, was reported by Cooley and DeBakey in 1956. The ongoing improvements in the 1960s of perfusion techniques, myocardial protection, brain protection and hypothermia brought tremendous innovations in procedures dealing with the replacement of the thoracic aorta.

### 23.2.1 Aortic Root Procedures

In 1963, Albert Starr reported the first replacement of an incompetent aortic valve with a concomitant graft replacement of the ascending aorta [11]. The subsequent year, Myron Wheat completed a subtotal resection of the aortic root by leaving solely a ridge of aorta compromising the coronary artery buttons [11]. In 1967, Hugh Bentall and Anthony de Bono sewed a mechanical valve with a Teflon tube graft to replace the entire root (composite aortic graft replacement). The coronary arteries were re-implanted within the aortic graft [12]. To minimise the dissection of the coronary arteries and to lessen perioperative bleeding the inclusion technique was used by which the coronary ostium were re-implanted to the graft from within the aneurysm. Furthermore, the aneurysm wall was wrapped around the graft to reduce the bleeding often encountered through the porous graft of the time. The accumulation of blood between the graft and the aneurysm wall occasionally led to formation of a pseudo-aneurysm by suture line disruption of the coronary or distal aortic anastomosis. Christian Cabrol described a technique using an 8-mm Dacron graft to re-implant the coronary ostia to the main graft by an end-to-end anastomosis on the coronary ostium and a side-to-side anastomosis on the main graft [13]. As a modification of the Bentall inclusion technique and a means of decreasing perioperative bleeding, Cabrol created a fistula between the closed aneurysm space and the right atrial appendage, hoping the fistula would close spontaneously with time. However, significant complications were related to a persistent shunt. To minimise the risk of pseudo-aneurysm at the coronary anastomosis, Nicholas Kouchoukos proposed a complete mobilisation of the coronary arteries with full thickness wall incorporation within the anastomosis. In addition, the treatment of Dacron grafts with gelatine or collagen rendered the graft impermeant, thus eliminating the necessity to wrap the aneurysm wall around the graft.

Although the concept of the Cabrol's procedure allows a tension-free anastomosis between the coronary ostia and the composite graft, early and long-term results were reported to be inferior to the Bentall procedure. Modifications of the Cabrol's procedure, such as the use of separate grafts to each coronary ostium ensured better graft patency and still remain indicated in complex re-operations. With the experience gained with the Bentall procedure using a composite mechanical valved graft, other aortic root substitutes were developed such as homografts, stentless valves and stented biological valve conduits. Donald Ross proposed a challenging operation employing the patient's own pulmonary artery root to replace the diseased aortic root and native pulmonary replaced with homograft [14]. The operation gained acceptance predominantly in the paediatric population owing to the growth potential of the pulmonary autograft.

In 1989, Tirone David operating on a young woman with Marfan syndrome reconstructed the aortic root within a graft while preserving the patient's native aortic valve [15]. The aortic valve-sparing operation described was initially proposed for Marfan patients. Subsequently, the procedure was applied to young patients with annuloecstasia or bicuspid aortic valves. Many techniques and modifications have been described and debates still persist such as the importance of creating "neosinuses" of Valsalva or the necessity to add a procedure to stabilise the aortic annulus.

### 23.2.2 Arch Replacement

The first complete replacement of the aortic arch was performed by Cooley in 1955 [16]. While maintaining perfusion in the arch vessels with a shunt between the ascending and the descending aorta, Cooley replaced the arch with a prosthetic graft. Although novel and innovative, this technique was abandoned with the introduction of cardiopulmonary bypass [17]. In 1957, DeBakey first reported an arch replacement using cardiopulmonary bypass. The procedure performed under normothermia was complex because of the use of four different arterial pumps. Subsequently, different surgeons proposed methods of replacing the arch using normothermic cardiopulmonary bypass with different modalities to perfuse the arch vessels. In 1975, the Stanford group, under Randall Griepp [18], reported the use of hypothermia as an adjunct to replacing the aortic arch. This led to a significant advancement in arch surgery owing to the possibility of operating in a bloodless field without clamping the aorta while preserving brain functions through hypothermia. However, further studies proved that cerebral consumption even at 8 °C was still 5 % of baseline. With solely hypothermic circulatory arrest (HCA) recommended between 15 and 18 °C, safe duration of circulatory arrest was uncertain after 30 min. Furthermore, the long duration of the cardiopulmonary bypass needed to complete these operations was associated with a significant systemic inflammatory response with significant coagulation disorders. To increase the safe duration of HCA, retrograde cerebral perfusion (RCP) and antegrade cerebral perfusion (ACP) were investigated. RCP, introduced by Yuichi Ueda [19], consists of perfusing the brain retrogradely through a cannula in the superior vena cava. Although experimental studies suggested that circulatory arrest could be extended to 60 min, clinical studies failed to confirm these findings. ACP, on the other hand, is based on the principal of bringing metabolism to the brain during HCA by perfusing blood through the arch vessels [20]. ACP prolongs significantly the safe duration of HCA. Many techniques of arch vessel perfusion, such as temperature and flow of perfusate as well as level of systemic hypothermia, have been studied and proposed with ACP. The use of the axillary artery as an arterial perfusion site during the last decade has facilitated the initiation of ACP during HCA. Combined with the advances in brain protection, new operative techniques were developed to improve surgical outcomes. The trifurcated arch graft and the "arch first technique" described by Griepp and colleagues have contributed to reducing the morbidity and mortality linked to arch reconstruction [21]. For aneurysms involving the aortic arch and descending aorta, Hans Borst proposed leaving a vascular graft free-floating within the descending aorta to facilitate the second stage of the procedure [22].

## 23.3 Replacement of the Descending Aorta: Open Approach and Thoracic Stent Grafting

### 23.3.1 Open Approach

As stated previously, the first attempts to replace the descending aorta with a substitute were performed to repair an aortic coarctation. In 1953, Cooley and DeBakey reported the first replacement of a descending thoracic aneurysm with a homograft [23]. A year later, Stephen Etheredge described the first successful thoracoabdominal repair [24]. In 1965, Stanley Crawford initiated what would become the benchmark of thoracoabdominal aneurysm surgery describing the inclusion and "clamp and sew" technique. However, morbidity, especially in terms of spinal cord ischemia, led surgeons to investigate new strategies to reduce the risks of post-operative paraplegia [25]. Although beyond the scope or this chapter, during the last three decades, major advances in perfusion techniques such as left-heart bypass and partial cardiopulmonary bypass, cerebrospinal fluid drainage and neuromonitoring have contributed to lessening the morbidity and mortality linked to thoracoabdominal repairs. With this progress, techniques to replace the entire intra-thoracic aorta during one operation were proposed by Lars Svensson and Kouchoukos during the 1990s; procedures requiring either a bi-thoracotomy or a separate thoracic incision in addition to the sternotomy [26, 27]. Nowadays, with the advent of thoracic stent grafts, one may consider replacing the entire intra-thoracic aorta through a sternotomy using the "elephant trunk" technique combined with a distal stent graft extension.

### 23.3.2 Thoracic Stent Graft

In 1991, Juan Parodi reported the use of an endograft to treat an abdominal aneurysm [28]. This new concept revolutionised the treatment of aneurismal disease during the next decade. The Stanford team was the first to apply the concept of endograft to treat aneurysms of the thoracic aorta. First-generation thoracic stent-grafts were custom-made, bulky and required large and rigid introducers. Through ongoing engineering efforts, the next generations of endografts were mounted on smaller introducers, were more conformable to the aortic wall and allowed for more precise deployment. In addition to aneurismal diseases, thoracic stent grafts were used to treat a diversity of pathologies of the descending aorta such as dissections, complicated penetrating ulcers, transection tears, and post-operative pseudoaneurysms. Owing to the rapidity of the procedure, thoracic stent grafts have been shown to significantly decrease the morbidity and mortality of patients presenting with acute type B dissection and severe malperfusion. In an attempt to increase the length of treatment with thoracic stent grafts, different surgeons proposed combining the use of stent-grafts and extra-anatomical bypasses to cover visceral and arch vessels with stent-grafts. With these hybrid techniques, complete arch and/or thoracoabdominal replacement procedures were performed. More recently, new custom-fitted branch grafts (Cook Medical) were designed to treat high-risk patients with thoracoabdominal aneurysms. A similar technology has been applied to treat a subset of arch aneurysms totally endovascularly.

## 23.4 Conclusion

The surgery of the thoracic aorta has evolved tremendously during the past 60 years. In the pre-cardiopulmonary era pioneers have progressively perfected anastomotic techniques. The introduction of cardiopulmonary bypass facilitated the replacement procedures of the thoracic aorta. Experimental and clinical evaluations have led to better grafts, safer duration of brain and spinal cord ischemia, better perfusion techniques and operative techniques. More recently, thoracic stent-grafts dramatically reduced the mortality of high-risk patients requiring resection of the descending aorta, albeit with the presence of favourable endovascular anatomy. Nowadays, dedicated multidisciplinary teams evaluate and treat patients with thoracic diseases with excellent outcomes owing to the skills and knowledge transmitted from their predecessors.

## References

1. Thompson JE (1998) Early history of aortic surgery. J Vasc Surg 28:746
2. Castiglioni A (1941) A History of medicine. (trans: Krmbhaar EB). Alfred A. Knopf, New York, p 370
3. Cooley DA (1999) The history of surgery of the thoracic aorta. Cardiol Clin 17(4):609–613
4. Harrison PW, Chandy J (1943) A subclavian aneurysm cured by cellophane fibrosis. Ann Surg 118:478
5. Tuffier T (1902) Intervention chirurgicale directe pour un aneurysme de la crosse de l'aorte, ligature du sac. Presse Med 1:267
6. Carrel A (1907) The surgery of blood vessels. John Hopkins Hosp Bull 18:18
7. Crafoord C, Nylin G (1945) Congenital coarctation of the aorta and its surgical treatment. J Thorac Surg 14:347–361
8. Ochsner A (1952) Discussion of "surgical considerations of intrathoracic aneurysms of the aorta and great vessels", by Cooley DA and DeBakey ME. Ann Surg 135:686
9. Gross RE, Bill AH Jr, Pierce ED II (1949) Methods for preservation and transplantation of arterial grafts; observations on arterial grafts in dogs. Report of transplantation of preserved arterial grafts in 9 human cases. Surg Gynecol Obstet 88:689–701
10. Voorhees AB Jr, Jaretski A IV, Blakemore AH (1952) The use of tubes constructed from vinyon-"N" cloth in bridging arterial defects. Ann Surg 135:322–326
11. Westaby S, Bertoni GB (2007) Fifty years of thoracic aortic surgery: lessons learned and future directions. Ann Thorac Surg 83:S832–S834
12. Bentall H, De Bono A (1968) A technique for complete replacement of the ascending aorta. Thorax 23:338
13. Cabrol C, Pavie A, Gandjbakhch I et al (1981) Complete replacement of the ascending aorta with reimplantation of the coronary arteries: new surgical approach. J Thorac Cardiovasc Surg 81:309–315
14. Ross D (2007) Pioneers of cardiology: Donald Ross, DSc, FRCS. Interview by Mark Nicholls. Circulation 115(9):f33–f34
15. David TE (2011) The aortic valve-sparing operation. J Thorac Cardiovasc Surg 141:613–615
16. Cooley DA, Mahaffey DE, DeBakey ME (1955) Total excision of the aortic arch for aneurysm. Surg Gynecol Obstet 101(6):667–672
17. DeBakey ME, Crawford ES, Cooley DA, Morris GC Jr (1957) Successful resection of fusiform aneurysm of aortic arch with replacement by homograft. Surg Gynecol Obstet 105(6):657–664
18. Griepp RB, Stinson EB, Hollingsworth JF, Buehler D (1975) Prosthetic replacement of the aortic arch. J Thorac Cardiovasc Surg 70(6):1051–1063
19. Ueda Y, Miki S, Kusuhara , Okita Y, Tabata T, Yamanoka K (1992) Deep hypothermic systemic circulatory arrest and continuous retrograde cerebral perfusion for surgery of aortic arch aneurysm. Eur J Cardiothorac Surg 6:36–42
20. Guilmet D, Roux PM, Bachet J, Goudot B, Tawil N, Diaz F (1986) Nouvelle technique de protection cérébrale: chirurgie de la crosse aortique. Presse Med 15:1096–1098
21. Strauch JT, Spielvogel D, Lauten A, Galla JD, Lansman SL, McMurthy K, Griepp RB (2004) Technical advances in total aortic arch replacement. Ann Thorac Surg 77:581–590
22. Borst HG, Walterbusch G, Schaps D (1983) Extensive aortic replacement using "elephant trunk" prosthesis. Thorac Cardiovasc Surg 81:309–315
24. DeBakey MEm, Creech O, Morris GC (1956) Aneurysm of the thoracoabdominal aorta involving celiac superior mesenteric and renal arteries. Report of four cases treated by resection and homograft replacement. Ann Surg 144:549–572

24. Stanley G (1990) A history of aneurysm surgery. In: Greenhalgh RM, Mannick JA, Powell JT (eds) The cause and management of aneurysm. Saunders, London, pp 1–18
25. Crawford ES (1974) Thoracoabdominal and abdominal aortic aneurysm involving renal, superior mesenteric, and celiac arteries. Ann Surg 188:404–422
26. Svensson LG, Shahian DM, Davis FG et al (1994) Replacement of entire aorta from aortic valve to bifurcation during one operation. Ann Thorac Surg 58:1164–1166
27. Kouchoukos NT, Mauney MC, Masetti P, Castner CF (2004) Single-stage repair of extensive thoracic aortic aneurysms: experience with the arch-first technique and bilateral anterior thoracotomy. J Thorac Cardiovasc Surg 128:669–676
28. Parodi JC, Palmaz JC, Barone HD (1991) Transfemoral intraluminal graft implantation for abdominal aortic aneurysms. Ann Vasc Surg 5(6):491

# Surgical Treatment of Atrial Fibrillation

# 24

Gino Gerosa, Carlo Dal Lin and Vincenzo Tarzia

*Oh, that Einstein, always skipping lectures…I certainly never would have thought he could do it.*

Hermann Minkowski


**Abstract**

Because of disappointing results with medical strategies of rate and rhythm control, there has been strong interest in the nonpharmacological treatment of atrial fibrillation (AF), leading to the development of various interventional catheter and surgical therapies. In 1980, Williams et al. developed the "left atrial isolation procedure" confining the AF to the left atrium and restoring the remainder of the heart to sinus rhythm. In 1982 Scheimnman et al. described the "catheter fulguration of the His bundle," thus confining the arrhythmia to the atria and implanting a pacemaker to restore a normal ventricular rhythm. After Guiraudon et al. description of the "Corridor procedure" (1985), Cox et al. developed the "atrial transection procedure" in a canine model of AF, observing that a single long incision across both atria down into the septum cured AF. Nowadays, the Cox-Maze III procedure represents the gold standard for surgical management of AF and has recently given way to a variety of simpler operations that employ alternative energy sources and lesion sets to treat AF.


Atrial fibrillation (AF) is associated with detrimental clinical consequences that include reduced survival, stroke, thromboembolism, tachycardia-induced cardiomyopathy, and symptoms related to rapid and irregular heart rates. Because of


G. Gerosa (✉) · V. Tarzia
Division of Cardiac Surgery, Department of Cardiac Thoracic and Vascular Sciences, University of Padova, Padua, Italy
e-mail: gino.gerosa@unipd.it

C. Dal Lin
Division of Cardiology, Department of Cardiac Thoracic and Vascular Sciences, University of Padova, Padua, Italy



M. Picichè (ed.), *Dawn and Evolution of Cardiac Procedures*,
DOI: 10.1007/978-88-470-2400-7_24,© Springer-Verlag Italia 2013

disappointing results with medical strategies of rate and rhythm control there has been strong interest in the nonpharmacological treatment of AF leading to the development of various interventional catheter and surgical therapies. In 1980, Williams et al. developed the "left atrial isolation procedure" [1] confining the AF to the left atrium and restoring the remainder of the heart to sinus rhythm. In 1982 Scheimnman et al. [2] described the "catheter fulguration of the His bundle" thus confining the arrhythmia to the atria and implanting a pacemaker to restore a normal ventricular rhythm. After Guiraudon et al. [3] description of the "corridor procedure" Cox et al. [4] developed the "atrial transection procedure" in a canine model of AF observing that a single long incision across both atria down into the septum cured AF.

Nowadays, the Cox-Maze III [5, 6] procedure represents the gold standard for surgical management of AF. This procedure has recently given way to a variety of simpler operations that employ alternative energy sources and lesion sets to treat AF.

## 24.1 Development of the Cox-Maze Procedure

Cox in 1987 designed the so-called "Cox-Maze procedure" [7–10] to interrupt any of all macroreentrant atrial circuits in order to prevent the possibility of the atrium fibrillating or fluttering. The operation aims to create many incisions across both the right and left atria in order to direct the sinus impulse throughout both atria, preserving the atrial transport function in most patients.

The original technique (Maze I procedure), introduced in 1991, was soon modified as the Maze II [5] procedure because of late chronotropic incompetence and the high number of pacemaker implantations. The Maze II was then modified again because of its complexity and became the Cox-Maze III [5] procedure as it is performed today (Fig. 24.1).

Reported late freedom from AF ranges from 75 to 98 % at 5–10 years after surgery. Disparities in results from different groups may be related to different follow-up methodologies and different definitions of success. Risk factors for recurrent AF after a Cox-Maze procedure include:

1. Longer duration of preoperative AF and left atrial enlargement.
2. Pattern of AF (paroxysmal, persistent or permanent).
3. Need for concomitant procedures that do not affect results.

In addition to restoring sinus rhythm, the Cox-Maze procedure virtually eliminates the risk of late stroke. This beneficial effect may relate in part to excision of the left atrial appendage [11].

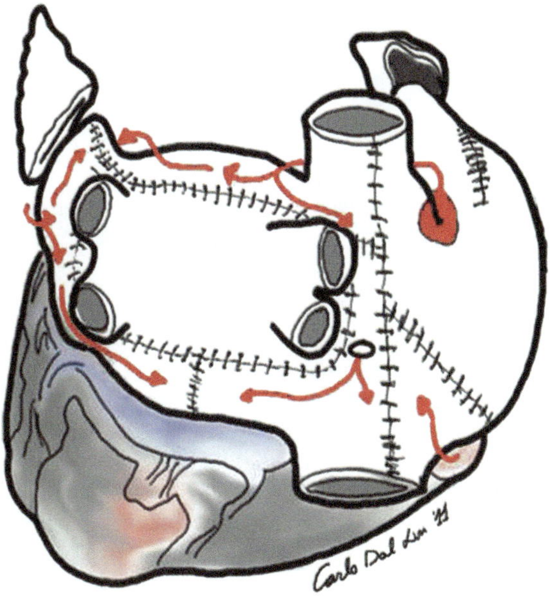

**Fig. 24.1** The Cox-Maze III. The procedure is performed on cardiopulmonary bypass with cardioplegic arrest. It consists of encircling and isolation of the pulmonary veins and excision of both left and right atrial appendages. The pulmonary veins are encircled by surgical incision, and there is a connecting incision towards the mitral valve annulus. The left atrial appendage is excised, and this incision is connected to the pulmonary vein-encircling incision

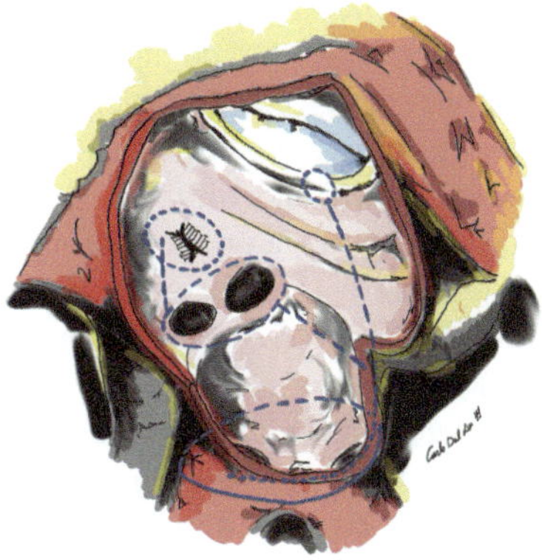

**Fig. 24.2** The Cox-Maze IV. Left atrial lesion set performed through a standard left atriotomy. *Continuous line* surgical incision, *dashed lines* RF ablation. On the mitral anulus: criothermy lesion. The left atrial appendage is excised

## 24.2 New Surgical Ablation Technology

The Cox-Maze III procedure still remains complex and technically difficult and did not reach widespread application despite its proven efficacy. At most centers, the Maze III surgical incision lines have been replaced by linear lines of ablation using different energy sources including radiofrequency, microwave, cryoablation, laser, and high frequency ultrasound (Cox-Maze IV procedure; Fig. 24.2). These modifications shortened the operation time, maintaining the success rate of the traditional cut and sew Cox-Maze III technique [12–14]. Improvement in the ablation technologies allowed the development of minimally invasive procedures for AF performed through small incisions or ports and on beating hearts.

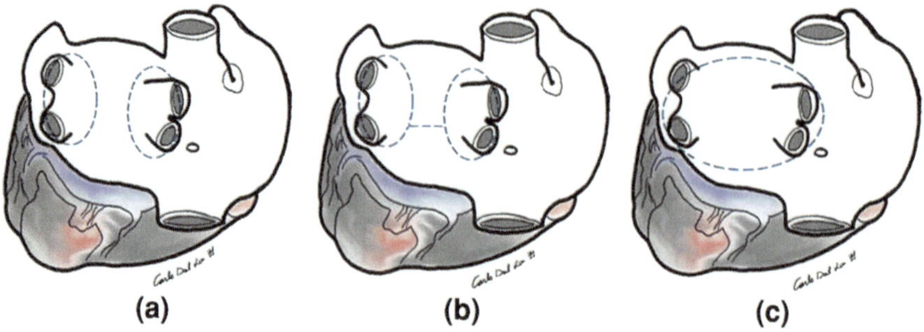


**Fig. 24.3** Alternative approaches to surgical ablation. **a** Pulmonary vein isolation (PVI), **b** PVI with connection, **c** box lesion

An ablation device must meet several crucial requirements:

1. The capability to produce transmural lesions in order to interrupt micro- and macroreentrant circuits and isolate trigger foci.
2. The safety of the device in terms of intensity and localization of the energy delivered.
3. The device should be simple to handle and be adaptable to a minimally invasive approach.

The various technologies can be divided into two major groups: unipolar energy source and bipolar clamp. The unipolar energy sources (cryosurgery, unipolar radiofrequency energy, microwave, laser, ultrasound) radiate either heat or cold from a unifocused single source (with the ultrasound exception). Unipolar energy sources have had difficulties creating transmural lesions when used from the epicardial surface on the beating heart. Ultrasound is the only unipolar source that results in a focused delivery of energy. Thus, it potentially has the ability to create transmural lesions on the beating heart. Ultrasound has the disadvantage of having a fixed depth of penetration [15].

Bipolar radiofrequency ablation has been able to overcome some of these shortcomings [16–19]. Energy is delivered between two closely approximated electrodes embedded in a jaw of a clamp device, the energy is focused and results in discrete lesions. The energy is confined within the jaws of the clamp, eliminating the possibility of collateral cardiac or extracardiac damage. Bipolar ablation has the advantage of shorter ablation times ensuring in the mean time the transmurality of the lesion. The weakness of these devices is that they can only ablate tissue that can be clamped within the jaws of the device [15].

## 24.3 Alternative Approaches to Surgical Ablation

A number of alternative approaches have been proposed to cure AF. These procedures could be divided into two main groups:

1. Isolated left atrial lesion set [20–22]: pulmonary vein isolation either separately with a connecting lesion or as a box (Fig. 24.3b, c). These approaches are

associated with mitral annulus lesion and amputation of the left atrial appendage and are indicated for persistent/permanent AF treatment. When applied to patients with permanent AF and mitral valve disease, this approach is associated with approximately 80 % freedom from AF at 1 year. Adjunctive measures, such as left atrial reduction in those with left atrial enlargement, may improve results.
2. Exclusive pulmonary vein isolation either separately or as a box [23–25] (Fig. 24.3a, c). Paroxysmal AF originates from pulmonary veins in 94 % of cases; thus, this procedure is indicated for the treatment of this form of AF.

## 24.4 Pulmonary Vein Isolation

A variety of energy sources have been employed to perform pulmonary vein isolation. The pulmonary veins can be isolated with two separate oval-shaped lesions (Fig. 24.3a) or, alternatively, as a single, large, boxlike lesion (Fig. 24.3c). Either approach is acceptable.

With the use of bipolar radiofrequency, pulmonary vein isolation is simple. A bipolar radiofrequency clamp is applied around the pulmonary veins isolating as much atrial tissue as possible and ensuring that energy is not delivered directly to pulmonary vein tissue because this may cause pulmonary vein stenosis. Each set of pulmonary veins is isolated with two parallel applications of the bipolar radiofrequency clamp to ensure that there are no gaps.

The "box lesion" represents a continuous circular lesion, encircling the pulmonary veins, produced by different energy sources.

Pulmonary vein isolation with a connecting lesion could be made linking the two oval shaped lesions encircling the pulmonary veins using a radiofrequency source [11].

## 24.5 Isolated Atrial Fibrillation and Minimally Invasive Epicardial Ablation

Several minimally invasive approaches have been devised to surgically manage isolated AF. All have in common the use of thoracoscopy, small incisions and the avoidance of cardiopulmonary bypass.

Current surgical techniques for minimally invasive AF surgery include [26–28]:

1. Totally endoscopic robotic-guided epicardial pulmonary vein isolation performed on a beating heart using a microwave probe [29].
2. Off-pump bilateral or monolateral, closed-chest thoracoscopic pulmonary vein isolation using microwave [30, 31].
3. Off-pump monolateral or bilateral video-assisted thoracoscopic surgery (VATS) utilizing high-intensity focused ultrasonography, monopolar or bipolar RF clamps [32–34].
4. Subxyphoid approach for closed-chest epicardial microwave atrial ablation [35].

Usually, in minimally invasive approaches, the ablation line is a continuous circular lesion, encircling the pulmonary veins (box lesion; Fig. 24.3c).

## 24.6 Indications for Surgical Treatment of AF

The main indications for surgical treatment of AF are:

1. Failure of medical/percutaneous treatment and persistence of patient symptoms.
2. Tachycardia-induced cardiomyopathy.
3. Patients with associated AF who undergo elective cardiac surgery.

## 24.7 Future Directions

Advances in AF understanding and improvement of current ablation technologies will refine surgical techniques and outcomes. Real-time, intraoperative electrophysiological mapping will enable precise targeted (rather than empiric) ablation based on patient's particular electrophysiological pathophysiology. Intraoperative electrophysiological assessment of lesions created will guide the surgeon, enabling more confident creation of lesions that effectively block conduction.

Furthermore, a minimally invasive surgical pulmonary vein isolation (box lesion) could be associated with a percutaneous electrophysiological ablative procedure [36]. This kind of hybrid approach involving cardiac surgeons and electrophysiologists as a heart team, is extremely innovative, probably representing the most comprehensive therapeutical strategy for the cure of AF, either paroxysmal or permanent, providing the highest success rates along with the best care for patients' health.

The future technological improvements are directed at developing more friendly devices that allow safe and direct epicardial delivery of ablation energy through ports or very small incisions. Additionally, surgical/percutaneous management of the left atrial appendage could be part of the procedure.

## References

1. Williams JM, Ungerleider RM, Lofland GK et al (1980) Left atrial isolation: new technique for the treatment of supraventricular arrhythmias. J Thorac Cardiovasc Surg 80(3):373–380
2. Scheinman MM, Morady F, Hess DS et al (1982) Catheter-induced ablation of the atrioventricular junction to control refractory supraventricular arrhythmias. JAMA 248(7):851–855
3. Guiraudon GM, Campbell CS, Jones DL et al (1985) Combined sinoatrial node atrioventricular node isolation: a surgical alternative to his bundle ablation in patients with atrial fibrillation. Circulation 72 [Suppl 3]:220
4. Smith PK, Holman WL, Cox JL (1985) Surgical treatment of supraventricular tachyarrhythmias. Surg Clin North Am 65(3):553–570
5. Cox JL, Boineau JP, Schuessler RB et al (1995) Modification of the Maze procedure for atrial flutter and atrial fibrillation. I. Rationale and surgical results. J Thorac Cardiovasc Surg 110(2):473–484

6. Prasad SM, Maniar HS, Camillo CJ et al (2003) The Cox Maze III procedure for atrial fibrillation: long-term efficacy in patients undergoing lone versus concomitant procedures. J Thorac Cardiovasc Surg 126(6):1822–1828
7. Cox JL (2011) The first Maze procedure. J Thorac Cardiovasc Surg 141(5):1093–1097
8. Cox JL, Canavan TE, Schuessler RB et al (1991) The surgical treatment of atrial fibrillation. II. Intraoperative electrophysiologic mapping and description of the electrophysiologic basis of atrial flutter and atrial fibrillation. J Thorac Cardiovasc Surg 101(3):406–426
9. Cox JL, Schuessler RB, D'Agostino HJ Jr et al (1991) The surgical treatment of atrial fibrillation. III. Development of a definitive surgical procedure. J Thorac Cardiovasc Surg 101(4):569–583
10. Cox JL (1991) The surgical treatment of atrial fibrillation. IV. Surgical technique. J Thorac Cardiovasc Surg 101(4):584–592
11. Marc Gillinov A (2007) Surgical treatment of atrial fibrillation. In: Kaiser L, Kron I, Spray T (eds) Mastery of cardiothoracic surgery. Lippincott Williams & Wilkins, Philadelphia, pp 606–611
12. Gaynor SL, Diodato MD, Prasad SM et al (2004) A prospective, single-center clinical trial of a modified Cox Maze procedure with bipolar radiofrequency ablation. J Thorac Cardiovasc Surg 128(4):535–542
13. Lall SC, Melby SJ, Voeller RK, Zierer A, Bailey MS, Guthrie TJ, Moon MR, Moazami N, Lawton JS, Damiano RJ Jr (2007) The effect of ablation technology on surgical outcomes after the Cox-Maze procedure: a propensity analysis. J Thorac Cardiovasc Surg 133(2):389–396
14. Damiano RJ Jr, Schwartz FH, Bailey MS, Maniar HS, Munfakh NA, Moon MR, Schuessler RB (2011) The Cox Maze IV procedure: predictors of late recurrence. J Thorac Cardiovasc Surg 141(1):113–121
15. Damiano RJ Jr, Schuessler RB, Voeller RK (2007) Surgical treatment of atrial fibrillation: a look into the future. Semin Thorac Cardiovasc Surg 19(1):39–45
16. Prasad SM, Maniar HS, Schuessler RB et al (2002) Chronic transmural atrial ablation by using bipolar radiofrequency energy on the beating heart. J Thorac Cardiovasc Surg 124(4):708–713
17. Prasad SM, Maniar HS, Diodato MD et al (2003) Physiological consequences of bipolar radiofrequency energy on the atria and pulmonary veins: a chronic animal study. Ann Thorac Surg 76(3):836–841
18. Gaynor SL, Ishii Y, Diodato MD et al (2004) Successful performance of Cox Maze procedure on beating heart using bipolar radiofrequency ablation: a feasibility study in animals. Ann Thorac Surg 78(5):1671–1677
19. Khargi K, Deneke T, Haardt H et al (2001) Saline-irrigated, cooled-tip radiofrequency ablation is an effective technique to perform the Maze procedure. Ann Thorac Surg 72(3):S1090–S1095
20. Kottkamp H, Hindricks G, Autschbach R et al (2002) Specific linear left atrial lesions in atrial fibrillation: Intraoperative radiofrequency ablation using minimally invasive surgical techniques. J Am Coll Cardiol 40(3):475–480
21. Gaita F, Riccardi R, Caponi D et al (2005) Linear cryoablation of the left atrium versus pulmonary vein cryoisolation in patients with permanent atrial fibrillation and valvular heart disease: correlation of electroanatomic mapping and long-term clinical results. Circulation 111(2):136–142
22. Kondo N, Takahashi K, Minakawa M et al (2003) Left atrial Maze procedure: a useful addition to other corrective operations. Ann Thorac Surg 75(5):1490–1494
23. Salenger R, Lahey SJ, Saltman AE (2004) The completely endoscopic treatment of atrial fibrillation: report on the first 14 patients with early results. Heart Surg Forum 7(6):E555–E558
24. Tada H, Ito S, Naito S et al (2005) Long-term results of cryoablation with a new cryoprobe to eliminate chronic atrial fibrillation associated with mitral valve disease. Pacing Clin Electrophysiol 28 [Suppl 1]:S73–S77
25. Geidel S, Lass M, Boczor S et al (2004) Monopolar and bipolar radiofrequency ablation surgery: 3 year experience in 90 patients with permanent atrial fibrillation. Heart Surg Forum 7(5):E398–E402

26. Saltman AE (2007) Minimally invasive surgery for atrial fibrillation. Semin Thorac Cardiovasc Surg 19(1):33–38
27. Sales VL, McCarthy PM (2010) Minimally invasive surgery for atrial fibrillation. Tex Heart Inst J 37(6):660–661
28. Wolf RK (2007) Minimally invasive surgical treatment of atrial fibrillation. Semin Thorac Cardiovasc Surg 19(4):311–318
29. Gerosa G, Bianco R, Buja G, di Marco F (2004) Totally endoscopic robotic-guided pulmonary veins ablation: an alternative method for the treatment of atrial fibrillation. Eur J Cardiothorac Surg 26(2):450–452
30. Saltman AE, Rosenthal LS, Francalancia NA, Lahey SJ (2003) A completely endoscopic approach to microwave ablation for atrial fibrillation. Heart Surg Forum 6(3):E38–E41
31. Bisleri G, Muneretto C (2005) Innovative monolateral approach for closed-chest atrial fibrillation surgery. Ann Thorac Surg 80(5):e22–e25
32. Klinkenberg TJ, Ahmed S, Ten Hagen A, Wiesfeld AC, Tan ES, Zijlstra F, Van Gelder IC (2009) Feasibility and outcome of epicardial pulmonary vein isolation for lone atrial fibrillation using minimal invasive surgery and high intensity focused ultrasound. Europace 11(12):1624–1631
33. Speziale G, Bonifazi R, Nasso G, Bartolomucci F, Caldarola P, Fattouch K, Martines G, Tavazzi L, Chierchia SL (2010) Minimally invasive radiofrequency ablation of lone atrial fibrillation by monolateral right minithoracotomy: operative and early follow-up results. Ann Thorac Surg 90(1):161–167
34. Wolf RK, Schneeberger EW, Osterday R, Miller D, Merrill W, Flege JB et al (2005) Video-assisted bilateral pulmonary vein isolation and left atrial appendage exclusion for atrial fibrillation. J Thorac Cardiovasc Surg 130(3):797–802
35. Lecoq RR, Gracia JM, Sureda C, Igual A (2006) Subxyphoid approach for closed-chest atrial fibrillation surgery: the one hand operation. Interact Cardiovasc Thorac Surg 5(6):669–671
36. Krul SP, Driessen AH, van Boven WJ, Linnenbank AC, Geuzebroek GS, Jackman WM, Wilde AA, de Bakker JM, de Groot JR (2011) Thoracoscopic video-assisted pulmonary vein antrum isolation, ganglionated plexus ablation, and periprocedural confirmation of ablation lesions: first results of a hybrid surgical-electrophysiological approach for atrial fibrillation. Circ Arrhythm Electrophysiol 4(3):262–270

# Catheter Ablation of Atrial Fibrillation

# 25

Alessio Marinelli and Domenico Corrado

*I believe in Spinoza's God who reveals himself in the orderly harmony of what exists, not in a God who concerns himself with the fates and actions of human beings.*

Albert Einstein

**Abstract**

Atrial fibrillation (AF) is the most common sustained arrhythmia encountered in clinical practice, leading to more hospital admissions than any other arrhythmia. AF is commonly associated with structural heart disease such as valvular disease, coronary artery disease or cardiomyopathies. As with any other procedure in clinical medicine, potential risks and benefits need to be considered in deciding what to recommend for a particular patient. Balloon-based ablation systems are an attractive method of performing pulmonary vein isolation. Cryoballoon ablation appears to be the most completely tested. In 2011 ACCF/AHA/HRS Focused Update on the management of patients with AF state that "catheter ablation performed in experienced centers is useful in maintaining sinus rhythm in selected patients with significantly symptomatic, paroxysmal AF who have failed treatment with an anti-arrhythmic drug and have normal or mildly dilated left atria, normal or mildly reduced LV function, and no severe pulmonary disease". (Level of evidence: A; class of recommendation changed from IIa to I and level of evidence changed from C to A). Furthermore, the authors have added a new recommendation that state "Catheter ablation is reasonable for treating symptomatic persistent AF" (class IIa, level of evidence: A).

A. Marinelli (✉) · D. Corrado
Department of Cardiac Thoracic and Vascular Sciences,
University of Padua Medical School, Padova, Italy
e-mail: alessio.marinelli2@tin.it

M. Picichè (ed.), *Dawn and Evolution of Cardiac Procedures*,
DOI: 10.1007/978-88-470-2400-7_25, 

## 25.1 Introduction

Atrial fibrillation (AF) is the most common form of sustained arrhythmia encountered in clinical practice, leading to more hospital admissions than any other form. AF is commonly associated with structural heart disease such as valvular disease, coronary artery disease or cardiomyopathies [1]. However, AF may occur, in approximately 5 % of cases, in the absence of a clinically evident heart disease. Molecular, ionic, and genetic influences have all been implicated in AF [2].

In patients with significant structural heart disease the associated atrial dilatation and fibrosis play an important role in creating intra-atrial conduction defects, which predispose to both the initiation and perpetuation of AF [3, 4].

Usually, AF is initiated by a focal source, which is usually located in the pulmonary veins (PV) [5]. The underlying anatomical substrate is the presence of striated atrial muscle around the pulmonary veins. These myocardial–venous sleeves may extend as far as the lung border and beyond it. Some studies [6] showed that myocardial sleeves did not form discrete sphincters, but were continuous with the atrial myocardium. The anisotropic characteristics of myocardial sleeves in the veins may facilitate the escape of a focus with subsequent atrial activation [7].

Over the past 20 years, catheter ablation for the treatment of AF has evolved from an investigational procedure to one that is now performed on thousands of patients annually in many large medical centers.

## 25.2 Historical Consideration

In 1982 the era of catheter ablation therapy for cardiac arrhythmias began [8]. The source of ablative energy was DC shock and the target was the ablation of the atrioventricular junction in patients with intractable supraventricular tachyarrhythmias [9]. In the late 1980s and early 1990s, radiofrequency (RF) energy replaced DC shocks as a source of ablative energy, allowing safer and more controlled lesion formation. This technical advance led to more widespread use of catheter ablation, with higher success rates and lower complication rates [10].

At the same time Cox developed a series of techniques for the surgical interruption of AF [11]. The idea behind the Maze procedure was that by dividing the atria into electrically isolated subsections that were small enough, maintenance of AF could be prevented regardless of the mode of initiation.

## 25.3 Catheter Ablation for AF

The success of the Maze III procedure in the early 1990s led some interventional cardiac electrophysiologists to attempt to reproduce the surgical approach with RF catheter lesions. Although the efficacy was modest, complication rates were high, and procedures and fluoroscopy times were exceedingly long. However, this demonstrated a proof of concept that led others to try to improve the catheter-based approach.

### 25.3.1 Linear Ablation Approach

In 1996, Haissaguerre et al. [12] reported the technique and outcomes of linear catheter ablation in 45 patients undergoing right and/or left atrial ablation for paroxysmal AF. The right atrial lesion sets consisted of an intercaval line along the interatrial septum and a cavotricuspid isthmus line to prevent atrial flutter. Left atrial lesions were designed to connect the four PVs to each other and to the mitral annulus. An additional line from the right PVs to the interatrial septum was made in 23 patients. The authors concluded that safety, efficacy, and applicability needed to be improved. Other trials were terminated prematurely owing to high complication rates and poor efficacy [13].

On the basis of these observations and the rapid advances in the ablation of focal triggers, the only catheter-based linear approach to AF has been largely abandoned.

### 25.3.2 Focal Approach

One important observation that came from the study of Haissaguerre et al. [14] from their work on the ablation of AF was the fact that some patients with paroxysmal AF appeared to have a focal source of electrical activity triggering the arrhythmias.

They published findings in a larger series of 45 patients in a landmark publication in 1998 [5]. Patients had frequent paroxysms of drug-refractory AF. They also had at least 700 isolated premature atrial beats. All underwent intracardiac mapping of premature atrial ectopic beats. Sixty-nine foci were found and targeted for ablation. Ninety-four percent of these originated within PVs, most within 2–4 cm of the ostium. AF was initiated with a burst of pacing from the foci and was interrupted with RF ablation at the site of origin. After a follow-up period of $8 \pm 6$ months, 28 patients (62 %) were free of AF and off anti-arrhythmic drugs. These findings were soon replicated by other groups [15].

With further research, it was also observed that non-PV foci were an important source of AF in some patients. Among the sources identified were the vein of Marshall (a remnant of the fetal left superior vena cava on the posterior left atrial wall), the coronary sinus, and the superior vena cava [16, 17].

With increasing use of the focal ablation of PV triggers, the problem of stenosis quickly became recognized owing to its serious sequelae, including hemoptysis, pulmonary edema, and pulmonary hypertension [18]. Another problem with the focal approach was the recognition that after successful ablation, recurrence rates were high and remapping usually showed new foci in the ablated vein or in other veins. A final major limitation of this approach is that it requires atrial premature beats triggering AF to be observed during the ablation procedure, limiting it to patients with frequent spontaneous or inducible atrial premature beats [5].

### 25.3.3 Segmental Ostial Approach

The evidence of these major limitations of focal ablation led to development of the PV isolation (PVI) technique. Recognizing that PV musculature conducts to the left atrial wall by discrete connections allowed investigators to target those connections using multipolar catheters shaped into rings or baskets [19]. After defining PV anatomy with contrast-enhanced venography, a circular mapping catheter was placed at the ostium of the targeted PV. Ablation was performed with a separate catheter through the second trans-septal sheath at the site of earliest activation sequentially until PV electrical activity disappeared or became dissociated from left atrium activity [20]. Using this strategy, between 20 and 60% of the PV circumference was targeted for ablation [21].

The technique of segmental ostial PV isolation represented an important advance in the catheter treatment of AF over the focal approach. Studies have shown good success for patients with paroxysmal AF, but generally poor results for persistent and permanent AF.

### 25.3.4 Circumferential Approach

Concurrently with the development of the segmental approach to PV isolation, Pappone et al. [22] developed the circumferential approach using electroanatomical mapping. After placement of one or more electrophysiological catheters, a single trans-septal puncture was performed, and a long sheath was placed in the left atrium. Using a magnetic-based electroanatomical mapping system, an anatomical shell was constructed with the mapping/ablation catheter, including the PVs. RF ablation was then performed circumferentially around each vein with the end point of ablation being the absence or marked reduction (80 %) in the amplitude of electrical signals within the encircling lesions (Fig. 25.1).

If the inferior and superior veins were closely spaced or shared a common ostium, a single large circumferential RF lesion set was performed (Figs. 25.2, 25.3). Despite the lack of evidence showing that PVs treated in this way were electrically isolated from the left atrium, this group began reporting results for paroxysmal AF that were just as good or better than those working with the ostial segmental approach. Furthermore, patients with persistent/permanent AF treated with the circumferential approach achieved freedom from AF nearly as good as those with paroxysmal AF and far better than reports of patients treated with segmental PV isolation.

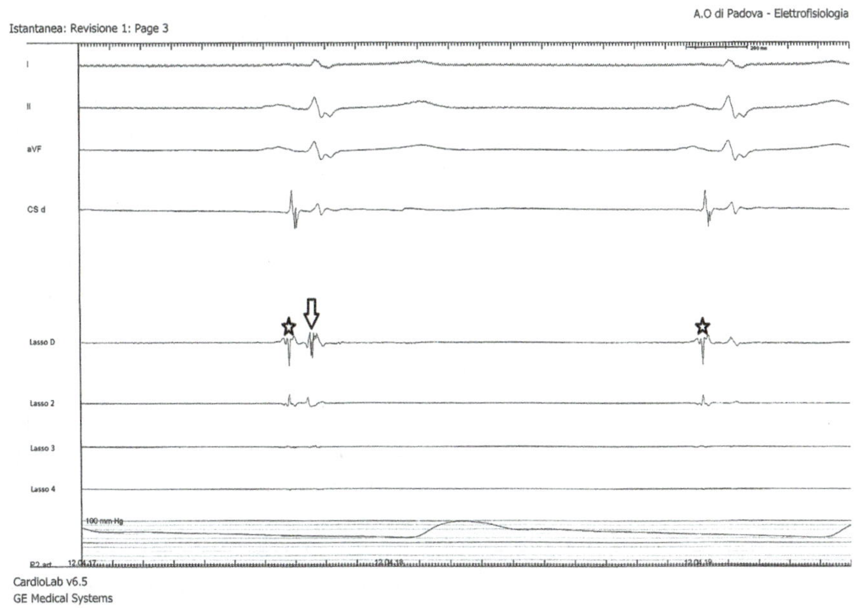


**Fig. 25.1** Pulmonary vein (PV) isolation: the *star* is the left atrial electrogram, the *arrow* the PV potential that disappears during RF ablation

Thus, the relative simplicity in the technique and the reportedly equivalent or greater efficacy have led many centers to adopt the circumferential approach to PV ablation [23].

### 25.3.5 Hybrid Approach

The reported success of the circumferential approach has raised several important questions in the field of ablation for AF and has led investigators to attempt modifications to the standard circumferential lesion set, resulting in hybrid approaches to AF ablation. The first question is whether complete electrical isolation of the PVs is necessary to achieve clinical success. Ouyang et al. [24] treated 41 patients with paroxysmal AF with a modified circumferential ablation approach. In each patient, a single large extraostial circumferential lesion set was placed around inferior and superior PVs on each side, while a circular mapping catheter was present in each of the two ipsilateral veins. Ablation was continued until complete electrical isolation was achieved in all four PVs. Ten patients had early recurrence and 9 underwent a second procedure. All these patients showed recurrent conduction from a previously isolated PV and underwent reisolation of that. At about 6 months' follow-up, 39 out of 41 patients (95 %) were free of AF without anti-arrhythmic drugs. Major complications were limited to one patient with asymptomatic PV stenosis in a single PV.

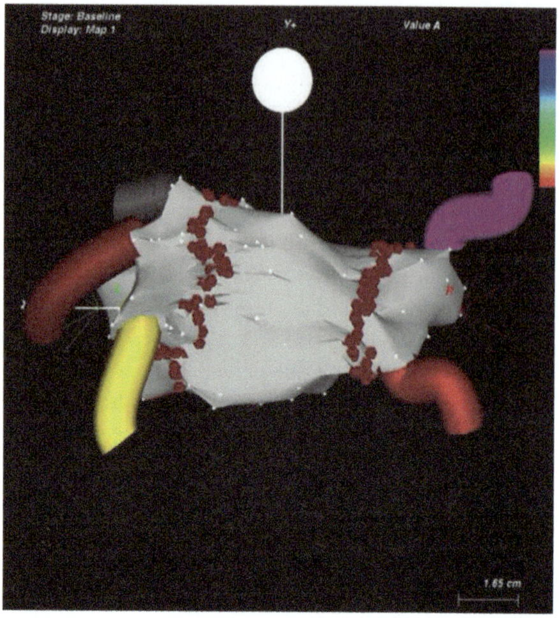


**Fig. 25.2** PV isolation: a single large extraostial circumferential lesion set was placed around inferior and superior PVs on each side, using a magnetic-based electroanatomical mapping system

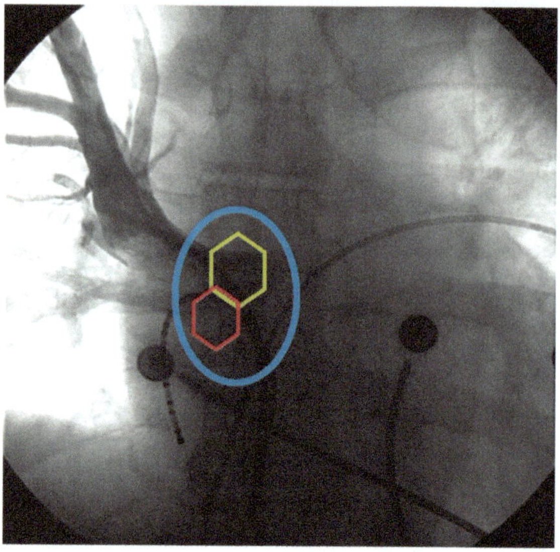

**Fig. 25.3** RF ablation performed circumferentially around each ostium vein (*yellow and red hexagons*) or a single large extraostial circumferential lesion placed around inferior and superior PVs (*blue circle*). Note the angiography of the right superior PV

A second important question concerns the safety and efficacy of adding left atrial linear lesions to the basic circumferential PV ablation lesion set. The two linear lesions most commonly added are a line connecting the right and left superior veins, the so-called "roof" line, and a line connecting the left inferior PV to the mitral valve annulus, the so-called "mitral isthmus" line. These lesion sets are designed to further modify electrical substrate to prevent AF as well as to prevent left atrial flutter, which might be formed by the large circumferential lines of block. Jais et al. [25] have shown that achieving block with the mitral isthmus line in particular is technically challenging and sometimes requires ablation deep within the coronary sinus.

In 2004 Nademanee et al. [26] studied 121 patients with drug-refractory paroxysmal (57 patients) and persistent/permanent (64 patients) AF and used a novel approach to mapping of AF substrate and performing ablation. During AF in all patients biatrial electroanatomical mapping was performed. Areas of complex fractionated electrical potentials (so-called "CFAE", complex fractionated atrial electrogram) were noted and tagged. Complex fractionated atrial electrograms were found in 7 of the 9 regions of both atria, but were mainly confined to the interatrial septum, pulmonary veins, roof of the left atrium, the left posteroseptal mitral annulus, and the coronary sinus ostium. At the 1-year follow-up, 110 patients (91 %) were free of arrhythmia and symptoms, 92 after one ablation and 18 after two.

## 25.4 New Approaches to Catheter Ablation of AF

Like many other medical procedures, technological innovation is likely to be a contributing factor in making atrial fibrillation ablation a more commonplace and widely practiced therapy.

Navigating the complex anatomy of the left atrium is also difficult to master. With fluoroscopy alone, it is difficult to determine anterior versus posterior orientation or the presence of the catheter in a pulmonary vein versus the left atrial appendage. Intracardiac echocardiography (ICE) provides two-dimensional navigation assistance and excellent anatomical detail; however, it is difficult to locate the catheter tip at all times in the echocardiography field. Electroanatomical mapping (EAM) systems offer a 3D view and nearly real-time catheter tip localization within a created construct of the left atrium, but the data are heavily dependent on the input of the operator and cartographer. Newer technology has merged these two imaging modalities to offer the best of both worlds [27].

Remotely obtained computed tomography (CT) imaging of the left atrium has been performed to define the complex anatomy of the left atrium. This can be integrated into EAMs or imaging systems to aid in navigation and procedure planning. However, conditions at the time of CT may be different from those at the time of ablation. New fluoroscopic systems allow the performance of rotational angiography, which can be used to re-create CT-like images of the left atrium for use in the procedure at the same time.

Another method of tackling the challenge of the dexterity required for atrial fibrillation ablation is remote navigation. The two currently available technologies include remote robotic navigation and remote magnetic navigation [28]. A reduction in radiation exposure for the operator and the patient has also been nearly universally reported [29]. The close interaction with the EAM system is likely the main reason for the reduction in fluoroscopy. These navigation technologies hold great promise, but require adaption to the newer ablation technologies for long-term survival.

Another method of performing large-area ablations for pulmonary vein isolation is using multielectrode radiofrequency ablation catheters. The catheters used for pulmonary vein isolation are circular and mesh array-shaped. Ablation at specific poles could allow pinpoint-type ablation without the requirement of large-area lesions. Currently, these catheters do not appear to be as maneuverable as the circular mapping catheters, limiting their use outside the pulmonary veins [30].

It is difficult for an operator to accurately determine the force at the catheter tip. New force-sensing technologies have been developed to aid the operator in applying appropriate force to deliver optimal lesions without risking pressure-related complications. The angle of the catheter in relation to the tissue may also be displayed. Early data have shown that this information may reduce pressure-related complications [31, 32]

### 25.4.1 Balloon-Based Ablation System

Balloon-based ablation systems are an attractive method of performing pulmonary vein isolation. The balloon system should fit the pulmonary vein anatomy and offer a method of performing electric isolation with a minimum number of lesions. It is conceivable that pulmonary vein stenosis might be eliminated because the energy could be directed away from the center of the vein. The thousands of movements required to isolate all of the pulmonary veins could be replaced by placing a single catheter in each vein and making a large-area lesion.

Balloon-based ablation systems offer the ability to deliver other ablation technologies such as cryoablation, laser, and high-frequency ultrasound. Each of these ablation technologies has different potential benefits. High-frequency ultrasound may offer transmural ablation without the complete occlusion of the vein required with other technologies [33]. Laser therapy can be combined with endoscopic visualization, and cryoablation may carry less risk of esophageal injury or ablation-induced perforation [34].

Balloon-based ablation has had limited success. Balloons offer only pulmonary vein isolation and do not address areas such as the posterior wall, septum, roof, mitral valve isthmus, coronary sinus, base of the left atrial appendage, or other areas that may harbor complex fractionated electrograms. Different catheters and possibly different ablation technologies are needed to address these areas.

Cryoballoon ablation appears to be the most completely tested [35]. The left atrium is accessed via the trans-septal route. After angiography each PV is mapped. The balloon is then advanced toward the PV ostium and inflated. During cryoablation the balloon reaches temperatures around −50 °C for about 300 s (Fig. 25.4).

Testing on the high-frequency ultrasound balloon system has stopped [36].

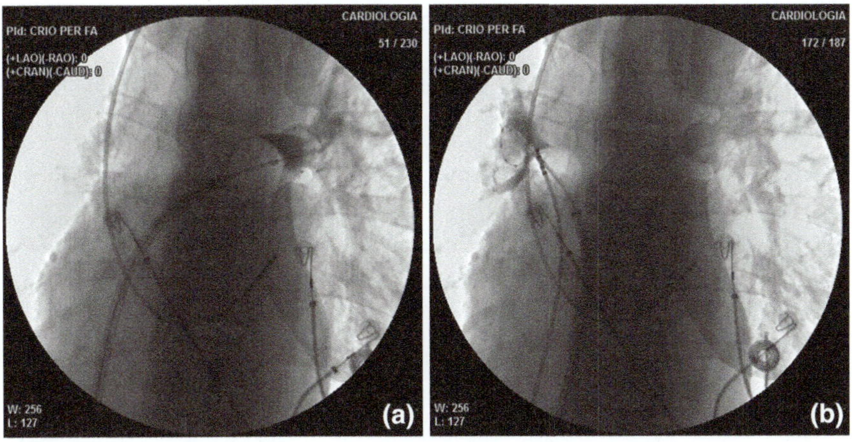


**Fig. 25.4** Cryoballoon ablation. **a** The balloon was inflated in the left superior PV. **b** Ablation of the right superior PV. The degree of balloon occlusion was excellent in both. Note the circular mapping catheter inside the PV and the electrophysiological catheter in the right atrium for the phrenic nerve stimulation during the ablation of the right PV

The laser balloon has been evaluated [37]and is undergoing a design change to address some of the issues, including complications and the inability to isolate all veins. If these obstacles can be overcome, balloon-based ablation may become part of the armamentarium for atrial fibrillation ablation [38].

## 25.5 Current Approach to Catheter Ablation of AF

In 2011 ACCF/AHA/HRS Focused Update [39] on the management of patients with AF state that "catheter ablation performed in experienced centers is useful in maintaining sinus rhythm in selected patients with significantly symptomatic, paroxysmal AF who have failed treatment with an anti-arrhythmic drug and have normal or mildly dilated left atria, normal or mildly reduced LV function, and no severe pulmonary disease. (Level of evidence: A; class of recommendation changed from IIa to I and level of evidence changed from C to A). Furthermore, the authors have added a new recommendation that states that "Catheter ablation is reasonable for treating symptomatic persistent AF" (class IIa, level of evidence: A).

## 25.6 Risks and Benefits of Catheter Ablation for AF

As with any other procedure in clinical medicine, potential risks and benefits need to be considered in deciding what to recommend for a particular patient (Table 25.1).

**Table 25.1** Major complications in the overall population (total population was 16,309 patients. Major complications occurred in 741 patients 4.54%) [40]

| Type of complications | Rate (%) |
|---|---|
| Tamponade | 1.31 |
| Femoral pseudoaneurysm | 0.93 |
| Transient ischemic attack | 0.71 |
| Arterio-venous fistulae | 0.54 |
| Pulmonary vein stenoses requiring intervention | 0.29 |
| Stroke | 0.23 |
| Permanent diaphragmatic paralysis | 0.17 |
| Death | 0.15 |
| Pneumothorax | 0.09 |
| Valve damage/requiring surgery | 0.07 |
| Atrium-esophageal fistulae | 0.04 |
| Sepsis, abscesses or endocarditis | 0.01 |
| Total | 4.54 |

In 2008 Jais, Haissaguerre et al. [41] in "The A4 Study" demonstrated the superiority of catheter ablation over anti-arrhythmic drugs in patients with AF with regard to maintenance of sinus rhythm and improvement in symptoms, exercise capacity, and quality of life. Symptom score, exercise capacity, and quality of life were significantly higher in the ablation group.

In 2011 Jais et al. [42] describes 5-year follow-up results of catheter ablation for AF. Patients with long-standing persistent AF experienced a higher recurrence rate than those with paroxysmal or persistent forms. Thus, the conclusion of this study is that in selected patients with AF, a catheter ablation strategy with repeat intervention as necessary provides acceptable long-term relief. Although most recurrences transpire over the first 6–12 months, a slow but steady decline in arrhythmia-free survival is noted thereafter.

## References

1. Falk RH (2001) Atrial fibrillation. N Engl J Med 344:1067–1078
2. Corrado D, Leoni L, Basso C, Buja G, Iliceto S, Thiene G (2003) Anatomic substrates of atrial fibrillation: do they play a role in clinical practice? CEPI
3. Allessie MA, Ausma J, Schotten U (2002) Electrical, contractile and structural remodeling during atrial fibrillation. Cardiovasc Res 54:230–246

4. Hordof AJ, Edie R, Malm JR, Hoffman BF, Rosen MR (1976) Electrophysiologic properties and response to pharmacologic agents of fibers from diseased human atria. Circulation 54:774–779
5. Haissaguerre M, Jais P, Shash DC et al (1998) Spontaneous initiation of atrial fibrillation by ectopic beats originating in the pulmonary veins. N Engl J Med 339:659–666
6. Ho SY, Anderson RH, Sanchez-Quintana D (2002) Atrial structure and fibres: morphologic bases of atrial conduction. Cardiovasc Res 54:325–336
7. Cheung DW (1981) Electrical activity of the pulmonary vein and its interaction in the right atrium in the guinea-pig. J Physiol 314:445–456
8. Marine JE, Dong J, Calkins H (2005) Catheter ablation therapy for atrial fibrillation. Prog Cardiovasc Dis 48:178–192
9. Scheinman MM, Morady F, Hess DS et al (1982) Catheter induced ablation of the atrioventricular junction to control refractory supraventricular arrhythmias. JAMA 248:851–855
10. Calkins H, Sousa J, Atassi R et al (1991) Diagnosis and cure of the Wolff-Parkinson-White syndrome or paroxysmal supraventricular tachycardias during a single electrophysiologic test. N Engl J Med 324:1612–1618
11. Cox JL, Schuessler RB, Lappas DG et al (1996) An 8 ½ year clinical experience with surgery for atrial fibrillation. Ann Surg 224:267–275
12. Jais P, Shah DC, Haissaguerre M et al (1999) Efficacy and safety of septal and left linear ablation for atrial fibrillation. Am J Cardiol 84:139R–146R
13. Calkins H, Hall H, Ellenbogen K et al (1999) A new system for catheter ablation of atrial fibrillation. Am J Cardiol 83:227D–236D
14. Haissaguerre M, Marcus FI, Fischer B et al (1994) Radio-frequency catheter ablation in unusual mechanisms of atrial fibrillation: report of three cases. J Cardiovasc Electrophysiol 5:743–751
15. Chen SA, Hsieh MH, Tai CT et al (1999) Initiation of atrial fibrillation by ectopic beats originating from the pulmonary veins: electrophysiological characteristic, pharmacological responses an effects of radiofrequency ablation. Circulation 100:1879–1886
16. Tsai CF, Tai CT, Hsieh MH et al (2000) Initiation of atrial fibrillation by ectopic beats originating from the superior vena cava. Circulation 102:67–74
17. Hwang C, Wu TJ, Doshi RN et al (2000) Vein of Marshall cannulation for the analysis of electrical activity in patient with focal atrial fibrillation. Circulation 101:1503–1505
18. Saad EB, Rossillo A, Saad CP et al (2003) Pulmonary vein stenosis after radiofrequency ablation of atrial fibrillation: functional characterization, evolution and influence of the ablation strategy. Circulation 108:3102–3107
19. Haissaguerre M, Shah DC, Jais P et al (2000) Electrophysiological breakthroughs from the left atrium to the pulmonary veins. Circulation 102:2463–2465
20. Hocini M, Sanders P, Jais P et al (2004) Techniques for curative treatment of atrial fibrillation. J Cardiovasc Electrophysiol 15:1467–1471
21. Marchlinski FE, Callans D, Dixit S et al (2003) Efficacy and safety of targeted focal ablation versus PV isolation assisted by magnetic electroanatomic mapping. J Cardiovasc Electrophysiol 14:358–365
22. Pappone C, Rosanio S, Oreto G et al (2000) Circumferential radiofrequency ablation of pulmonary vein ostia: a new anatomic approach for curing atrial fibrillation. Circulation 102:2619–2628
23. Oral H, Scharf C, Chugh A et al (2003) Catheter ablation for paroxysmal atrial fibrillation: segmental pulmonary vein ostia ablation versus left atrial ablation. Circulation 108:2355–2360
24. Ouyang F, Baensch D, Ernst S et al (2004) Complete isolation of the left atrium surrounding the pulmonary veins: new insights from the double-lasso technique in paroxysmal atrial fibrillation. Circulation 110:2090–2096
25. Jais P, Hocini M, Hsu LF et al (2004) Technique and results of linear ablation at the mitral isthmus. Circulation 110:2996–3002

26. Nademanee K, McKenzie J, Kosar E et al (2004) A new approach for catheter ablation of atrial fibrillation: mapping of the electrophysiologic substrate. J Am Coll Cardiol 43: 2044–2053
27. Burkhardt JD, Natale A (2009) New technologies in atrial fibrillation ablation. Circulation 120:1533–1541
28. Reddy VY, Neuzil P, Malchano ZJ, Vijaykumar R, Cury R, Abbara S, Weichet J, McPherson CD, Ruskin JN (2007) View-synchronized robotic image-guided therapy for atrial fibrillation ablation: experimental validation and clinical feasibility. Circulation 115:2705–2714
29. Pappone C, Santinelli V (2008) Safety and efficacy of remote magnetic ablation for atrial fibrillation. J Am Coll Cardiol 51:1614–1615
30. Kistler PM (2008) Multielectrode ablation for paroxysmal atrial fibrillation: pulmonary vein isolation made easy? Heart Rhythm 5:1643–1644
31. Di Biase L, Natale A, Cummings JE et al (2009) Relationship between catheter forces, lesion characteristics, "popping", and char formation: experience with robotic navigation system. J Cardiovasc Electrophysiol 20:436–440
32. Schmidt B, Kuck KH, Shah D, Reddy V, Saoudi N, Herrera C, Hindricks G, Natale A, Jais P, Lambert H (2009) Toccata multi-center clinical study using irrigated ablation catheter with integrated contact force sensor: first results. Heart Rhythm 6:S536
33. Okumura Y, Kolasa MW, Johnson SB, Bunch TJ, Henz BD, O'Brien CJ, Miller DV, Packer DL (2008) Mechanism of tissue heating during high intensity focused ultrasound pulmonary vein isolation: implications for atrial fibrillation ablation efficacy and phrenic nerve protection. J Cardiovasc Electrophysiol 19:945–951
34. Evonich RF III, Nori DM, Haines DE (2007) A randomized trial comparing effects of radiofrequency and cryoablation on the structural integrity of esophageal tissue. J Interv Card Electrophysiol 19:77–83
35. Chun KR, Schmidt B, Metzner A, Tilz R, Zerm T, Koster I, Furnkranz A, Koektuerk B, Konstantinidou M, Antz M, Ouyang F, Kuck KH (2009) The "single big cryoballoon" technique for acute pulmonary vein isolation in patients with paroxysmal atrial fibrillation: a prospective observational single centre study. Eur Heart J 30:699–709
36. Neven K, Schmidt B, Metzner A, Chun KRJ, Ouyang F, Kuck KH et al (2010) Fatal end of a safety algorithm for pulmonary vein isolation with use of high-intensity focused ultrasound. Circ Arrhythm Electrophysiol 3:260–265
37. Reddy VNP, Themistoclakis S, Bonso A, Rossillo A, Raviele A, Natale A et al (2007) Visually-guided pulmonary vein isolation using a balloon ablation catheter to treat patients with paroxysmal atrial fibrillation: one-year clinical outcome following a single ablation procedure. Circulation 116 [Suppl II]:II-536. Abstract
38. Schmidt B, Chun KR, Metzner A, Ouyang F, Kuck KH (2008) Balloon catheters for pulmonary vein isolation. Herz 33:580–584
39. Wann LS, Curtis AB, January CT et al (2011) ACCF/AHA/HRS focused update on the management of patients with atrial fibrillation (updating the 2006 guideline): a report of the American College of Cardiology Foundation/American Heart Association task force on practice guidelines. Circulation 2011(123):104–123
40. Cappato R, Calkins H, Chen S, Davies W, Iesaka Y, Kalman J, Kim Y, Klein G, Natale A, Packer D, Skanes A, Ambrogi F, Biganzoli E (2010) Updated worldwide survey on the methods, efficacy and safety of catheter ablation for human atrial fibrillation. Circ Arrhythmia Electrophysiol 3:32–38
41. Jais P, Clementy J, Haissaguerre M et al (2008) Catheter ablation versus antiarrhythmic drugs for atrial fibrillation: the A4 study. Circulation 118:2498–2505
42. Weerasooriya R, Haissaguerre M, Jais P et al (2011) Catheter ablation for atrial fibrillation: are results maintained at 5 years of follow-up? J Am Coll Cardiol 57:160–166

# The History of Cardiac Pacemakers and Defibrillators

# 26

Serge Boveda, Stéphane Garrigue and Philippe Ritter

> *A knowledge of the existence of something we cannot penetrate, of the manifestations of the profoundest reason and the most radiant beauty—it is this knowledge and this emotion that constitute the truly religious attitude; in this sense, and in this alone, I am a deeply religious man.*
>
> Albert Einstein

**Abstract**

Cardiac pacing has hugely and rapidly improved in just over 50 years, thanks to advances in electronics, computing, nanotechnology, and medicine. Engineers and physicians are committed to reproducing, as closely as possible, the physiological cardiac cycle and the mechanical activity of the right and left ventricles. The history of the implantable cardioverter defibrillator (ICD) is unique because it relies on the bold project of one man, Mirowski. In 1985, the first implantable cardioverter defibrillator was marketed. This system allowed the ventricle to be paced and provided better detection, which improved the percentage of appropriate shocks. We can imagine that, in the future, progress will continue toward further miniaturization and longevity, but also perhaps the research of new and more compatible biological materials. Research into cardiac pacing and ICDs has been motivated by huge medical and economic issues, and will continue, although we are still amazed by these small but fascinating metal boxes!

S. Boveda (✉)
Arrhythmia Department, Clinique Pasteur, Toulouse, France
e-mail: s.boveda@clinique-pasteur.com

S. Garrigue
Cardiology Department, Clinique St. Agustin, Bordeaux, France

P. Ritter
Cardiology Department, CHU de Haut-Lévêque, Pessac, France

M. Picichè (ed.), *Dawn and Evolution of Cardiac Procedures*,
DOI: 10.1007/978-88-470-2400-7_26, © Springer-Verlag Italia 2013

## 26.1 Pacing Hearts: The Beginning of a Success Story

The first conference on cardiac pacing was organized in September 1958, in the United States, by the Rockefeller Institute (now Rockefeller University). A total of 24 engineers, surgeons, and cardiologists attended the event. Companies were absent from this meeting of pioneers, and most innovations were reported by small teams of researchers within University Hospitals. Yet, already in 1958, crucial questions were being asked [1], such as:

- Was long-term pacing possible in patients with chronic heart disease?
- How could pacemakers be inhibited automatically in cases of spontaneous cardiac activity?
- Was miniaturization of the generator, and its implantation inside the body, feasible?
- What was the ideal pacing rate and how could this be changed after implantation of the generator?
- Sensing the atrium with synchronous pacing and maintenance of the physiological atrio-ventricular sequence was also of major concern.

This fascinating venture (Fig. 26.1) was begun in 1871 when Steinert paced animal hearts, and Greene, in 1872, did the same in humans. John McWilliam, Professor at Aberdeen University, published, in 1889 "...the repeated electrical pacing should be used to maintain the heart rate in patients with bradycardia..." [2].

However, everything really began in 1952 (Table 26.1) when Zoll, of Boston's Beth Israel Hospital, described how he had resuscitated a patient, who was in cardiac arrest, using subcutaneous electrodes connected to an external generator [3]. During the 1950s, several hospitals equipped themselves with external pacemakers. Transient external cardiac pacing for emergency resuscitation was the main condition from which patients could benefit until 1957.

In 1957, Walton Lillehei and his colleagues, at the University of Minnesota, took the first step of suturing the distal part of an electrode, coated with copper and silver and insulated with Teflon, onto the right ventricular myocardium, while the other end was connected to a generator through the chest wall. The patient had a postoperative complete atrioventricular (AV) block [4].

The first external generators were bulky, but were soon "miniaturized" to allow patients to carry them around (Fig. 26.2). The same year, a group of European researchers devised a generator that could be inhibited when it sensed QRS complexes.

In 1958, two patients from the Montefiore Hospital in New York, received a pacemaker as an external device, thanks to a lead that, for the first time, was endocardially placed in the right ventricle (RV) via a venous approach. Yet, despite this rapid progress, Parsonnet and Bernstein reported in 1958: "...Nobody has shown that cardiac pacing could help routinely to save lives..." [1]. In September 1958, Zoll presented a cohort of over a 100 patients who had undergone this technique. Lillehei and colleagues paced 57 patients, most for less than 2 weeks [5, 6], although one patient was treated for 21 days. In Montefiore

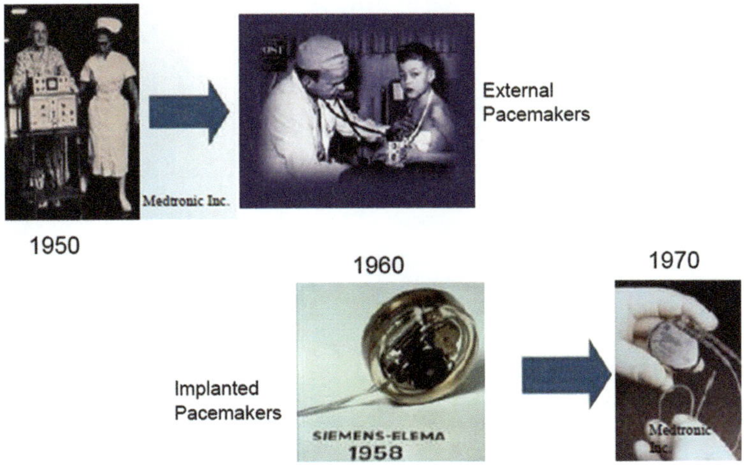


**Fig. 26.1** The history of pacemakers at a glance

**Table 26.1** Key dates in the story of cardiac pacing and defibrillation

| |
|---|
| 1952 Zoll PB—Resuscitation of the heart in ventricular standstill by external electrical stimulation [3] |
| 1958 Elmquist R, Senning A—An implantable pacemaker for the heart [8] |
| 1969 Berkovits BV et al.—Bifocal demand pacing [12] |
| 1980 Mirowski M et al.—Termination of malignant ventricular arrhythmias with an implanted automatic defibrillator in human beings [26] |
| 1994 Cazeau S et al.—Four chamber pacing in dilated cardiomyopathy [21] |
| 2010 Bardy GH et al.—An entirely subcutaneous implantable cardioverter defibrillator [27] |

Hospital, Furman had paced a patient for 23 days continuously, and intermittently for a total of 96 days [7]. Several groups of researchers at the time were also working on implantable asynchronous pacemakers (VOO) designed for chronic cardiac pacing. However, these research groups were not invited to a conference at the Rockefeller Institute as they were unknown in 1958 because of their lack of publication. Among these "forgotten" researchers were Senning (Stockholm), Chardack (Buffalo), and William Glenn (Yale).

In 1959, two groups who were non-guests at the Rockefeller Institute, Senning and his colleague Elmqvist in Sweden [8], and Chardack associated with Greatbatch in the United States [9], realized, in parallel, the first complete implantation (generator and lead) of a pacemaker in humans: the implantable pacemaker was born.

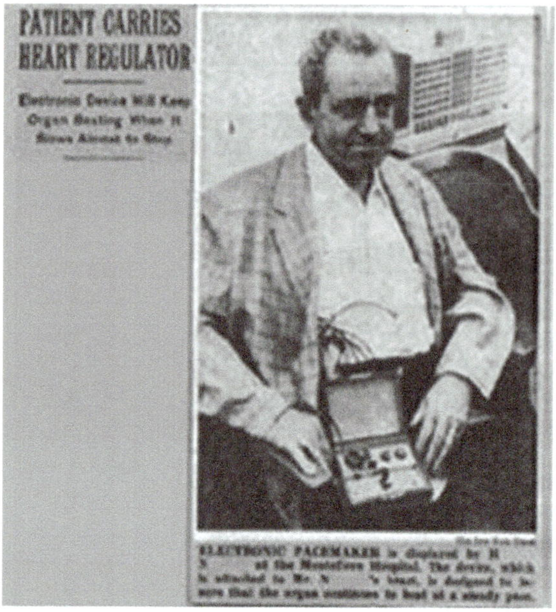


**Fig. 26.2** Starting miniaturization. Patient carrying a generator (New York Times June 23, 1959)

Since the glorious 1950s, pacing has steadily evolved:

- The 1960s was devoted to miniaturization of the generator, which was implanted abdominally, and improvement in its longevity thanks to lithium batteries [10].
- The 1970s brought sophisticated dual-chamber pacemakers (DDD) [11, 12].
- The 1980s offered the rate-responsive pacemaker (VVIR, DDDR), capable of increasing its rate according to effort, coupled with physical activity of the patient, body temperature, variation in thoracic impedance, and duration of QT [13, 14].
- The 1990s gave the opportunity to implant very small generators (Fig. 26.3), with greater longevity ($\sim$7 years), sophisticated algorithms such as the fallback system (DDD–VVIR) in cases of paroxysmal atrial fibrillation, adaptable AV delays, and hysteresis. At the same time, programmers were more powerful and easy to use.

Nevertheless, one of the most important improvements in the era of cardiac pacing took place at the end of the last century with the development of cardiac resynchronization. This technique allowed pacing of the left ventricle (LV) through the coronary sinus to treat heart-failure patients who were refractory to conventional treatments.

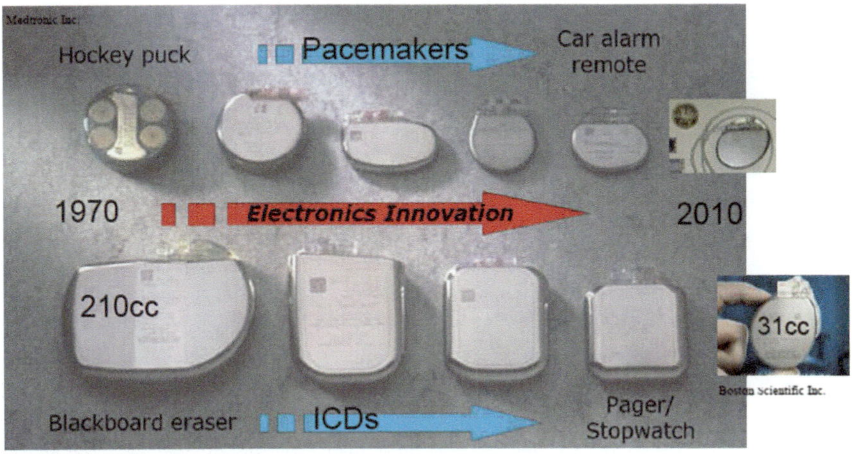


**Fig. 26.3** Miniaturization of pacemakers and defibrillators over time

## 26.2 Cardiac Resynchronization: Pacing and More

The idea of biventricular pacing, or cardiac resynchronization therapy (CRT) as it is more commonly known today, most likely came from a variety of animal studies performed in the late 1980s and early 1990s. Most notable among these was the 1986 study on canine pacing in which Burkhoff and colleagues noted that left ventricular pressure decreased linearly as QRS duration increased [15]. It was noted in further studies that there was a high prevalence of left-bundle-branch block (LBBB) or intraventricular conduction delay in chronic heart-failure [16]. The hemodynamic effects of LBBB in chronic heart failure include reduced left ventricular ejection fraction, reduced cardiac output, reduced mean arterial pressure, and reduced dP/dt [17, 18]. Following the Burkhoff study, Lattuca and colleagues [19] hypothesized that, by simultaneously pacing the LV along with the RV, more synchronous ventricular activation (QRS) plus a resultant improvement in synchronous ventricular-contraction pattern could be achieved by reducing the duration of QRS, thereby reducing intraventricular asynchrony.

Pacing systems were initially implanted via a thoracotomy using an epicardial lead system. This approach was associated with significant morbidity and a theoretical risk of mortality. Subsequent investigators realized that the coronary sinus could provide an alternative transvenous approach to LV pacing via one of its LV venous branches (Fig. 26.4). Yee [20], Cazeau, and Ritter [21] were among the first to realize this approach through their investigations. Over the past two decades, CRT has evolved from concept to clinical application.

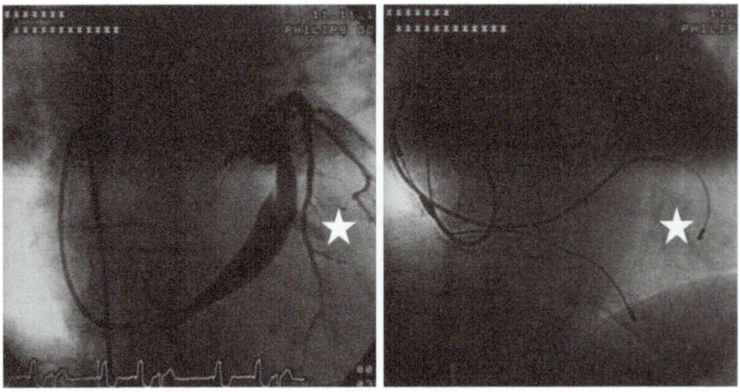

**Fig. 26.4** Cardiac resynchronization device. Coronary sinus angiogram before implantation (*left*). Chest radiography (*right*) showing the three leads placed endocardially through the subclavian vein, inside the right atrium, the right ventricle, and the lateral vein of the coronary sinus in order to pace epicardially the left ventricle (*star*)

## 26.3 An Implantable Cardioverter Defibrillator to Prevent Sudden Death

The survival of patients with a cardiac arrest outside a medical environment is extremely low, and does not exceed 5 %. In this context, the implantable cardioverter defibrillator (ICD) is the standard treatment for sudden death.

In 1899, in Geneva, Jean-Louis Prevost and Frederic Battelli discovered, in animals, that they could induce ventricular fibrillation by applying an electrical stimulus of low energy, and reduce it by applying an alternate electric current of high intensity to the skin [22]. This discovery was crucial because it introduced the concept of nonpharmacological and nonsurgical treatment, which is still used today. However, it was not until the 1920s that Prevost and Battelli's results were re-examined [22].

In 1926, Kouwenhoven was an electrical engineer working at Johns Hopkins Hospital in Baltimore, in the department of William H. Howell (this department is now called Biomedical). In 1933, Kouwenhoven confirmed Prevost and Battelli's theory: a current of high-voltage can reduce ventricular fibrillation and, therefore, can theoretically save a person who has been electrocuted or is inanimate. This was the first time that the application of a high-voltage current was called a "defibrillation current." Yet in 1937, when Kouwenhoven published his first article on this subject, no clinician would embark on the adventure, and defibrillation remained in the experimental stages. However, his work did inspire many "competing" teams, such as that led by Dr. Beck, a cardiac surgeon at Case Western Reserve University in Cleveland, Ohio, USA.

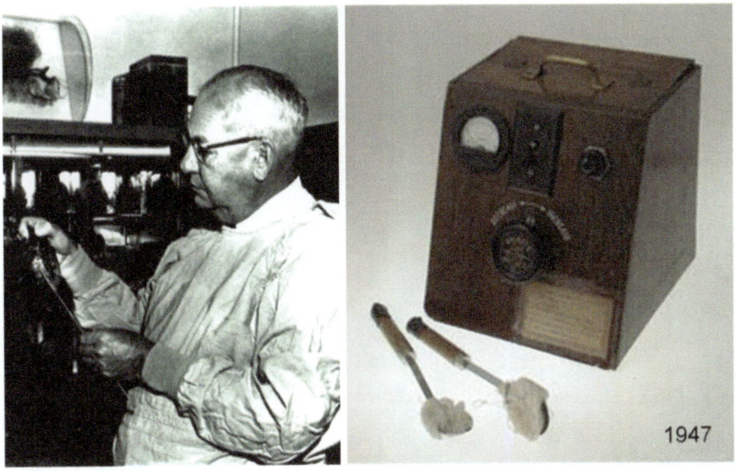


**Fig. 26.5** Claude Schaeffer Beck (1894–1971) and the first AC internal defibrillator used to convert ventricular fibrillation occurring during open-heart surgery

In 1947, Dr. Beck developed a defibrillator with paddles that could be placed directly on the heart (Fig. 26.5). It delivered the first electric shock on the open-chest of a 14-year-old patient suffering ventricular fibrillation during surgery for a thoracic deformity [23]. The young man was saved and Dr. Beck traveled the world equipping all cardiac surgery services with a defibrillator to reduce mortality during surgery. However, this technique remained unused outside the operating theater as it required a thoracotomy to be performed.

Kouwenhoven also developed an open-chest defibrillator for the Johns Hopkins Hospital. Then, in 1951, the Edison Electric Institute strongly encouraged Kouwenhoven to design the famous closed-chest transportable defibrillator, which he did, and developed a defibrillator with capacitance [24].

In 1952, an already cited cardiac surgeon joined the race to develop an external defibrillator. Zoll, at the Beth Israel Hospital Boston and a Harvard professor, was the father of the external pacemaker and the external portable defibrillator. Zoll was inspired by the work of Kouwenhoven and published a paper in 1956 describing the first closed-chest external defibrillator [25]. Based on the same box as the external pacemaker, the defibrillator was able to deliver 750 V (AC) for 150 ms via two copper electrodes (7.5 cm diameter). The first ECG tracings reported in the scientific community were rapidly disseminated.

In the late 1950s, the closed-chest external defibrillator was in existence but suffered several restrictions. First, the charging time was very long, the current used was alternate, was particularly arrhythmogenic, and had low efficacy (30 %). In addition, there was no battery storage. It was Bernard Lown who added the final adaptations: he began work on a DC version and the use of capacitors to store charge, which allowed the defibrillator to use battery power, rendering the device portable and more convenient for cardiac emergencies.

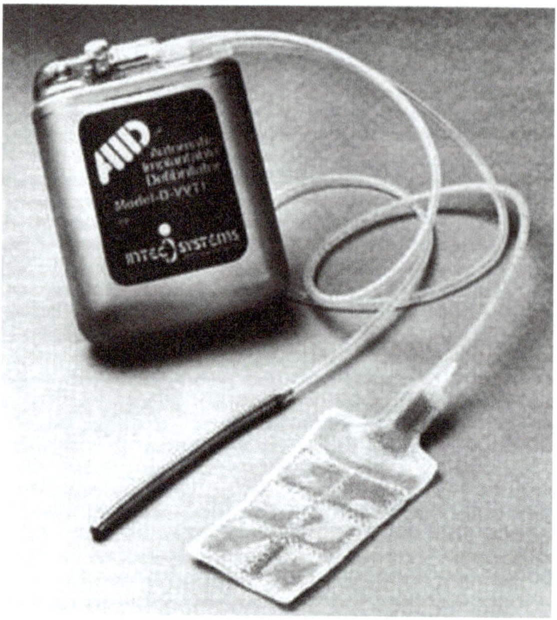

**Fig. 26.6** First model of an implantable defibrillator (1980)

A new type of external defibrillator was then developed with the help of Berkovits, an engineer working for the American Optical Company. This device delivered a sinusoidal shock wave called a "Lown wave", and was more efficient and safer, with capacitors capable of storing and delivering 1,000 V.

In the mid-1960s, external defibrillators were used within virtually all cardiac intensive-care units, but now no-one pauses to realize the progress that was made to make cardiac defibrillators implantable and automatic. Yet these researchers needed to retain mental perseverance and strength despite the skepticism of peers, including the designers of the original external defibrillator.

The history of the implantable defibrillator is unique because it relies on the bold project of one man, Mirowski. In 1975, the first prototype of an ICD was evaluated in dogs. The first implantation took place in a human on 4 February 1980, at the Johns Hopkins Hospital in Baltimore. It used a mixed system of endocardial electrodes in the superior vena cava and an epicardial patch next to the LV (Fig. 26.6) [26]. At this time, eligible patients had to have survived at least two resuscitated sudden deaths.

Unfortunately, Mirowski was often criticized by some of his contemporaries who compared the defibrillator to "a bomb inside the heart". Nevertheless, his concept was developed, and technological advances enabled an efficient electrical treatment to be developed.

In 1980, the first automatic defibrillator implanted in a human showed very limited technological capability, and only delivered a high-amplitude monophasic electric shock, without any atrial or ventricular pacing options. Electric shocks

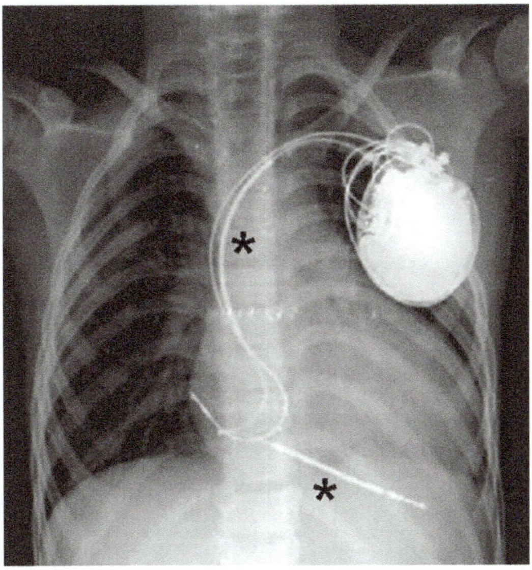


**Fig. 26.7** Chest radiography with an implantable dual-chamber defibrillator. Atrial and ventricular leads are placed endocardially through the subclavian vein (*star*: defibrillation coils)

were delivered between a patch sewn directly onto the epicardial surface after a thoracotomy, and a coil was located in the superior vena cava. Because the defibrillator was positioned in the abdomen, the system's patch and leads were implanted epicardially (and always via a thoracotomy).

In 1985, the first ICD was marketed. This system allowed the ventricle to be paced and gave better detection, which improved the percentage of appropriate shocks: that is to say, it gave a shock in response to a real ventricular arrhythmia. However, defibrillation and ventricular pacing thresholds remained high; in addition, fibrosis around the epicardially placed electrodes caused reliability problems in the medium term. In addition, the need for a thoracotomy was still impeding diffusion of this technique, especially in patients whose hemodynamic status was impaired. It was in 1991 that the first ICD, with endocardial pacing and a defibrillation lead, was placed at the apex of the RV (Fig. 26.7).

This development meant that a thoracotomy was no longer needed if the box was placed in the epigastric region. The defibrillation lead could then be inserted through the jugular or left subclavian vein, and then tunneled through the ICD. A year or two later, clinicians realized that if the ICD was located in the left subclavian region it was much simpler to implant and long-term management was improved. The shock was then delivered between the coil of the endocardial lead (negative pole) and the defibrillation box itself (positive pole): i.e., it could become an active electrode when giving a shock. However, when this technique was first used, very high defibrillation thresholds were not uncommon, which exceeded the capacity of the ICD. Therefore, it was often necessary to add a subcutaneous patch (as Mirowski had conceived at the beginning), so that the LV (accounting for >70 % of the heart's weight) was centered in the generated electric field.

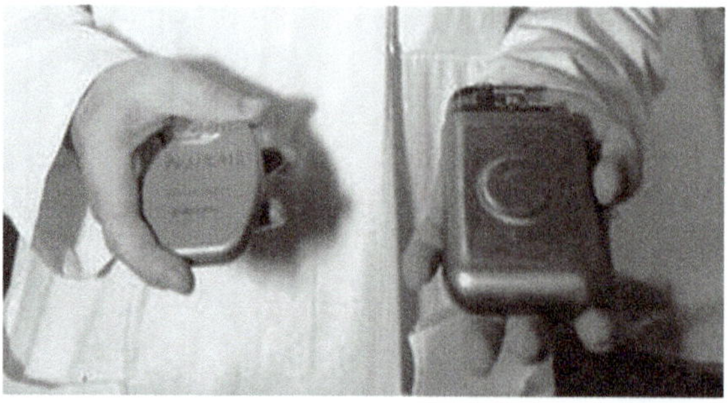


**Fig. 26.8** Dimensions of the latest (*left*) and first (*right*) generation of defibrillators

In 1995, the first dual-coil leads were developed, and the shock was then delivered between the can and the two coils, making installation of the subcutaneous patch exceptional, and thus simplifying and shortening the operative procedure. Also in 1995, the first dual-chamber ICD was marketed. ICDs with biventricular pacing for cardiac resynchronization first appeared in 1998.

The volume of the first ICDs was also a problem compared with the impressive progress made today in miniaturization. Little by little, the developmental size of a single pacemaker is being refined (Fig. 26.8).

Another major step forward during the last decade has been the development of remote monitoring for pacemakers, ICDs, and cardiac resynchronization devices. Thanks to this technology, patients can be better monitored without needing to go as frequently to a hospital.

## 26.4 What Does the Future Hold?

Cardiac pacing has hugely and rapidly improved in just over 50 years, thanks to advances in electronics, computing, nanotechnology, and medicine. Engineers and physicians are committed to reproducing, as closely as possible, the physiological cardiac cycle and the mechanical activity of the right and left ventricles. We can imagine that, in the future, progress will continue towards further miniaturization and longevity, but also perhaps the research of new and more compatible biological materials.

Curiously, the leads have remained relatively unchanged all these years, and it is likely that improvements will be made in this area. An interesting line of research concerns the suppression of current leads, and their replacement with receptors, which could then be implanted in multiple locations inside the heart cavities. This could prevent cardiac lead damage, such as ruptures or infections, which are life-threatening and very difficult to treat.

Future devices will not only incorporate cardiac resynchronization, but may vary the pacing of timing sequences of the left and right ventricles and incorporate other adjunctive therapies (atrial fibrillation suppression algorithms), and perhaps even drug-delivery systems. In addition, companies have been investigating long-term implantable of sensors to monitor a patient's physiological state (i.e., risk of increasing heart failure or hemodynamic compromise) with the goal of providing an appropriate electrical and/or pharmacological intervention to optimize myocardial performance.

We are at the dawn of the third millennium and, concerning the defibrillator, we can say that it starts with a bang as we are now reaching the concept of a leadless defibrillator [27]. This new type of ICD has a generator positioned in the left subclavian region and a subcutaneous patch next to the LV.

Research into cardiac pacing and ICDs has been motivated by huge medical and economic issues, and will continue; although we are still amazed by these small but fascinating metal boxes!

## References

1. Jeffrey K (1992) The next step in cardiac pacing: the view from 1958. Pacing Clin Electrophysiol 15(6):961–967
2. Bloomfield P, Boon NA (1989) A century of cardiac pacing. BMJ 298(6670):343–344
3. Zoll PM (1952) Resuscitation of the heart in ventricular standstill by external electric stimulation. N Engl J Med 247:768–771
4. Allen P, Lillehei CW (1957) Use of induced cardiac arrest in open heart surgery. Minnesota Med 40:672–676
5. Zoll PM, Linenthal AJ, Norman LR et al (1954) Treatment of stokes-adams disease by external electric stimulation of the heart. Circulation 9:482–493
6. Lillehei CW, Gott VL, Hodges PC et al (1960) Transistor pacemaker for treatment of complete atrioventricular dissociation. JAMA 172:2006–2010
7. Furman S, Robinson G (1959) Stimulation of the ventricular endocardial surface in control of complete heart block. Ann Surg 150:841–845
8. Elmqvist R, Senning A (1960) An implantable pacemaker for the heart. In: Smyth CN (ed) Proceedings of the Second International Conference on Medical Electronics, 24–27 June 1959, Iliffe & Sons, Paris, London, pp 253–254
9. Chardack WM, Gage AA, Greatbatch W (1960) A transistorized, self contained implantable pacemaker for the long-term correction of complete heart block. Surgery 48:643–654
10. Schneider A, Moser J, Webb THE et al (1970) A new high energy density cell with a lithium anode. In: Proceedings of the US Army Signal Corps Power Sources Conference, Atlantic City
11. Nathan DA, Center S, Wu C-Y et al (1963) An implantable synchronous pacemaker for the long term correction of complete heart block. Circulation 27:682–685
12. Berkovits BV, Castellanos A Jr, Lemberg L (1969) Bifocal demand pacing. Circulation 40 [Suppl III]:44
13. Donaldson RM, Rickards AF (1983) Rate responsive pacing using the evoked QT principle. A physiological alternative to atrial synchronous pacemakers. Pacing Clin Electrophysiol 6(6):1344–1349
14. Shapland JE, MacCarter D, Tockman B, Knudson M (1983) Physiologic benefits of rate responsiveness. Pacing Clin Electrophysiol 6(2 Pt 2):329–332
15. Burkhoff D, Oikawa RY, Sagawa K (1986) Influence of pacing site on canine left ventricular contraction. Am J Physiol 251:H428–H435
16. Grines CL, Bashore TM, Boudoulas H et al (1989) Function abnormalities in isolated left bundle branch block: The effect of interventricular asynchrony. Circulation 79:845–853

17. Ziao HB, Lee CH, Gibson DG (1991) Effect of left bundle branch block on diastolic function in dilated cardiomyopathy. Br Heart J 66:443–447
18. Kerwin WF, Botvinick EH, O'Connell JW et al (2000) Ventricular contraction abnormalities in dilated cardiomyopathy: effect of biventricular pacing to correct interventricular dyssynchrony. J Am Coll Cardiol 35:1221–1227
19. Lattuca JJ, Cohen TJ, Mower MM (1990) Biventricular pacing to improve cardiac hemodynamics. Clin Rev 38:882A
20. Saxon LA, Boehmer JP, Hummels H, et al. (1999) For the VIGOR CHF and VENTAK CHF Investigators. Biventricular pacing in patients with congestive heart failure: two prospective randomized trials. Am J Cardiol 83:120D–123D
21. Cazeau S, Ritter P, Bakdach S, Lazarus A, Limousin M, Henao L, Mundler O, Daubert JC, Mugica J (1994) Four chamber pacing in dilated cardiomyopathy. Pacing Clin Electrophysiol 17(11 Pt 2):1974–1979
22. Prevost JL, Battelli F (1899) La mort par les décharges électriques. J Physiol 1:1085–1100
23. Beck CS, Pritchard WH, Feil HS (1947) Ventricular fibrillation of long duration abolished by electric shock. JAMA 135:985–986
24. Kouwenhoven WB, Milnor WR (1954) Treatment of ventricular fibrillation using a capacitor discharge. J Appl Physiol 7:253–257
25. Zoll PM, Linenthal AJ, Gibson W et al (1956) Termination of ventricular fibrillation in man by externally applied electric countershock. N Engl J Med 254:727–736
26. Mirowski M, Reid PR, Mower MM et al (1980) Termination of malignant ventricular arrhythmias with an implanted automatic defibrillator in human beings. N Engl J Med 303:322–332
27. Bardy GH, Smith WM, Hood MA et al (2010) An entirely subcutaneous implantable cardioverter-defibrillator. N Engl J Med 363:36–44

# The History of Surgery for Ischemic Heart Disease and Mechanical Complications of Myocardial Infarction After the Advent of CPB

# 27

Roland G. Demaria and Mohammed Al Yamani

*Any intelligent fool can make things bigger and more complex...It takes a touch of genius—and a lot of courage to move in the opposite direction.*

Albert Einstein

**Abstract**

The birth of modern coronary surgery was not possible before two separate innovations: cardiopulmonary bypass (CPB) in 1953 and coronarography in 1958. After that, coronary endarterectomies with pericardial or venous patches were replaced by venous bypasses, and finally internal mammary artery (IMA) bypasses. Myocardial protection was improved. Sternotomy became the standard approach and surgeons used more and more microsurgical techniques. The co-existence of both techniques in large centers like the Cleveland Clinic Foundation, Ohio, USA allowed large clinical studies and rapid development of this surgery worldwide. One of the greatest developments in surgery is thanks to the use of two new tools, one diagnostic and one therapeutic, at the same time, and in the same place, and to the work and imagination of great pioneers, in these very favorable conditions.

## 27.1 Introduction

The history of heart surgery is divided into two totally different parts: the period before and the period after the use of the heart–lung machine, or cardiopulmonary bypass (CPB). The year separating the two periods is officially 1953 (the first successful open

R. G. Demaria (✉) · M. A. Yamani
Department of Thoracic and Cardio-Vascular Surgery,
Montpellier University Hospital Arnaud de Villeneuve, Montpellier, France
e-mail: r-demaria@chu-montpellier.fr

M. Picichè (ed.), *Dawn and Evolution of Cardiac Procedures*,
DOI: 10.1007/978-88-470-2400-7_27, 

heart surgery was carried out on 6 May by J.H. Gibbon with his own heart–lung machine), but the 1960s represent the real period of expansion and development of heart surgery under CPB in different countries and cities in the world, allowing heart arrest and open-heart surgery and introducing a new era in the field of cardiac surgery.

Concerning ischemic heart diseases, the initial period without CPB was principally represented by surgery for anginal pain using the neurectomy approach (Franck, Arnulf) [1], then by the improvement of non-direct coronary artery circulation (Beck, Vineberg, Sen), and finally by direct coronary surgery with endarterectomy followed by coronary bypass (Bailey, Sabiston, Kolessov). Indeed, Bailey performed the first coronary endarterectomy in 1956, then Sabiston in 1962 performed the first aortocoronary venous bypass graft in a human. Kolessov in 1966, in Leningrad, performed the first left internal thoracic artery to left anterior descending (LAD) artery graft. All these operations were performed on a beating heart [2].

At the end of the 1960s, Favaloro and the Cleveland Clinic cardiac surgical team, directly used the advantage of having the coronarography developed by Mason Sones in 1958, and together they opened the era of modern direct coronary artery bypass surgery. Rapidly, CPB without and finally with cardioplegic arrest, was used almost universally in coronary bypass surgery to obtain an optimal bloodless and motionless operative field, allowing more secure and also more precise surgery. In France, Alain Sisteron in Lyon with Daniel Guilmet and Charles Dubost from Paris [3], and Paul-André Chaptal in Montpellier were among the pioneers of direct coronary surgery. The majority of coronary operations were soon performed using this technique and beating heart coronary revascularization was abandoned except in selected situations or certain countries such as Brazil [4] and Argentina [5], in part for economic reasons.

Thus, coronary bypass surgery under CPB and cardioplegic arrest, guided by coronary angiogram, became the gold standard in coronary surgery and also allowed, in optimal conditions, the repair of the mechanical complications of acute myocardial infarction. Coronary bypass surgery under CPB represents one of the major developments of surgery in the last century, according to both the number of patients operated on and the satisfactory results obtained.

## 27.2 The History of Direct Coronary Surgery After the Advent of CPB

### 27.2.1 Cine Coronary Arteriography: 1958

The history of direct coronary artery surgery after the advent of CPB in 1953 and the coronaro-angiography in 1958 is in fact the history of modern coronary surgery. The two dates are closely associated and allowed the development of a new approach to coronary surgery. Indeed, surgery under CPB, theoretically possible since 1953, allowed a bloodless and motionless field, but surgeons were obliged to explore epicardial coronary vessels with their fingers to find the endarterectomy or anastomosis sites, and the accuracy of this exploration was sometimes very poor, inducing some disastrous mistakes. In 1958, Sones and Shirey performed an unexpected right coronary angiogram during a ventriculography [6]. This discovery, associated with the use of CPB in cardiac surgery, was the true starting point of modern direct coronary surgery because surgeons were able to plan their intervention exactly according to the coronary lesions, with the security and comfort of CPB.

### 27.2.2 Coronary Endarterectomy Under CPB with Venous Patch Enlargement: 1958

In the same year, 1958, but published 3 years later, probably the first case of direct coronary artery surgery under CPB and guided by preoperative coronary angiography was performed, by Ake Senning, from Sweden. At 20 °C, after dissection and clampage with snares of the left main, the LAD, and the circumflex coronary arteries, these arteries were split longitudinally and reconstructed with great saphenous veins split lengthwise, to obtain an enlargement of the artery diameter. A post-operative control coronarography was carried out and the follow-up 3 months after surgery was satisfactory [7].

### 27.2.3 Ostial Endo-Aortic Disobliteration: 1960

In 1960, a case of coronary artery surgery under CPB was performed in France by Charles Dubost, from Broussais hospital in Paris, with an endo-aortic disobliteration of a syphilitic ostial right coronary obstruction, corrected under CPB with profound hypothermia at 10 °C [1, 8, 9]. However, this pathology was less frequent than atheroma; thus, the first operation routinely performed directly on the coronary arteries under CPB was the "coronary Senning operation" described previously.

Starting around 1962 at the Cleveland Clinic, the cardiac surgical team with Effler and Favaloro operated on 76 selected patients using this technique, under CPB and wearing binocular loupes with magnification of 1.5–2 times. The heart was arrested by regional hypothermia. They published their technique and results in 1967 [10]. However, and despite a rigorous surgical technique, hospital mortality was around 23 %. Another surgical option had to be developed.

### 27.2.4 Venous Aorto-Coronary Bypass Under CPB: 1964

After experimental development by De Bakey of aorto-coronary bypass grafting, published in 1961 [11], and using polyester grafts, the first aorto-coronary bypass was performed by Edward Garrett on 23 November 1964, at Baylor University hospital, Houston, Texas [1]. This case was published 9 years later [12]. After an attempt to perform the coronary Senning operation, he was obliged to perform a bypass graft between the aorta and coronary artery with a saphenous vein. He performed first the anastomosis of the aorta, then a distal anastomosis on the LAD. The time taken to perform that distal anastomosis was 23 min. The patient was cannulated, but CPB was not started because the patient was stable. However, this operation must be considered the first coronary artery bypass with CPB technology available, and was in part used, because the patient was cannulated. Seven years later, a coronary angiogram was carried out, showing the venous graft and the occlusion of the LAD above the anastomosis. The patient died 1 year later of a myocardial infarction [13].

### 27.2.5 René Favaloro and the Cleveland Clinic: Modern Direct Coronary Surgery: 1967

This operation was developed and regularly performed in the Cleveland Clinic, Ohio, the prestigious institution where the coronary angiogram was discovered by Mason Sones almost 10 years before, and where the development of new strategies was facilitated by the huge number of patients treated at the institution. Bypasses were first performed on the right coronary artery, and then on the LAD and circumflex artery. Technique and results were published in 1968 by René Favaloro involving 15 patients with replacement of the right coronary artery with a saphenous autograft inserted distally with end-to-end anastomosis on the coronary artery [14]. Proximal anastomosis was performed on the lower portion of the ascending aorta. The 15 patients were operated upon without any mortality. Six of these patients benefited from a postoperative right coronary angiographic control showing excellent function of the venous bypass. For the first 55 patients operated on by this technique of bypass under CPB at the Cleveland Clinic, hospital death was less than 3.7 %. The competition between coronary bypass and endarterectomy was over.

Direct coronary artery bypass with a saphenous vein, under CPB became the gold standard among other coronary operations and was developed in a lot of centers all around the world [15]. Sternotomy was also progressively preferred to the thoracotomy, allowing more complete treatment of the coronary disease.

### 27.2.6 Mammary Artery Coronary Bypass Under CPB: 1968

In 1968 also, Reed performed the first arterial bypass on the LAD using the internal mammary artery (IMA) [16], under CPB without cardioplegic arrest, on a fibrillating heart to avoid motion. This bypass represents the keystone of modern direct coronary surgery. The end of this story is represented by the large clinical studies carried out by the Cleveland Clinic [17], showing the results of coronary artery bypass graft and the interest in using one and finally two IMAs.

## 27.3 The History of Surgery for Mechanical Complications of Myocardial Infarction After the Advent of CPB

There were three complications: left ventricular free wall rupture, ischemic interventricular communication, and acute papillary muscle rupture of the mitral valve.

### 27.3.1 Left Ventricular Free Wall Rupture

The left ventricular free wall rupture is the most frequent complication (around 85 %) of myocardial infarction and it also has the highest mortality rate, which makes it the most feared of all mechanical complications. This pathology was first reported by William Harvey, the discoverer of blood circulation, in 1649. The first surgical procedure reported seems to be from Hatcher in 1970 [18]. A recent evolution is to perform this salvage surgery on a beating heart and sometimes without CPB, with an external application of a hemostatic device.

### 27.3.2 Ischemic Interventricular Communication

Described by Latham in 1847 on cadavers, the first surgical case was performed by Denton Cooley in 1957 [19]. Despite some successful reported cases, mortality was very high, and was progressively improved by the introduction of the intra-aortic balloon pump, the extensive use of felt and glue, and the earlier surgical intervention. However, despite all the progress made, this pathology remains of high surgical risk.

### 27.3.3 Acute Mitral Papillary Muscle Rupture

This is a rare complication of acute myocardial infarction [20]. The surgery of acute papillary muscle rupture of the mitral valve was first described in 1965 by Austen [21]. The first surgical technique used was mitral valve replacement, rapidly followed by attempt at papillary muscle reattachment [22]. Repair is better than replacement, but, in this pathology, the fragility of acute ischemic tissues, and the associated cardiogenic shock calls for rapid mitral valve replacement, with conservation of subvalvular apparatus if possible, to avoid unsatisfactory consequences.

## 27.4 Conclusions

The birth of modern coronary surgery was not possible before two separate innovations: CPB in 1953 and coronarography in 1958. After that, coronary endarterectomies with pericardial or venous patches were replaced by venous bypasses, and finally by IMA bypasses. Myocardial protection was improved. Sternotomy became the standard approach and surgeons used more and more microsurgical techniques. The co-existence of both techniques in large centers like the Cleveland Clinic Foundation, Ohio, USA, had allowed large clinical studies and rapid development of this surgery worldwide. One of the greatest developments in surgery was thanks to the use of two new tools, one diagnostic and one therapeutic, at the same time, and in the same place, and to the work and imagination of great pioneers, in these very favorable conditions.

In mid 1990s, off-pump coronary surgery was rediscovered, following some surgeons who had continued using this technique for 25 years with satisfactory results, and helped by news tools such as stabilizers, intra-coronary shunts, and $CO_2$ applicators. After an increase in the number of patients undergoing off-pump surgery all around the world, the proportion seems to be stabilized at around 15 % in a lot of countries. On-pump direct coronary surgery remains the gold standard for the majority of cardiac surgeons, but off-pump direct coronary surgery has created an improvement for a selected group of patients. Finally, today, on- and off pump direct coronary surgery are both optimized and represent two technical possibilities, both of which may be very helpful for the cardiac surgeon and his patient. It is not opposition but complementary. This is another example of the revival of an old technique with new tools, and good results.

If only one surgeon has to be promoted as the "Father" of modern coronary surgery, the name René Geronimo Favaloro will be probably the more frequently cited. Born on 12 July 1923 in Argentina, he started off as a rural doctor. Then, he moved in 1962 to Cleveland, Ohio, to join the prestigious Cleveland Clinic with Sones and Effler. He performed as a pioneer numerous saphenous vein bypasses under CPB starting from May 1967, and also performed the first bypass for acute myocardial infarction [23]. In 1970, Dr. Favaloro performed at the National Heart Hospital in London, with the help of Dr. Ross, the first coronary artery bypass in the UK [24, 25]. In 1971, He returned home and created the Favaloro foundation, based on the model of the Cleveland Clinic. Secondary to financial and other difficulties, he sadly took his own life on 29 July 2000, at the age of 77. He performed in his career more than 17,000 coronary bypasses.

## References

1. Cachera JP (1985) Historique de la chirurgie coronaire. In: La Maladie coronaire, 2nd edn. Flammarion Médecine-Sciences Editions, Paris, pp 551–555
2. Demaria RG, Perrault LP (2004) Effects of vascular interrupting and hemostatic devices on coronary artery endothelial function in beating heart coronary artery bypass surgery. In: Cartier R (ed) Off pump coronary artery bypass surgery. Chapter 7, Landes Bioscience, Austin, TX, pp 1–8
3. Guilmet D (1997) Le cœur qui bat. Editions de Fallois, Paris
4. Buffolo E, Silva de Andrade JC, Rodrigues Branco JN et al (1996) Coronary artery bypass grafting without cardiopulmonary bypass. Ann Thorac Surg 61:63–66

5. Benetti FJ (1985) Direct coronary surgery with saphenous vein bypass without either cardiopulmonary bypass or cardiac arrest. J Cardiovasc Surg 26:217–222
6. Sones FM, Shirey EK (1962) Cine coronary arteriography. Mod Concept Cardiovasc Dis 31:735–738
7. Senning A (1961) Strip grafting in coronary arteries report of a case. J Thorac Cardiovasc Surg 41:542–549
8. Dubost C, Blondeau P, Piwnica A et al (1960) Syphilitic coronary obstruction: correction under artificial heart-lung and profound hypothermia at 10°C. Surgery 48:540–547
9. Blondeau P, Dubost C (1962) Surgical treatment under deep hypothermia of syphilitic ostial coronaritis. Apropos of 2 cases operated on with success. Ann Chir Thorac Cardiovasc 1:802–806
10. Effler DB, Groves LK, Suarez EL et al (1967) Direct coronary artery surgery with endarterectomy and patchgraft reconstruction. Clinical application and technical consideration. J Thorac Cardiovasc Surg 53:93–101
11. De Bakey ME, Henly WS (1961) Surgical treatment of angina pectoris. Circulation 23:111–120
12. Garrett HE, Dennis EW, De Bakey ME (1973) Aortocoronary bypass with saphenous vein graft. JAMA 223:792–794
13. Liotta D (1984) La leçon de l'histoire de la chirurgie coronaire. In: Maloine (ed) La chirurgie cardiaque d'aujourd'hui, Paris, pp 215–224
14. Favaloro RG (1968) Saphenous vein autograft replacement of severe segmental coronary artery occlusion operative technique. Ann Thorac Surg 5:334–339
15. Favaloro RG, Effler DB, Groves LK et al (1970) Direct myocardial revascularization by saphenous vein graft. Present operative technique and indication. Ann Thorac Surg 10:97–111
16. Reed GE, Stertzer SH, Reppert EH (1968) Coronary arterial bypass graft. Ann Thorac Surg 5:443–450
17. Lytle BW, Loop FD, Cosgrove DM et al (1985) Long term (5 to 12 years) serial studies of IMA and saphenous vein coronary bypass graft. J Thorac Cardiovasc Surg 89:248–258
18. Hatcher CR, Mansour K, Logan WD Jr et al (1970) Surgical complications of myocardial infarction. Am Surg 36:163–170
19. Cooley DA, Belmonte VA, Zeiss LB et al (1957) Surgical repair of ruptured interventricular septum following acute myocardial infarction. Surgery 41:930–937
20. Loisance D, Vouhé P, Cachera JP (1985) Traitement chirurgical des complications mécaniques de l'infarctus du myocarde. In: La Maladie coronaire, 2nd edn. Flammarion Médecine-Sciences Editions, Paris, pp 611–626
21. Austen WG, Sanders CA, Averill JH (1965) Ruptured papillary muscle: report of a case with successful mitral valve replacement. Circulation 32:597–601
22. Horlick L, Merriman JE, Robinson LN (1966) A case of mitral insufficiency following myocardial infarction with rupture of a papillary muscle: improvement following reattachment of papillary muscle and placation of the mitral valve. Can Med Ass J 94:192–195
23. Cooley DA (2000) Memoriam: tribute to René Favaloro, pioneer of coronary bypass. Tex Heart Inst J 27:231–232
24. Favaloro RG (1998) Landmarks in the development of coronary artery bypass surgery. Circulation 66:1106–1109
25. Captur G (2005) René Géronimo Favaloro. Pioneer of cardiac surgery. Malta Med J 17:55–61

# Progress and Milestones in the Treatment of Deep Sternal Wound Infections

# 28

Richard Baillot and Daniel Cloutier

*Let us go through the results of our predecessors and we will see that sometimes they have done more than we did…*
B. Sawicki

**Abstract**

Numerous advances have been made during the last half century in the treatment of deep sternal wound infection following sternotomy for open heart surgery. In the early years of cardiac surgery debridement and wound packing was the mainstay of therapy until closed chest drainage with mediastinal irrigation with antibiotics and/or antiseptics was later recommended. Treatment failure and mortality were still high with these techniques until wound coverage with viable tissues such as the greater omentum and the pectoralis major myocutaneous flap began to be applied. During the last 10 years another step ahead has been taken with the introduction of negative wound pressure therapy. This treatment modality is now being proposed following debridement to limit further the extension of sternal osteomyelitis and preserve the sternum for later chest wall reconstruction with horizontal titanium plating.

In 1897, Milton [1] was the first to demonstrate the feasibility of median sternotomy using cadavers and goats, and prophetically stated that "If it be established that median thoracic incision is a fairly safe procedure, I have no doubt that it will constitute the most generally useful route to thoracic organs. Heart surgery is still

R. Baillot (✉)
Department of Cardiac Surgery, Institut Universitaire de Cardiologie et Pneumologie de Québec Hôpital Laval, Quebec, Canada
e-mail: richard.baillot@chg.ulaval.ca

D. Cloutier
Department of Plastic Surgery, Centre Hospitalier Universitaire de Québec CHUL, Quebec, Canada
e-mail: Daniel.cloutier@crchul.ulaval.ca

M. Picichè (ed.), *Dawn and Evolution of Cardiac Procedures*,
DOI: 10.1007/978-88-470-2400-7_28, 

quite in its infancy but it requires no great stretch of fancy to imagine the possibility of plastic operations in some at all events of its valvular lesions" [2]. Heart valve replacement and coronary artery surgery had not even been thought of at the time, but decades later, median sternotomy, or Milton's operation, would prove to be the most frequently used incision in cardiac surgery. Julian et al. [3], in a landmark paper published in 1957, popularized the approach with techniques using caval occlusion procedures using the newly introduced heart–lung machine.

A few years after these developments, reports began to appear of deep sternal wound infections (DSWI) following sternotomies, including complications such as severe hemorrhaging, superinfections, and significant mortality as surgeons struggled to manage these new hospital-acquired infections (HAI). It is our intent in this chapter to chronologically situate the most significant advances in understanding and treating these HAI.

## 28.1 Physiopathology and Definition

The DSWI (Fig. 28.1) are HAI that present following sternotomies for open-heart surgery (OHS). Their prevalence is estimated to be 0.5–5 %. They are inversely correlated with cardiac surgical volume [4] and usually present 10–15 days post-surgery [5]. They are characterized by fever, chest pain, purulent discharges, significant leucocytosis, and bacteremia, especially when the infection is associated with *Staphylococcus aureus*, Sternal dehiscence with various degrees of osteomyelitis, as per CDC criteria [6, 7], is also present, and early surgical debridement is usually warranted (Fig. 28.2).

Hematogenous seeding of wounds is rarely associated with DSWI, which is more often related to *sternal instability* in patients at risk. As stated by Gottlieb, "...early sternal instability creates an inflammatory exudate which, in the presence of foreign body like bone wax and small amounts of devitalized tissues from the motion and squeezing of the tissues by the wire, establishes a locus minus resistance for bacteria leading to a secondary infection" [8].

## 28.2 Risk Factors and Microbiology

Major risk factors for DSWI have been identified in numerous studies and are categorized as pre-, per-, and post-operative (Table 28.1). The main pre-operative predictors include male gender, obesity, diabetes, renal failure, smoking and COPD, immunosuppression (steroids), poor dental hygiene, and nasal carriage of *Staphylococcus*. Intra-operative predictors include failure to implement in-time administration of antibioprophylaxis and mismanagement of hyperglycemia. Poor surgical technique and hemostasis, inadvertent paramedian sternotomy, overuse of cautery, indiscriminate use of bilateral internal mammary arteries, and use of bone wax all contribute to sternal instability and the development of DSWI. Post-operative predictors include hemodynamic instability, prolonged intubation, overuse of

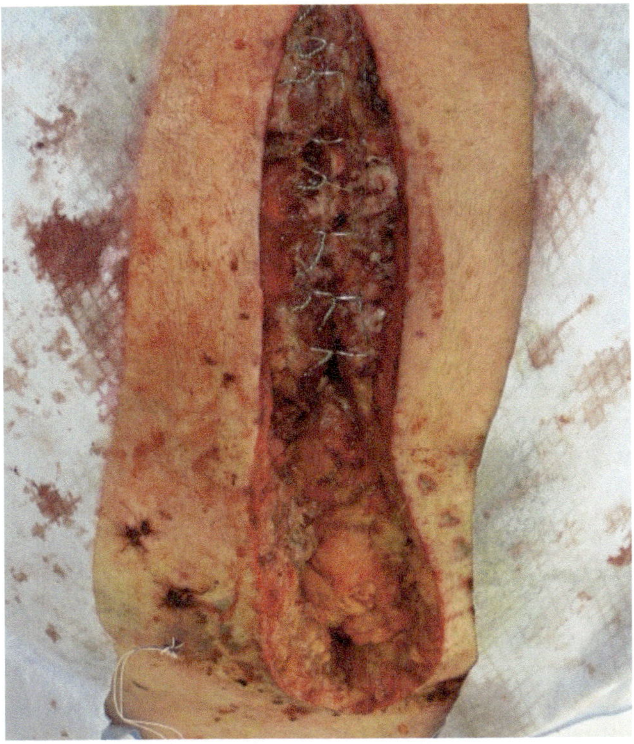

**Fig. 28.1** Deep sternal wound infection

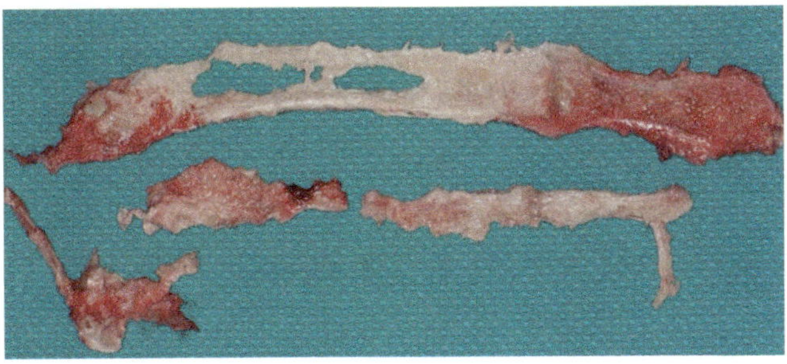

**Fig. 28.2** Sternal osteomyelitis

blood transfusions, renal failure, re-operation for bleeding, and prolonged ventilation and ICU stays. A study [9] performed at the Institut Universitaire de Cardiologie et de Pneumologie de Québec (IUCPQ) showed that skin inhabitants such as staphylococcal species are common in patients with DSWI, unlike patients with a prolonged ICU stay, who are more likely to carry Gram-negative *Enterobacter*, *Pseudomonas*, and *Klebsiella* species as well as *Candida* [10].

**Table 28.1** Major risk factors

| Pre-operatively | Intra-operatively | Post-operatively |
|---|---|---|
| Smoking/COPD | Off-center sternotomies | Transfusions |
| Redo surgery | Long CPB (> 2 h) | Retained foreign bodies |
| Renal failure | Transverse sternal FX | Ventilation |
| Diabetes | BIMA grafting | ICU stay |
| Steroids | Intra-aortic balloon pump | Tracheostomy |
| BMI > 30 | Concomitant surgery | |
| Congestive heart failure/shock | Duration of pacing wires | |
| H/O radiation | Hyperglycemia | |
| Male sex | Electrocautery/bone wax | |
| MRSA status | Antibiotics within 30 min | |
| HIV/cancer | | |
| AF/high CRP | | |
| Low albumin | | |

## 28.3 Evolution of Mortality Rates and Surgical Therapy

Despite numerous advances in anesthesiology and cardiac surgical care, the morbidity and mortality associated with DSWI has remained significant over the years. This appears to be related to delays in initial debridement. Historically, two techniques have been used to treat DSWI [4].

### 28.3.1 The Open Technique

This technique was used when OHS was in its infancy and is now only of historical interest. Conventional treatments involved drainage of purulent exudates, debridement of sternal necrotic wounds, and open packing of the mediastinum with coarse mesh gauze. Primary closure of sternal wounds was never performed, and wounds healed by secondary intention with granulation tissue formation. Further debridement was carried out when dressings were changed. Complete healing could take as long as a year. Major complications included life-threatening hemorrhaging from suture lines and major vascular structures including the right ventricle, secondary fungal infections, and mediastinal herniation of the heart with poor functional and cosmetic results [11]. This technique was initially recommended for more extensive mediastinal suppuration involving the entire sternum, including the cartilage. Mortality ranging from 20 to 45 % has been reported [12–14].

### 28.3.2 The Closed Technique

Closed retrosternal irrigation was initially proposed by Shumacker and Mandelbaum in 1963 and was later modified by Bryant et al. in 1968. This technique reduced mortality to 20 % [15, 16]. It was recommended for patients with less extensive infections. Following debridement, fenestrated chest tubes were inserted into the anterior mediastinum for drainage and antibiotic irrigation. The sternum was immediately rewired, and the subcutaneous tissues were closed or allowed to heal by secondary intention. Repeat bacterial cultures were performed on chest tube drainage fluids, and irrigation was discontinued 7–10 days later. Grossi et al. later recommended longer irrigation times (10–20 days) until repeat cultures of the drainage fluids were negative [17]. The mediastinum was usually irrigated with saline, Dakin's solution, dilute iodine solution, or antibiotics. Parenteral antibiotics were also given at the same time. The advantages of this technique included better cosmetic and functional results with less pulmonary insufficiency, shorter lengths of ICU stay, and fewer complications such as major bleeding. Disadvantages included occasional irrigant-related toxicity, superinfections with resistant microorganisms, and recurring deep suppurative mediastinitis and costochondritis.

Mortality rates as high as 28 % have been reported with this technique, although Molina et al. [18], who studied a cohort of 114 patients treated with debridement, irrigation, and primary sternal rewiring with lateral reinforcement, did not report any treatment failures or mortalities. However, such results have never been reported by other investigators. More recently, surgical experience with closed chest techniques using continuous irrigation and strong negative pressure described earlier for the treatment of long bone ostemyelitis (−700 mmHg/Redon catheters) has been summarized by Calvat et al. [19] and compared with standard closed chest irrigation. Treatment failure (13 %) and mortality (17 %) are still being reported as significant with the use of the Redon catheters, but lower than the percentage seen in the standard continuous irrigation regimens as summarized by these authors. From 1974 to 1991, 14 studies were reported with standard closed chest irrigation in this review, mean failure rate of 34 % and mortality of 24 %.

## 28.4 Vascularized Tissue

Jurkiewicz reported, in his seminal 1979 publication, the successful use of vascularized tissues to treat DSWI. This was one of the most important developments in the field of contemporary thoracic surgery [20]. Following debridement with or without total sternectomy, depending on the extent of the osteomyelitis, delayed obliteration of the anterior mediastinum was performed using the pectoralis muscles. This development followed in the footsteps of the report by Lee in 1976 describing intra-thoracic omental transposition [21], which was also used by Jurkiewicz in 1975 for patients in whom catheter irrigation had failed [22]. These approaches were the first alternatives to open granulation [23].

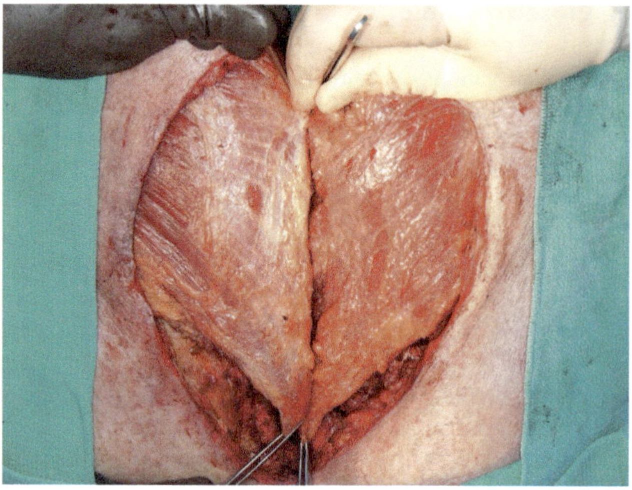

Fig. 28.3 Pectoralis major muscle flaps

### 28.4.1 Muscle Flaps

The idea of using muscle flaps and vascularized tissues to treat chronic wounds was not new, but their application for treating DSWI rapidly gained acceptance following these reports. The use of muscle flaps greatly improved morbidity, which decreased to less than 10 % [24]. The use of muscle flaps for chest wall repair was first reported in 1896 by Tansini [25], who used the latissimus dorsi for breast reconstruction following Halstead radical mastectomy. This contribution was ignored for years by surgeons who preferred thinned breast skin grafting and observation of the wound to diagnose tumor recurrence [26]. Muscle flaps were also used in the late 19th century to treat osteomyelitis of the lower limbs, while Sawicki was among the first to propose the use of the gastrocnemius to treat tibial osteomyelitis [27]. The proximity of the pectoralis major to the sternotomy site led to its widespread use in the treatment of DSWI and in oncological head and neck reconstruction surgery [28]. These flaps are vascularized by the thoracoacromial artery and the mammary artery perforators. They lead to fewer complications than other transposed muscles, result in less local contamination [29], and can be used with or without humeral detachment or in a turnover fashion. One muscle can often be used to cover the entire open chest wound, fill intra-thoracic defects, and treat empyemas and bronchopleural fistulas. If additional wound coverage is required, the rectus can be used as a rotation flap or bipedicle–rectus unit [23]. The sacrifice or mobilization of these two muscles is not associated with a functional deficit when the humeral attachment is left intact, since the nerve supply from the lateral pectoral nerves is preserved, which prevents secondary atrophy (Fig. 28.3).

Immediate closure [30] or single-stage management of DSWI with muscle flaps has also been reported to be associated with mortality of less than 10 %.

However, recent reports in the literature favor repeat debridement for deep suppurative mediastinitis [31].

### 28.4.2 The Greater Omentum

The greater omentum has been used in the past to fill abdominal abscesses and pancreatic pseudocysts, cover thoracic defects following breast amputation and osteoradionecrosis of the chest wall, treat bronchopleural fistulae, chronic lymphedema of the arm, and repair vesicovaginal and rectal communications. Kiricuta [32] is mainly credited with the use of the greater omentum for surgical reconstruction [22]. Because of its rich blood supply, the omentum has also been used to revascularize the heart and treat angina [33]. In 2002, Hultman et al. published a report on donor-site complications in which they used the omentum to treat extraperitoneal wounds [34]. They managed 135 patients with scalp, intracranial, and head and neck pathologies using the omentum as a free flap and performed sternal and chest wall reconstructions in 52 of the patients using a pedicled flap transposed through the diaphragm of the abdominal wall. They reported complications with 25 patients (18.5 %), including 9 (6.7 %) with abdominal wall infections and 8 (5.9 %) with ventral hernias. Other investigators have reported that the omentum is associated with lower mortality rates, better overall success, and low flap failure [35, 36]. Laparoscopic harvesting of the omentum has also recently been proposed as an alternative to formal laparotomy to decrease abdominal wall complications [37]. Milano et al. reported that patients managed with an omental flap had lower hospital mortality (4.8 vs 10.5 %), a shorter ICU stay, and fewer early complications (9.5 vs 27.7 %) than patients managed with muscle flaps [38]. According to Milano, this surgical option in probably underused. The results with the omentum can be explained by its neovascularization potential, which Cartier et al. demonstrated using a rabbit cornea model [39]. Cartier injected one cornea with autologous omental fat and the other with perirenal fat. Neovascularization was three-fold greater with the omental fat extract, suggesting that it has an angiogenic effect on tissues. Angiographic studies of the gastroepiploic artery by Krabatsch et al. also showed that the omentum was well vascularized and anastomosed with mediastinal vessels within 26–82 weeks of thorax transposition. The neovascularization potential and the ability to fight off infections have been associated with the presence of active immunological active cells such as macrophages, monocytes, and T and B lymphocytes [40].

## 28.5 Newer Therapeutic Modalities

Despite numerous advances in the treatment of DSWI using vascularized tissues, there is a lack of consensus regarding the optimal surgical management approach. It has been suggested that prospective randomized trials are required in this context [41]. Recently, negative pressure wound therapy has been proposed to

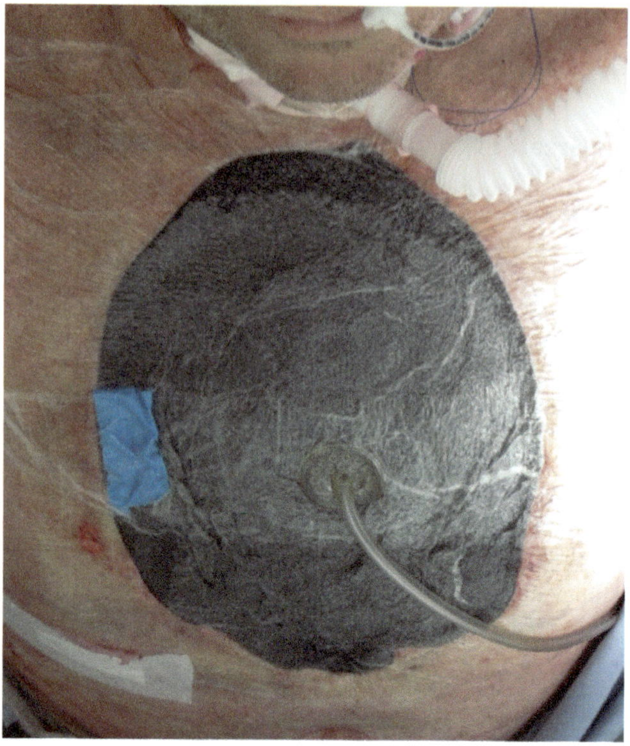

Fig. 28.4 Negative pressure wound therapy

manage these difficult to treat wounds. This treatment modality was introduced by Morykwas et al. in 1997 following successful animal studies (Fig. 28.4) [42].

## 28.5.1 Negative Pressure Wound Therapy

Negative pressure or subatmospheric pressure wound therapy (vacuum-assisted wound therapy/VAC®) was initially developed to expedite wound healing in debilitated patients. In a pig wound model, evenly applying a constant negative pressure through a sterile sponge resulted in a four-fold increase in blood flow to tissues, sustained growth of granulation tissue, and a significant reduction of the number of bacteria, which dropped below $10^5$ cfu per gram of tissue [43]. The mechanical deformation of the tissues caused by negative pressure wound therapy (NPWT) [44] increases arteriolar dilation and tissue oxygenation, even after internal thoracic artery harvesting, resulting in fewer recurrent infections than the open and closed techniques [45, 46]. Wound pre-conditioning with NPWT also reduces bony and cartilaginous destruction, making it possible to plan sternal reconstruction, which should now be a formal objective. Lower sternal instability and sternal reconstruction are associated with better cosmetic and functional

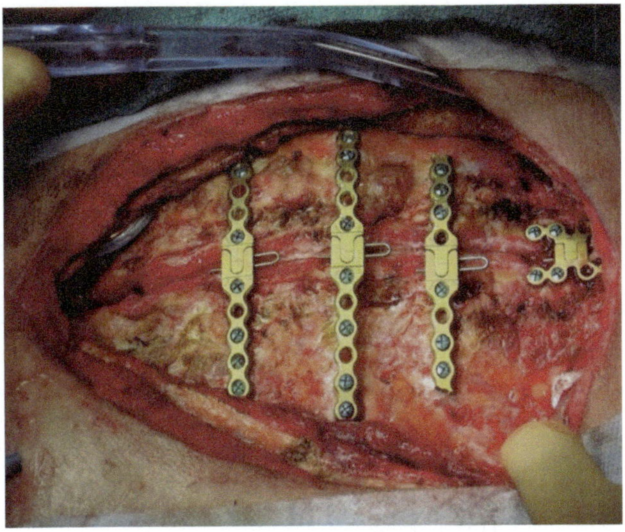

**Fig. 28.5** Sternal osteosynthesis

results. While no prospective randomized trials comparing NPWT with other treatment modalities have been published, a summary of recently published studies has shown that NPWT is associated with lower morbidity and treatment failure rates, shorter hospital stays, better short and mid-term survival rates, and better quality of life than other therapies [47, 48].

### 28.5.2 Sternal Reconstruction with Osteosynthesis

When sternal wound cultures are negative, sternal reconstruction using titanium plates can be recommended, as proposed by Cicilioni et al. [48]. With NPWT, it usually takes three or four debridements over a 2-weeks period before sternal reconstruction can be planned. NPWT is used as a bridge to sternal reconstruction, which is usually indicated when there is pain and sternal instability, especially in younger and more active patients. Older patients can be managed conservatively using only muscle flaps when there is minimal discomfort and only a slight widening between each hemi-sternum (Fig. 28.5).

## 28.6 A Round Up: From Open Granulation to Primary Plating

Deep sternal wound infections remain a challenging complication following cardiac surgery. Mortality, despite significant progress, remains above 10 %, although since the advent of viable tissues, single-digit rates have been reported. We successfully used NPWT as a first-line therapy for the last 10 years with the goal of preserving the sternum for delayed osteosynthesis and pectoralis myoplasty. We rarely use the greater omentum, reserving it for total sternectomy patients in whom the great vessels are exposed. Prevention is a key factor as more and more obese and diabetic patients undergo OHS. Patients with a high BMI are at greater risk of DSWI, while sternal instability is a determining factor in the physiopathology of mediastinitis. In these patients, we recently used titanium plates to reduce the incidence of sternal complications during initial surgery [49, 50].

Over the past five decades, open granulation has given way to closed chest irrigation and then to viable tissues in the treatment of DSWI. NPWT has made it possible to preserve the sternum in many patients and proceed with delayed sternal osteosynthesis for better results. Our understanding of the physiopathology of DSWI has led us now to propose primary plating in high-risk patients as a measure to prevent sternal instability and DSWI.

## References


1. Dalton ML, Connally SR (1993) Median sternotomy. Surg Gynecol Obstet 176:615–624
2. Milton H (1897) Mediastinal surgery. Lancet 1:872–875
3. Julian OC, Lopez-Belio M, Dye WS, Javid H, Grove WJ (1957) The median sternal incision in intracardiac surgery with extracorporeal circulation; a general evaluation of its use in heart surgery. Surgery 42:753–761
4. Miller JI, Nahai F (1989) Repair of the dehisced median sternotomy incision. Surg Clin North Am 69:1091–1102
5. El Oakley RM, Wright JE (1996) Postoperative mediastinitis: classification and management. Ann Thorac Surg 61:1030–1036
6. Mangram AJ, Horan TC, Pearson ML, Silver LC, Jarvis WR (1999) Guideline for prevention of surgical site infection, 1999. Hospital infection control practices advisory committee. Infect Control Hosp Epidemiol 20:250–278
7. Horan TC, Andrus M, Dudeck MA (2008) CDC/NHSN surveillance definition of health care-associated infection and criteria for specific types of infections in the acute care setting. Am J Infect Control 36:309–332
8. Gottlieb LJ, Pielet RW, Karp RB, Krieger LM, Smith DJ Jr, Deeb GM (1994) Rigid internal fixation of the sternum in postoperative mediastinitis. Arch Surg 129:489–493
9. Baillot R, Cloutier D, Montalin L, Cote L, Lellouche F, Houde C, Gaudreau G, Voisine P (2010) Impact of deep sternal wound infection management with vacuum-assisted closure therapy followed by sternal osteosynthesis: a 15-year review of 23,499 sternotomies. Eur J Cardiothorac Surg 37:880–887
10. Modrau IS, Ejlertsen T, Rasmussen BS (2009) Emerging role of Candida in deep sternal wound infection. Ann Thorac Surg 88:1905–1909
11. Sarr MG, Gott VL, Townsend TR (1984) Mediastinal infection after cardiac surgery. Ann Thorac Surg 38:415–423
12. Culliford AT, Cunningham JN Jr, Zeff RH, Isom OW, Teiko P, Spencer FC (1976) Sternal and costochondral infections following open-heart surgery. A review of 2,594 cases. J Thorac Cardiovasc Surg 72:714–726
13. Grmoljez PF, Barner HH, Willman VL, Kaiser GC (1975) Major complications of median sternotomy. Am J Surg 130:679–681
14. Sutherland RD, Martinez HE, Guynes WA, Miller L (1977) Postoperative chest wound infections in patients requiring coronary bypass. A controlled study evaluating prophylactic antibiotics. J Thorac Cardiovasc Surg 73:944–947
15. Shumacker HB, Mandelbaum I Jr (1963) Continuous antibiotic irrigation in the treatment of infection. Arch Surg 86:384–387

16. Bryant LR, Spencer FC, Trinkle JK (1969) Treatment of median sternotomy infection by mediastinal irrigation with an antibiotic solution. Ann Surg 169:914–920
17. Grossi EA, Culliford AT, Krieger KH, Kloth D, Press R, Baumann FG, Spencer FC (1985) A survey of 77 major infectious complications of median sternotomy: a review of 7,949 consecutive operative procedures. Ann Thorac Surg 40:214–223
18. Molina JE, Nelson EC, Smith RR (2006) Treatment of postoperative sternal dehiscence with mediastinitis: twenty-four-year use of a single method. J Thorac Cardiovasc Surg 132:782–787
19. Calvat S, Trouillet JL, Nataf P, Vuagnat A, Chastre J, Gibert C (1996) Closed drainage using Redon catheters for local treatment of poststernotomy mediastinitis. Ann Thorac Surg 61:195–201
20. Jurkiewicz MJ, Bostwick J III, Hester TR, Bishop JB, Craver J (1980) Infected median sternotomy wound. Successful treatment by muscle flaps. Ann Surg 191:738–744
21. Lee AB Jr, Schimert G, Shaktin S, Seigel JH (1976) Total excision of the sternum and thoracic pedicle transposition of the greater omentum; useful strategems in managing severe mediastinal infection following open heart surgery. Surgery 80:433–436
22. Jurkiewicz MJ, Arnold PG (1977) The omentum: an account of its use in the reconstruction of the chest wall. Ann Surg 185:548–554
23. Nahai F, Rand RP, Hester TR, Bostwick J III, Jurkiewicz MJ (1989) Primary treatment of the infected sternotomy wound with muscle flaps: a review of 211 consecutive cases. Plast Reconstr Surg 84:434–441
24. Jones G, Jurkiewicz MJ, Bostwick J, Wood R, Bried JT, Culbertson J, Howell R, Eaves F, Carlson G, Nahai F (1997) Management of the infected median sternotomy wound with muscle flaps. The Emory 20-year experience. Ann Surg 225:766–776
25. Maxwell GP (1980) Iginio Tansini and the origin of the latissimus dorsi musculocutaneous flap. Plast Reconstr Surg 65:686–692
26. Perignon D, Qassemyar Q, Benhaim T, Robbe M, Delay E, Sinna R (2011) [From Tansini to Angrigiani: Improvement and refinement of the thoracodorsal flap.]. Ann Chir Plast Esthet 56:149–155
27. Noszczyk BH (1996) The origins of the concept of muscle flaps. Br J Plast Surg 49:107–110
28. Tobin GR (1989) Pectoralis major muscle-musculocutaneous flap for chest-wall reconstruction. Surg Clin North Am 69:991–1006
29. Chang N, Mathes SJ (1982) Comparison of the effect of bacterial inoculation in musculocutaneous and random-pattern flaps. Plast Reconstr Surg 70:1–10
30. Ascherman JA, Patel SM, Malhotra SM, Smith CR (2004) Management of sternal wounds with bilateral pectoralis major myocutaneous advancement flaps in 114 consecutively treated patients: refinements in technique and outcomes analysis. Plast Reconstr Surg 114:676–683
31. Pairolero PC, Arnold PG, Harris JB (1991) Long-term results of pectoralis major muscle transposition for infected sternotomy wounds. Ann Surg 213:583–589
32. Kiricuta I (1963) [The use of the great omentum in the surgery of breast cancer]. Presse Med 71:15–17
33. O'Shaughnessy L (1937) Surgical treatment of cardiac ischaemia. Lancet 1:185
34. Hultman CS, Carlson GW, Losken A, Jones G, Culbertson J, Mackay G, Bostwick J III, Jurkiewicz MJ (2002) Utility of the omentum in the reconstruction of complex extraperitoneal wounds and defects: donor-site complications in 135 patients from 1975 to 2000. Ann Surg 235:782–795
35. Shrager JB, Wain JC, Wright CD, Donahue DM, Vlahakes GJ, Moncure AC, Grillo HC, Mathisen DJ (2003) Omentum is highly effective in the management of complex cardiothoracic surgical problems. J Thorac Cardiovasc Surg 125:526–532
36. Schroeyers P, Wellens F, Degrieck I, De GR, Van PF, Vermeulen Y, Vanermen H (2001) Aggressive primary treatment for poststernotomy acute mediastinitis: our experience with omental- and muscle flaps surgery. Eur J Cardiothorac Surg 20:743–746
37. Van Wingerden JJ, Coret ME, van Nieuwenhoven CA, Totte ER (2010) The laparoscopically harvested omental flap for deep sternal wound infection. Eur J Cardiothorac Surg 37:87–92

38. Milano CA, Georgiade G, Muhlbaier LH, Smith PK, Wolfe WG (1999) Comparison of omental and pectoralis flaps for poststernotomy mediastinitis. Ann Thorac Surg 67:377–380
39. Cartier R, Brunette I, Hashimoto K, Bourne WM, Schaff HV (1990) Angiogenic factor: a possible mechanism for neovascularization produced by omental pedicles. J Thorac Cardiovasc Surg 99:264–268
40. Krabatsch T, Fleck E, Hetzer R (1995) Treating poststernotomy mediastinitis by transposition of the greater omentum: late angiographic findings. J Card Surg 10:46–51
41. Schimmer C, Sommer SP, Bensch M, Elert O, Leyh R (2008) Management of poststernotomy mediastinitis: experience and results of different therapy modalities. Thorac Cardiovasc Surg 56:200–204
42. Morykwas MJ, Argenta LC, Shelton-Brown EI, McGuirt W (1997) Vacuum-assisted closure: a new method for wound control and treatment: animal studies and basic foundation. Ann Plast Surg 38:553–562
43. Saxena V, Hwang CW, Huang S, Eichbaum Q, Ingber D, Orgill DP (2004) Vacuum-assisted closure: microdeformations of wounds and cell proliferation. Plast Reconstr Surg 114:1086–1096
44. Malmsjo M, Ingemansson R, Sjogren J (2007) Mechanisms governing the effects of vacuum-assisted closure in cardiac surgery. Plast Reconstr Surg 120:1266–1275
45. Fleck TM, Fleck M, Moidl R, Czerny M, Koller R, Giovanoli P, Hiesmayer MJ, Zimpfer D, Wolner E, Grabenwoger M (2002) The vacuum-assisted closure system for the treatment of deep sternal wound infections after cardiac surgery. Ann Thorac Surg 74:1596–1600
46. Sjogren J, Nilsson J, Gustafsson R, Malmsjo M, Ingemansson R (2005) The impact of vacuum-assisted closure on long-term survival after post-sternotomy mediastinitis. Ann Thorac Surg 80:1270–1275
47. Immer FF, Durrer M, Muhlemann KS, Erni D, Gahl B, Carrel TP (2005) Deep sternal wound infection after cardiac surgery: modality of treatment and outcome. Ann Thorac Surg 80:957–961
48. Cicilioni OJ Jr, Stieg FH III, Papanicolaou G (2005) Sternal wound reconstruction with transverse plate fixation. Plast Reconstr Surg 115:1297–1303
49. Raman J, Song DH, Bolotin G, Jeevanandam V (2006) Sternal closure with titanium plate fixation–a paradigm shift in preventing mediastinitis. Interact Cardiovasc Thorac Surg 5:336–339
50. Lee JC, Raman J, Song DH (2010) Primary sternal closure with titanium plate fixation: plastic surgery effecting a paradigm shift. Plast Reconstr Surg 125:1720–1724

# Engineering for IABP and ECMO

# 29

Roberto Lorusso, Attilio Renzulli and Sandro Gelsomino

*Those who are fond of pure practice without science are like the skipper who enters the harbour without any helm or compass, and has never certainty where he is going to.*

Leonardo da Vinci


## Abstract

The use of mechanical devices to compensate the acutely impaired contractile efficiency and power of the heart due to muscular, coronary or valvular diseases has been addressed for almost a century in the history of cardiovascular medicine. Indeed, it is well known that at the beginning of the 20th century, Alexis Carrel and Charles Lindbergh worked together to develop an alternative to the heart pump meant to support the failing circulation. Many other researchers and investigators from 1930 till 1960 investigated several forms and types of mechanical blood circulation and started their application in the clinical setting in the USA, Italy, France, Sweden, Russia, and elsewhere, and extracorporeal circulation (ECC) began to represent a major breakthrough in cardiovascular medicine allowing open heart interventions. The adverse events linked to prolonged ECC and the need for mechanical cardiocirculatory support outside the operating room prompted technicians and clinicians to explore alternative or modified systems to provide partial or full cardiac assistance that could function for several hours, days or weeks. This chapter will describe the development of two systems designed for that objective: a mechanically driven device to partially support the heart through an indirect action, named the intra-aortic balloon pump (IABP), and another system derived from conventional ECC to temporarily help the impaired heart and lung function, named extracorporeal membrane oxygenation (ECMO).



R. Lorusso (✉)
Cardiac Surgery Unit, Community Hospital, Brescia, Italy
e-mail: roberto_lorusso@iol.it

A. Renzulli
Cardiac Surgery Unit, Community Hospital, Catanzaro, Italy

S. Gelsomino
Cardiovascular Research Unit, Florence, Italy



M. Picichè (ed.), *Dawn and Evolution of Cardiac Procedures*,
DOI: 10.1007/978-88-470-2400-7_29, © Springer-Verlag Italia 2013

The use of mechanical devices to compensate the acutely impaired contractile efficiency and power of the heart due to muscular, coronary or valvular diseases has been addressed for almost a century in the history of cardiovascular medicine. Indeed, it is well known that at the beginning of the 20th century, Alexis Carrel and Charles Lindbergh worked together to develop an alternative to the heart pump meant to support the failing circulation. Many other researchers and investigators from 1930 till 1960 investigated several forms and types of mechanical blood circulation and started their application in the clinical setting in the USA [1–3], Italy [4], France [5], Sweden [6], Russia [7], and elsewhere, and extracorporeal circulation (ECC) began to represent a major breakthrough in cardiovascular medicine allowing open heart interventions. The adverse events linked to prolonged ECC and the need for mechanical cardiocirculatory support outside the operating room prompted technicians and clinicians to explore alternative or modified systems to provide partial or full cardiac assistance that could function for several hours, days or weeks. This chapter will describe the development of two systems designed for that objective: a mechanically driven device to partially support the heart through an indirect action, named the intra-aortic balloon pump (IABP), and another system derived from conventional ECC to temporarily help the impaired heart and lung function, named extracorporeal membrane oxygenation (ECMO).

## 29.1 IABP Development and Improvement

The first idea to augment diastolic blood flow mainly to increase coronary perfusion was provided by Kantrowitz in 1953 [8] and subsequently by Harken in 1958 [9]. Harken actually proposed the removal of blood through the femoral artery during ventricular systole and reinfusion of the same fluid volume during diastole. These observations were also addressed by Kantrowitz and McKinnon [10] in the search for auxiliary forms of left ventricular (LV) cardiocirculatory assistance in the presence of impaired cardiac contractility, proposing the attractive concept of improving the poor LV function by reducing the diastolic pressure and, hence, enhancing cardiac efficiency at a lower energetic and mechanical price. This innovative approach to depressed LV function found several supporters for pre-clinical and clinical applications, and reports about the use of such a mechanical assistance were published [11–14]. However, these initial experiences had several limitations, mainly related to the occurrence of haemolysis, the need for arteriotomies for device implantation, either at the femoral or the subclavian level, and by the observation that coronary blood flow was actually unchanged with femoral counterpulsation [15]. The change in counterpulsation configuration was addressed by Moulopoulos and associates [16] who proposed to place the counterpulsation in the descending thoracic aorta with balloon inflation just after the closure of the aortic valve in diastole and deflation before its opening in systole. The true and successful era of IABP then began.

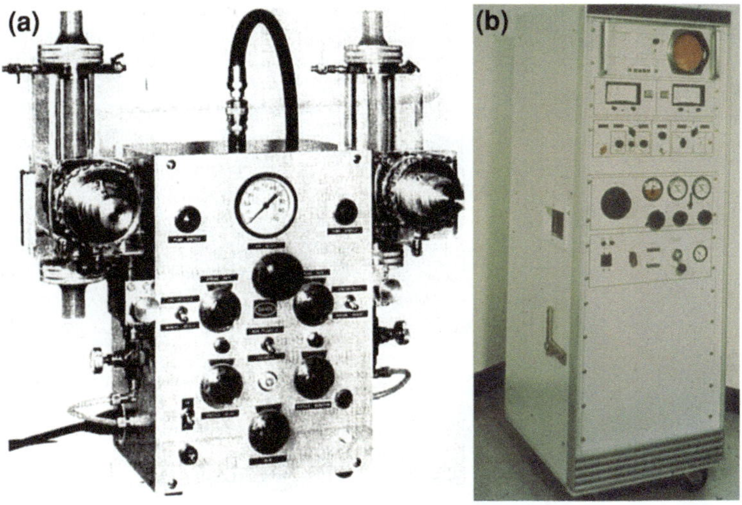


**Fig. 29.1** First prototypes: **a** Datascope (now Maquet AG, Hirrlingen, Germany) prototype. **b** Kontron (now Teleflex) prototype. By courtesy of Teleflex and Maquet AG

The use of IABP in the acute myocardial infarction scenario was carried out by Kantrowitz in 1968 [17], although subsequent clinical study did not show substantial reduction in patient mortality when IABP was applied [18]. The beneficial effects of IABP were, however, repetitively addressed and demonstrated by clinicians and researchers: increased coronary blood flow, reduced myocardial workload, reduced necrotic area during acute myocardial infarction, and opening of dormant intercoronary collateral beds were all effects clearly shown in many experimental or clinical studies.

From a technical and mechanistic IABP working mode standpoint, there were several key points along the IABP development. The first step referred to the use of a dual-balloon configuration (the distal one meant to occlude the distal aorta to let the augmented blood flow counterstream towards the proximal thoracic aorta and, hence, to the coronary arteries). The second step derived from the design of a single IABP balloon, thereby allowing blood flow to direct both proximally and distally. The third advancement related to the importance of IABP deflation to reduce end-diastolic pressure enhancing LV subsequent contraction. Finally, the application of sensoring and software updates allowed automatic IABP functioning, and enhanced pressure curve sensing owing to fibre optic adoption.

Regarding device features, the IABP world has been characterised from the beginning by a duopoly: Datascope (currently Maquet AG) and Kontron/Arrow (currently Teleflex). Datascope introduced the System 80 in 1971 (Fig. 29.1), which was replaced after a while by System 82 (followed by 83, 84, and 84A using the same device platform), which introduced the auto-filling feature in IABP management. At those times, the IABP balloons were surgically implanted through vascular cut-down, with a 12 F balloon size, high complication rate, and long

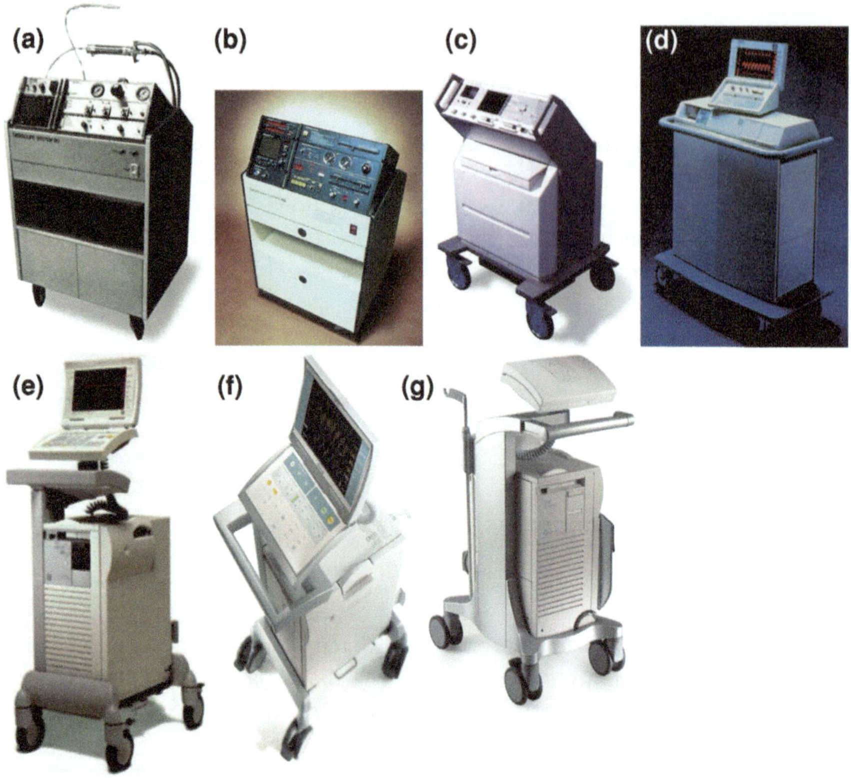


**Fig. 29.2** The progress of the Datascope (Maquet AG, Hirrlingen, Germany) intra-aortic balloon pump (IABP) device through time. **a** The System 80, **b** the system 82, **c** the system 90, **d** the system 95, **e** the system 93, **f** the system CS 100, **g** the system CS 300. By courtesy of Maquet AG, Hirrlingen, Germany

(1–2 h) insertion time. In 1979, Datascope introduced the percutaneous approach using the Seldinger technique, with a dramatic reduction in the vascular complication rate and significantly reduced insertion time (15 min).

Following the first prototypes (Fig. 29.2) and clinical systems in the 1970s, the advances in IABP components were substantial in the 1980s, and, besides the new IABP consoles, there was a relevant change in balloon configuration (development of the PERCOR DL balloon, with 10.5 F and then 9.5 F size, the launch of the paediatric balloon, and finally with the 34-$cm^3$ volume balloon for smaller patients introduced in 1989).

Subsequent IABP improvements enhanced IABP handling with more user-friendly consoles (System 90, 95, 93, and other 90s versions, including the Cardiosync software; Fig. 29.2), improved timing algorithm, pneumatic efficiency, inclusion of a modem for remote troubleshooting, pacemaker-based sensing, better screen-related display and other features. From the balloon standpoint, in 1997

**Table 29.1** Intra-aortic balloon pump (IABP)—historical milestones

| Year | Milestone |
|---|---|
| 1969 | The first commercially available IABP (the AVCO model 7) |
| 1971 | Datascope introduces the system 80 |
| 1976 | AVCO introduces the first microprocessor based IABP (the model 10) |
| 1979 | The first double-lumen surgical IABP catheter (the AVCO 14 F) |
| 1980 | Datascope introduces the first percutaneous IABP catheter |
| 1981 | Kontron introduces the first double-lumen percutaneous 12 F catheter |
| 1983 | Datascope introduces the 10.5 F double-lumen catheter |
| 1985 | Datascope introduces the first pre-wrapped 10 F double-lumen and 9.5 F double-lumen catheters |
| 1993 | Bard introduces the first hydrophilic IABP |
| 1998 | Arrow introduces the first 8 F IABP catheter |
| 1999 | Arrow introduces the first 7 F IABP catheter |
| 2003 | Arrow introduces the first fibre optic IABP catheter |

1980: AVCO Medical Products was acquired by Kontron Instruments. 1994: Kontron was acquired by Arrow International; 1998: Bard Division acquired by Arrow International; 2006: Arrow International acquired by Teleflex; 2009: Datascope acquired by Maquet AG

there was the introduction of the 25-cm$^3$ balloon for patients <1.5 m tall, in 1998 the profile 8 F IABP catheter was introduced, and the final, currently available version of the 7.5 F size, with the possibility of insertion through the brachial arteries, was launched in 2005.

In 2007, the fibre optic pressure monitoring capability and new software for fully automatic operation and IABP catheter sensoring were introduced.

The second company dealing with IABP manufacturing was Kontron, subsequently acquired by Arrow International, finally merging into Teleflex Company. The major contributions and milestones in IABP development of Kontron/ARROW/Teleflex are reported in Table 29.1, and may be summarized by the search for smaller catheter sizes and high-quality arterial pressure curve sensing and analysis, as shown by the fibre optic-based IABP catheter recently released.

As is clearly shown, these two companies contributed significantly to the constant and high-standard process of miniaturizing catheters and IABP consoles, together with increasingly reliable pressure sensoring as well as implantability, particularly with the current "sheathless" implantation technique, which reduced dramatically the IABP-related complication rates, allowing a broader IABP application, mainly in cardiology patients.

## 29.2 Extracorporeal Life Support

Following the pioneering work of John Gibbon [1, 2] on the development of a cardiopulmonary support system whose first clinical application was carried out in 1951 [4], the subsequent major breakthrough was the concept of utilizing an ECC device outside the operating room and for a long period of time. Indeed, the first systems were characterized by a limited time-related use owing to the blood damage induced mainly by the direct exposure of the blood to oxygen gas [19, 20]. The breakthrough advance, something we could define a "broken barrier", was provided by the development of a spiral coil-type silicone rubber membrane oxygenator. Kolff and Kolobow independently studied these issues [21, 22], and the first experience of out-of-operating theatre application of the ECC system was reported in 1972 by Hill and associates in a patient suffering from ARDS after trauma [23]. Regarding the use of extracorporeal life support (ECLS) in newborns and neonates, Dorsons and White reported their own experience in 1969 and 1971 respectively [24, 25]. Bartlett, Gazzaniga and associates performed their first successful ECMO application in a 2 year old infant after a Mustard operation in 1972, followed by several other cases [26]. From three survivors among 16 patients treated by Bartlett and coworkers, there was a gradual improvement in clinical outcome [27], which promoted the interest and application in the surgical and intensive care community. After such a clinical attempt, many followed, culminating into the clinical trial endorsed by the NIH in 1975 comparing conventional respiratory therapies versus ECLS for ARDS in adults [28]. This trial was, as a matter of fact, a major threat for ECMO: the rather inexperienced centres that enrolled (only 3 out of 9 had experience in ECMO at the time of the trial start), the poorly performing technology available at that time, and the ventilatory techniques used in the patient while on ECMO did not lead to any improvement when comparing the two trial arms. These findings, although clearly underlining the complexity of the clinical scenario (66% mortality in the total population and 90% in severe ARDS patients), somewhat hampered the subsequent extension or even application of ECLS in respiratory failure and, to some extent, in acute cardiocirculatory impairment too.

In 1982, survival for ECMO in neonatal respiratory failure reached 55% [29], which rose to almost 90% in neonatal respiratory failure and 70% for diaphragmatic hernia by 1984. From that time on many neonatology and paediatric intensive care and surgical units worldwide established successful ECMO programmes.

In terms of the chronological reporting of ECLS, as shown in Table 29.2, after the development in 1950 of the flat-sheet membrane oxygenator in the laboratory, the first successful ECLS application was reported in 1972 in an adult patient [23], 1 year later in the first paediatric case, and in 1975 there was the first neonatal case. This was the beginning of much ECLS experience, particularly in USA. As mentioned, owing to the uncompelling evidence of the NIH study in the 1970s [28], ECLS witnessed a sort of slow-down. In the 1980s, only 18 centres worldwide were performing ECLS, and in the 1990s, thanks to technological advances, neonatal and paediatric application became common practice. In 1989, the Extra-Corporeal Life Support

**Table 29.2** Extracorporeal membrane oxygenation (ECMO) history: chronology

| Year | Milestone |
|---|---|
| 1954 | Cardiopulmonary bypass |
| 1960–1970 | Cardiopulmonary bypass modified for prolonged use |
| 1967 | ARDS diagnosis |
| 1971 | 1st successful extracorporeal life support case (adult ARDS) |
| 1972 | 1st successful extracorporeal life support cardiac case (paediatric post-operatively) |
| 1975 | 1st extracorporeal life support neonatal respiratory (newborn persistent fetal circulation) |
| 1979 | NIH-ARDS ECMO trial (zapol) |
| 1985–1990 | Neonatal ECMO trials |
| 1986 | 1st registry report 800 cases |
| 1989 | Extracorporeal life support established |
| 1993 | 3,000 cases |
| 2007 | ARDS ECMO CESAR trial |
| 2008 | 38,000 cases |

Organization (ELSO) was created in order to provide a more scientific and structured access to ECLS activity and to promote an international registry favouring well-designed and robust clinical investigations (Fig. 29.3).

The progress in ECLS (either in cardiocirculatory or respiratory impairment) has witnessed several major advancements and encompassed different fields. In terms of ECLS-related techniques, each field of ECLS application has gone through steps linked to pump and oxygenator components, ECLS circuit and configuration, vascular access, as well as indications, management and weaning protocols. As far as cardiac support is concerned, central or peripheral access represented a relevant aspect of ECLS improvement over the years. Femoro-femoral cannulation with reduced cannula sizes, the prevention of limb ischemia through selective distal perfusion, active drainage of the venous flow from the limb too, and the attention paid to LV unloading, have all played a critical role in the enhanced ECLS management, reduced complication rate and improved outcome. Regarding respiratory support, the knowledge and separation between oxygenation or $CO_2$ removal, vascular access and ECLS configuration, the availability of the double-lumen cannula with the neck approach, the new dedicated and biologically-friendly devices for $CO_2$ removal, the understanding of ventilation regimens during ECMO or $CO_2$ removal, and, obviously, the marked advances in technological components, have provided, once again, a major support for expanded application and favourable outcome in patients with respiratory distress [30, 31].

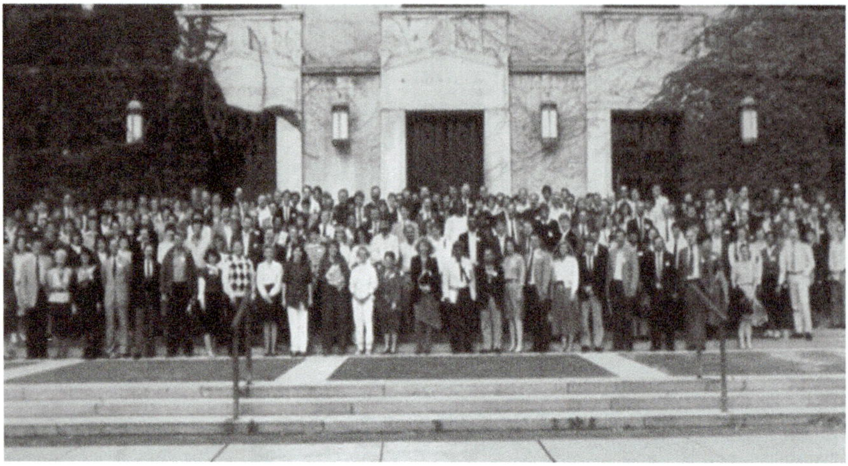

**Fig. 29.3** The ELSO (Extra-Corporeal Life Support Organization) charter meeting in Ann Arbor, Michigan, October 1989 (by courtesy of Robert Bartlett and the University of Michigan)

Vascular access, as mentioned, passed from surgical cut-down and insertion, usually centrally through the aorta and right atrium, of large-size cannulas, toward peripheral access, eventually achieved even with the Seldinger technique, with thin, small-sized, percutaneous cannulas, often characterized by non-thrombogenic surfaces. Needless to say, the most recent cannula design (double-lumen cannula for veno-venous ECMO [32] or low-profile cannula for arterial access) and the routine application of distal limb perfusion in the case of femoral artery cannulation for peripheral veno-arterial approach were additional breakthroughs for successful ECMO application with significant reduction of postprocedural complications.

From the circuit and pump standpoint, however, the most critical steps were provided by the development of the polymethylpentene membrane oxygenator, which allowed a low oxygenator pressure drop, high oxygenation efficiency, and long-lasting performance, currently achieving 30 days, to be achieved.

Finally, coating the circuit surfaces (heparin-bonded) [33], together with the miniaturization and integration of pump systems, led to the ultimate development of ECLS systems that were extremely simple, highly efficient, and portable, even for outside hospital applications.

In conclusion, in four decades, although with some difficulty, the advances in IABP technological systems, and, more remarkably, in the ECMO field, have provided new generations of catheters, circuit, oxygenators, pumps, and cannulas enhancing effective indirect and direct cardiocirculatory and respiratory support. Few fields in medicine have witnessed such a profound change with an incomparable impact on the clinical fate of patients affected by severe and sometimes refractory cardiocirculatory and respiratory disorders. Such an achievement must be recognized.

Additional ongoing technological improvements will certainly broaden IABP and ECMO applications, particularly with an earlier and more effective implantation and, maybe, for longer support times in an attempt to improve outcomes in patients who are most likely to be facing a fatal prognosis otherwise.

**Acknowledgments** The support, information, and documents provided by Maquet AG, Teleflex and Robert H. Bartlett, are gratefully acknowledged.

## References

1. Stokes TL, Gibbon JH Jr (1950) Experimental maintenance of life by a mechanical heart and lung during occlusion of the venae cavae followed by survival. Surg Gynecol Obstet 91:138–156
2. Gibbon JH Jr (1954) Application of a mechanical heart and lung apparatus to cardiac surgery. Minn Med 37:171–185
3. Dennis C, Spreng DS Jr, Nelson GE et al (1951) Development of a pump-oxygenator to replace the heart and the lungs: an apparatus applicable to human patients and application to one case. Ann Surg 134:709–721
4. Dogliotti AM, Costantini A (1951) First case of the human use of an apparatus for extracorporeal blood circulation. Minerva Chir 15:657–659
5. Dubost C, Lenfant C, Passelecq J et al (1956) Closure of an interventricular communication caused by an opening in the heart with extracorporeal circulation: the first French success. Mem Acad Chir 82:207–216
6. Bjork VO (1948) An artificial heart or cardiopulmonary machine: performance in animals. Lancet 2:491–493
7. Brukhonenko SS (1929) Circulation artificielle du sang dans l'organisme entrier d'un chien avec Coeur exclu. J Physiol Path Gen 27:257–272
8. Kantrowitz A (1953) Experimental augmentation of coronary flow by retardation of the arterial pressure pulse. Surgery 34:682–687
9. Harken DE (1958) Presentation at the International College of Cardiology meeting. Brussels, Belgium
10. Kantrowitz A, McKinnon WM (1958) The experimental use of the diaphragm as an auxiliary myocardium. Surg Forum 9:266–268
11. Willman VL, Cooper T, Riberi A, Hanlon CR (1961) Cardiac assistance by diastolic augmentation : hemodynamic evaluation in dogs with complete heart block. Tr Am Soc Artif Intern Organs 7:198–201
12. Jacobey JA, Craddock LD, Wolf PS, Beckwitt HJ (1968) Clinical experience with counterpulsation in coronary artery disease. J Thorac Cardiovasc Surg 56:846–857
13. Rosensweig J, Chatterjee S, Merino F (1970) Treatment of acute myocardial infarction by counterpulsation. Experimental rationale and clinical experience. J Thorac Cardiovasc Surg 69:243–250
14. Sugg WL, Webb WR, Ecker RR (1969) Reduction of extent of myocardial infarction by counterpulsation. Ann Thorac Surg 7:310–316
15. Dormandy JA, Goetz RH, Krippke DC (1969) Hemodynamics and coronary blood flow with counterpulsation. Surgery 65:311–320
16. Moulopoulos MD, Topas S, Kolff WJ (1962) Diastolic balloon pumping (with carbon dioxide) in the aorta: a mechanical assistance to failing circulation. Am Heart J 63:669–675
17. Kantrowitz A, Tionneland S, Freed PS, Phillips SJ, Butner AN, Sherman JL (1968) Initial clinical experience with intraaortic balloon pumping in cardiogenic shock. JAMA 203:135–140

18. Bregman D, Bailin M, Bowman FO Jr et al (1977) A pulsatile assist device (PAD) for improved myocardial protection during cardiopulmonary bypass. Ann Thorac Surg 24:574
19. Lee WH, Krumhaar D, Fonkalsrud EW et al (1961) Denaturation of plasma proteins as a cause of morbidity and death after intracardiac operations. Surgery 50:29–39
20. Dobell ARC, Mitri M, Galva et al (1965) Biological evaluation of blood after prolonged recirculation through film and membrane oxygenators. Ann Surg 161:617–622
21. Kolff WJ, Effler DB, Groves LK, Peereboom G, Moraca PP (1956) Disposable membrane oxygenator (heart-lung machine) and its use in experimental surgery. Cleve Clin Q. 23:69–97
22. Kolobow T, Spragg RG, Pierce JE, Zapol WM (1971) Extended term (to 16 days) partial extracorporeal blood gas excahnge with the spiral membrane lung in unesthetized lambs. Trans Am Soc Artif Intern Organs 17:350–345
23. Hill JD, O'Brien TG, Murray JJ et al (1972) Extracorporeal oxygenation for acute post-traumatic respiratory failure (shock-lung syndrome): use of the bramson membrane lung. N Engl J Med 286:629–634
24. Dorson W Jr, Baker E, Cohen ML et al (1969) A perfusion system for infants. Trans Am Soc Artif Intern Organs 15:155–160
25. White JJ, Andrews HG, Risemberg H et al (1969) Prolonged respiratory support in newborn infants with a membrane oxygenator. Surgery 70:288–296
26. Bartlett RH, Gazzaniga AB, Jefferies R et al (1976) Extracorporeal membrane oxygenation (ECMO) cardiopulmonary support in infancy. Trans Am Soc Artif Organ 22:80–88
27. Bartlett RH, Gazzaniga AB, Huxtable RF et al (1977) Extracorporeal circulation (ECMO) in neonatal respiratory failure. J Thorac Cardiovasc Surg 74:826–833
28. Zapol WM, Snider MT, Hill JD et al (1979) Extracorporeal membrane oxygenation in severe acute respiratory failure: a randomized prospective study. JAMA 242:2193–2196
29. Wang D, Zhou X, Liu X, Sidor B, Lynch J, Zwischenberger JB (2008) Wang-Zische double lumen cannula. Toward percutaneous and ambulatory paracorporeal artificial lung. ASAIO J 54:606–611
30. Matheis G (2003) New technologies for respiratory assist. Perfusion 18:238–243
31. Bartlett RH, Andrews AF, Tomasian JM, Haiduc NJ, Gazzaniga AB (1982) Extracorporeal membrane oxygenation for newborn respiratory failure: forty-five cases. Surgery 92:452–433
32. Peek G, Mugford M, Tiruvoipati R et al (2009) Efficacy and economic assessment of conventional ventilatory support versus extracorporeal membrane oxygenation for severe adult respiratory failure (CESAR): a multicentre randomised controlled trial. Lancet 374:1351–1363
33. Harig F, Feyrer R, Mahmoud FO et al (1999) Reducing the post-pump syndrome by using heparin-coated circuits, steroids, or aprotinin. Thorac Cardiovasc Surg 47:111–118

# The History of Research on Ventricular Assist Devices and Total Artificial Heart

# 30

Luc M. Jacquet

*It is only with one's heart that one can see clearly. What is essential is invisible to the eye.*

Antoine de Saint-Exupery, The Little Prince

**Abstract**

This chapter will focus on research specifically aimed at the total or partial replacement of the heart's function or that of one of its ventricles to support a failing heart for a prolonged period of time. The first report on the use a total artificial heart (TAH) to sustain life in an animal dates back to 1958. In 1969, the first human implantation of a pneumatic TAH was reported for bridge to transplantation and, after more than 10 years of research, a TAH as definitive therapy was used for the first time in 1982 without much success. About 20 years later, a totally implantable pump was released for clinical use. The initial feasibility study demonstrated that the device still needs improvements before a more widespread application can be expected. Most of the initial ventricular assist devices (VAD) were internal or paracorporeal pneumatically activated blood pumps and were temporarily used while waiting recovery of the heart's function or as a bridge to transplantation. For long-term support, however, an internal energy converter was necessary. An electrically activated LVAD was designed and used for the first time in 1984. In the 1990s, two implantable, electrically activated VAD were extensively used as a bridge to transplantation with excellent long-term results that opened the way to their use as destination therapy. Smaller continuous flow pumps, either centrifugal or axial, were created to overcome the problems of the pulsatile pumps. Some of these smaller pumps are nowadays used for extended duration with excellent

L. M. Jacquet (✉)
Cardiovascular Intensive Care Unit,
Saint-Luc University Hospital,
Brussels, Belgium
e-mail: luc-marie.jacquet@uclouvain.be

M. Pichè (ed.), *Dawn and Evolution of Cardiac Procedures*,
DOI: 10.1007/978-88-470-2400-7_30, © Springer-Verlag Italia 2013

results. Continuous flow technology is now integrated into TAH that are investigated in animals.

Before the advent of cardiopulmonary bypass, a brilliant student had already designed the first mechanical assist device, but had been ignored. For the first time in history, circulation was supported in a dog with the heart excised for 5.5 h. This was running in Russia by 1937, and the inventor's name was Vladimir Demikhov [1]. Since his publications were written in Russian, it took a considerable amount of time for his achievements to become known to the Western world.

## 30.1 Total Artificial Heart

In 1958, Kolff and Akutsu from the Cleveland Clinic reported at the American Society of Artificial Internal Organs their experience with a pneumatically driven plastic heart that had supported a living dog for 90 min. This was the first report of an artificial heart sustaining the life of an animal. During the same session, they presented the dummy of an electromagnetically driven artificial heart [2].

In the late 1950s, several teams around the world were developing pumps for cardiac replacement. One of the most active groups was at Baylor College in Houston where DeBakey had invited Liotta, previously assistant to Kolff at Cleveland. They worked on developing a cardiac prosthesis and were able to keep animals alive for more than 24 h [3].

In 1964, the National Heart, Lung and Blood Institute (NHLBI) in the United States established an artificial heart program with special congressional approval. Contracts were awarded to support the study and development of an artificial cardiac pump. However, DeBakey, who had played a major role in obtaining this funding, remained reluctant to proceed with a human trial of the artificial heart developed at Baylor College. Probably frustrated by this decision, Liotta approached Cooley, a surgeon at the nearby Texas Heart Institute, and convinced him to proceed with the first clinical use. In 1969, Cooley and Liotta implanted their artificial pump in the chest of a 47-year-old man who could not be weaned from bypass after a left ventricular aneurysmectomy. The Liotta–Cooley TAH supported the patient for 64 h when a cardiac transplantation could be performed. Unfortunately, the patient died shortly thereafter from infectious complications [4].

This first implantation demonstrated that it was possible to sustain human life with an artificial pump, but much improvement was clearly still mandatory. Progress continued in the field of pump design, biomaterials, and artificial valves with several pneumatic, electric, and even nuclear powered TAH being designed and used in animal studies. Akutsu and Cooley at Texas Heart Institute further developed new pumps and a second human implant of an Akutsu III TAH was performed in Houston in 1981 as a bridge to transplantation [5]. All around the world, teams were working on projects related to the artificial heart. In Germany, in Austria, in Japan, and even in the former USSR, animals were supported for several months with various TAH [6].

At the University of Utah in Salt Lake City, under the supervision of Kolff, Olsen, and Jarvik, a pneumatic TAH was developed with a uniconstructed smooth blood-contacting surface, tilting disk valves, and Dacron atrial cuffs [7]. After several years of animal studies, the designed Jarvik-7 TAH was implanted for the first time in a patient in December 1982 as a definitive therapy. The recipient, Barney Clark, survived 112 days [8]. The results of the initial Jarvik-7 trial were rather disappointing with a high rate of thromboembolic and infectious complications. Its use as a permanent TAH had to be abandoned. Nevertheless, with better medical expertise in patient management, the device continued to be used with success as a bridge to cardiac transplantation. The first of these planned interventions was performed by Copeland at the University of Arizona in 1985 [9]. The device was initially manufactured by Symbion Corporation and later by CardioWest Corporation, who renamed it CardioWest C-70, with very few changes to the initial design. The CardioWest C-70 received FDA approval as a bridge to transplantation and, after being acquired by Syncardia, Inc. is still in use in USA, Canada, France, and Germany. A portable driver called Freedom has now been released to power the device [10].

Meanwhile, the NHLBI continued to fund research into a totally implantable TAH. The Abiomed company, in conjunction with the Texas Heart Institute and the University of Louisville, was one of the NHLBI contractors and created a pump, the Abiocor, containing two ventricles and an energy converter situated between the ventricles. The energy converter contains a high efficiency miniature centrifugal pump that rotates to pressurize a low viscosity hydraulic fluid, which is moved between the right and left ventricles resulting in alternate left and right systole. The internal controller transmits device performance data to a bedside console via radiofrequency telemetry. An internal battery is capable of powering the device for brief periods of time and is recharged by transcutaneous energy transfer (TET) [11]. The first human implantation occurred in July 2001 at the Jewish Hospital, Louisville, Kentucky, USA [12]. The initial feasibility study included 14 patients, with the longest survival being 512 days. A relatively high rate of thromboembolic complications was observed requiring modifications of the pump. Research is still ongoing with several changes applied to improve the next generation Abiocor 2 (i.e., incorporation of technology acquired from Penn State University [13]).

New concepts have been elaborated to design original pumps, but they have not yet reached the level of clinical application. We will come back to some of the concepts later on.

## 30.2 Ventricular Assist Devices

Derived from the manual cardiac massage, some devices were created to act as a "pneumo-massage of the heart" (i.e., Bencini's cup described in 1956 [14]), but without much success. Most of the assist devices unload the natural heart by volume uptake and were, initially, derived from methods used in the heart–lung machines.

Dennis et al. had developed a pump-oxygenator to replace the heart and lung and used it in clinical practice for the first time in 1951. However, realizing that the oxygenator in the circuit limited the duration of possible support, Dennis and his co-workers pursued the idea of left heart bypass and demonstrated that left bypass could effectively decrease the workload of the normal heart in dogs [15]. They developed a cannula designed to access the left atrium (LA) by a transseptal approach. Oxygenated blood drained from the LA was circulated by means of a roller pump and reinfused in the femoral artery. In 1962, the first clinical application was reported in a patient suffering ventricular septal defect and cardiogenic shock after a myocardial infarction [16].

In the early 1960s, the cardiac surgery team at Baylor College in Houston, Texas, concentrated its research on prolonged support for cardiogenic shock following cardiotomy while awaiting recovery of the natural heart. A tubular, pneumatically activated intrathoracic LVAD was created by Liotta and Hall and implanted in 1963 by Crawford and DeBakey. However, the patient did not survive the surgical procedure [17]. In 1966, a paracorporeal Liotta–DeBakey LVAD was successfully implanted at the Methodist Hospital, Houston, in a patient who could not be weaned from bypass after double-valve replacement. The patient was supported for 10 days at a flow rate up to 1,200 ml/min and could be weaned from the LVAD. In this early version, the pump was lined with Dacron velour to create a pseudo neo-endocardium [18, 19].

In Boston, Bernhard and La Farge developed a series of axiosymetric double-valved blood pumps interposed between the left ventricular apex and the thoracic aorta. Their research work resulted in the approval of a Model X pump containing xenograft valves for use as a temporary clinical assist device [20]. At Texas Heart Institute in Houston, an abdominal LVAD (ALVAD) interposed between the apex and the infra-renal abdominal aorta was designed. This device was used for the first reported case of bridge to transplantation with an LVAD in 1975 by Norman, Cooley, and Frazier [21, 22].

Pierce and Donachy at Pennsylvania State University in Hershey worked on a paracorporeal, pneumatically activated pump, the Angle Port Pump [23]. They constructed a reliable pump that was acquired by Thoratec Corporation and became the Thoratec PVAD, which is still widely used nowadays. An internal version (IVAD), activated by an external air compressor, has existed since 2001.

For long-term application, however, an implantable LVAD was necessary, one of the most important components being an implantable energy converter. Portner at Stanford University renewed a concept of solenoid activator first described by Bindels in the early 1960s [24, 25]. The activator was incorporated into a dual pusher plate pump and by 1977, the first integrated LVAS had been designed. In 1982, Novacor Medical was created to commercialize this LVAS. The first human implantation of an electric VAD occurred in 1984 at Stanford University Medical Center [26]. A wearable controller and rechargeable batteries for power supply were released in 1993.

In the 1970s, the possibility of using other power sources was even contemplated and research into heat engine or nuclear power sources was initiated. The Department of Artificial Organs at the Cleveland Clinic (Whalen, Washizu, and Nosé) worked on a device that could be activated by a nuclear or an electrical system [27]. Outside the United States, the design of an LVAD was also the object of intense interest. In Europe, researchers from Vienna used parts of their total artificial heart to form the ellipsoid LVAD (E-LVAD) [28]. In Japan, teams in Hiroshima, Nagaya, and Tokyo also created innovative LVAD.

Thermedics Inc., a division of Thermo Electron Corporation, presented in the mid-1980s the results of their clinical experience with textured blood-contacting surfaces in a pneumatic ventricular assist device, the Thermedics Model 14 [29]. This surface results in the formation of a biologically active pseudoneointima that becomes nonthrombogenic. The technology was incorporated into the HeartMate, an implantable titanium alloy pump. The internal pneumatic HeartMate IP was implanted for the first time in 1986. A vented electric (VE) version, actuated by a low speed torque motor, came into clinical use in 1991. ThermoCardio systems merged with Thoratec Corporation in 2001.

In 1999, a totally implantable LVAD including internal batteries and controller, called the LionHeart, had been created by researchers at Penn State University in collaboration with Arrow Inc. Despite encouraging results, the company ended development and sales in 2005.

Both the Novacor and HeartMate were extensively used in the 1990s as a bridge to transplantation for long periods of time, sometimes exceeding 1 year. This opened a completely new avenue of research into the clinical application of this therapy. A landmark study was initiated in 1998, the Randomized Evaluation of Mechanical Assistance for the Treatment of Congestive Heart Failure (REMATCH), which demonstrated the superiority of the HeartMate VE over medical treatment in patients with terminal heart failure who were not candidates for heart transplantation [30].

Meanwhile, research teams were working on new technology to create safer devices that were less cumbersome and less noisy. Continuous flow pumps represented the most attractive alternative. In fact, back in 1960, Saxton and Andrews had already described a continuous flow pump for use as an artificial heart [31]. Since 1964, a combined team from the University of Minnesota, Medtronic Inc., and the University of California in San Diego, studied fundamental aspects of support with a centrifugal pump. They demonstrated in animal studies that pulseless flow was compatible with long-term survival [32]. Although intracorporeal implantation was the final goal, only extracorporeal pumps were developed for use during cardiac surgery or for short-term support.

In 1988, the concept of an axial pump appeared in clinical practice with the Hemopump. It had been developed by the Nimbus Corporation from the idea of Wampler who applied the principle of the Archimedes screw he had seen working in Egypt for water wells. Years of research had been necessary to create this miniaturized pump, mounted on a catheter and inserted through the femoral artery or in the ascending aorta. The feasibility of sustaining life with this type of pump without excessive blood damage was demonstrated and stimulated much interest, even though the Hemopump itself disappeared [33]. A catheter-mounted axial flow pump was later developed at the Helmholtz Institute in Aachen, the Impella pump, which has been acquired by Abiomed.

Axial flow pumps for long-term assistance were also widely investigated. The Baylor College of Medicine in Houston in collaboration with NASA developed the DeBakey–Noon pump, which was implanted clinically for the first time in Berlin in 1998 [34]. Jarvik and the Texas Heart Institute designed an intraventricular axial flow pump, the Jarvik 2000. With researchers in Oxford, a skull-mounted carbon pedestal was created to transmit fine electric wires through the scalp skin, which is resistant to infection [35]. The McGowan Center of the University of Pittsburgh with the Nimbus Company also initiated research into such a device. Nimbus was later acquired by Thermo Cardiosystems Inc., which merged with Thoratec. Their device, the HeartMate II, is nowadays the most widely implanted assist device for long-term support [36]. Recently published clinical trials have demonstrated the reliability of the device both as a bridge to transplantation and as destination therapy [37]. In Germany, the Berlin Heart GmbH worked with the German Heart Institute on a magnetically suspended impeller, which is the moving part of the Incor pump, implanted for the first time in 2002 [38].

Centrifugal pumps were also developed with hydrodynamic bearings (i.e., the Ventrassist pump developed in Australia, the Eva Heart from Sinu Medical in Japan), with magnetic bearings (the HeartQuest, a collaboration among the Utah Artificial Heart Institute, MedQuest Products, and the University of Virginia; the Dura Heart developed by Terumo Heart Inc.) or hybrid pumps with passive magnets and hydrodynamic thrust bearing (HeartWare HVAD, Miami) [39].

Efforts are now concentrated on further miniaturizing the devices, especially for use in children.

## 30.3 Conclusions

For years, projects have been conducted, aiming at the development of a permanently implantable continuous flow total artificial heart.

Owing to the excellent clinical results obtained with rotary pumps as LVAD, interest has increased in using two rotary pumps either as biventricular support or as a total artificial heart. Frazier at the Texas Heart Institute reported in 2006 the survival of a calf for 20 days using dual continuous flow pumps (Jarvik 2000) [40]. Biventricular continuous flow support has now reached clinical application with several devices.

Creating a reliable, totally implantable artificial heart is much more complex than anticipated by the first researchers in this field. After years of extensive laboratory and clinical research all around the world, reliable implantable assist devices can be used in daily clinical practice for short- and long-term support. Improvements are still required and research continues in several directions (miniaturization, total implantability, clinical management, total artificial heart), and the road is still long before we reach the Holy Grail.

## References


1. Konstantinov IE (2009) At the cutting edge of the impossible: a tribute to Vladimir P. Demikhov. Tex Heart Inst J 36:453–458
2. Akutsu T, Kolff W (1958) Permanent substitutes for valves and heart. Trans Am Soc Artif Intern Organs 4:230–234
3. Hall C, Akers W, O'Bannon W et al (1965) Intraventricular artificial heart. Trans Am Soc Artif Intern Organs 11:263–264
4. Cooley D, Liotta D, Hallman G et al (1969) Orthotopic cardiac prosthesis for two-staged cardiac replacement. Am J Cardiol 24:723–730
5. Cooley D, Akutsu T, Norman J et al (1981) Total artificial heart in two-staged cardiac transplantation. Cardiovas Dis Bull Texas Heart Instit 8:305–319
6. Unger F (1979) Assisted circulation. Springer, Berlin
7. Lawson J, Olsen D, Kolff W et al (1976) A three months survival of a calf with an artificial heart. J Lab Clin Med 87:848–858
8. DeVries W (1984) Clinical use of the total artificial heart. N Eng J Med 310:273–278
9. Copeland J, Smith R, Icenogle T et al (1989) Orthotopic total artificial heart bridge to transplantation: preliminary results. J Heart Lung Transplant 8:124–138
10. Discharge drivers at http://www.syncardia.com/Medical-Professionals/discharge-drivers-us.html. Accessed 22 May 2011
11. Dowling R, Etoch S, Stevens K et al (2001) Current status of the Abiocor implantable replacement heart. Ann Thorac Surg 71:S147–S149
12. Dowling R, Gray L, Etoch S (2003) The Abiocor implantable replacement heart. Ann Thorac Surg 75:S93–S99
13. Abiocor Frequently Asked Question at http://www.abiomed.com/assets/2010/11/AbioCor-FAQ-FINAL.pdf. Accessed 22 May 2011
14. Bencini A, Parola P (1956) The pneumomassage of the heart. Surgery 39:375–384
15. Dennis C, Hall D, Moreno J (1962) Reduction of the oxygen utilization of the heart by left heart bypass. Circ Res 10:298–305
16. Dennis C, Carlens E, Senning A (1962) Clinical use of a cannula for left heart bypass without thoracotomy: experimental protection against fibrillation by left heart bypass. Ann Surg 156:623–636
17. Liotta D, Crawford E, Cooley D et al (1962) Prolonged partial ventricular bypass by means of an intrathoracic pump implanted in the left chest. Trans Am Soc Artif Intern Organs 8:90–99
18. DeBakey M (1971) Left ventricular bypass pump for cardiac assistance. Am J Cardiol 27: 3–11
19. Liotta D, Hall C, Akers W et al (1966) A pseudoendocardium for implantable blood pumps. Trans Am Soc Artif Int Organs 12:129–138
20. Bernhard W, La Farge C, Robinson T et al (1968) An improved blood-pump interface for left ventricular bypass. Ann Surg 168:750–764
21. Norman J (1974) An abdominal left ventricular assist device (A-LVAD):perspectives and prospects. Cardiovasc Dis Bull Tex Heart Inst 1:251–264
22. Norman J, Brook M, Cooley D et al (1978) Total support of the circulation of a patient with post-cardiotomy stone-heart syndrome by a partial artificial heart (ALVAD) for 5 days followed by heart and kidney transplantation. Lancet 1:1125–1127
23. Pierce W, Brighton J, O'Bannon (1974) Complete left ventricular bypass with a paracorporeal pump: design and evaluation. Ann Surg 180:418–426
24. Bindels J, Grigsby L (1961) Considerations and calculations about the optimum solenoid to be used for an intrathoracic artificial heart. Trans Am Soc Artif Intern Organs 7:369–372
25. Portner P, Oyer P, Miller P et al (1978) Evolution of the solenoid-actuated left ventricular assist system: integration with a pusher-plate pump for intra-abdominal implantation in the calf. Artif Organs 2:402–412

26. Starnes V, Oyer P, Portner P et al (1988) Isolated left ventricular assist as bridge to cardiac transplantation. J Thorac Cardiovasc Surg 96:62–71
27. Whalen R, Molokhia F, Jeffery D et al (1972) Current studies with simulated nuclear-powered left ventricular assist devices. Trans Am Soc Artif Intern Organs 18:146–151
28. Wolner E, Deutsch M, Losert U et al (1978) Clinical application of the ellipsoid left heart assist device. Artif Organs 2:268–272
29. Dasse K, Chipman S, Sherman C et al (1987) Clinical experience with textured blood contacting surfaces in ventricular assist devices. Trans Am Soc Artif Intern Organs 10: 418–425
30. Rose E, Gelijns A, Moskowitz A et al (2001) Long term use of a left ventricular assist device for end-stage heart failure. N Engl J Med 345:1435–1443
31. Saxton G, Andrew C (1960) An ideal pump with hydrodynamic characteristics analogous to the mammalian heart. Trans Am Soc Artif Intern Organs 6:288–289
32. Rafferty E, Kletschka H, Wynyard (1968) Artificial heart I. Application of nonpulsatile force-vortex principle. Minn Med 51:11–16
33. Wampler R, Moise J, Frazier O et al (1988) In vivo evaluation of a peripheral vascular access axial flow blood pump. Trans Am Soc Artif Intern Organs 34:450–454
34. Potapov E, Loebe M, Nasseri B et al (2000) Pulsatile flow in patients with a novel nonpulsatile implantable ventricular assist device. Circulation 102(3):183–187
35. Westaby S, Katsumata Y, Evans R et al (1997) The Jarvik 2000 Oxford system: increasing the scope of mechanical circulatory support. J Thorac Cardiovasc Surg 114:467–474
36. Griffith B, Kormos R, Borovetz H et al (2001) HeartMate II left ventricular assist system: from concept to first clinical use. Ann Thorac Surg 71:S116–S120
37. Slaughter M, Rogers J, Milano C et al (2009) Advanced heart failure treated with continuous flow assist device. N Engl J Med 361:2241–2251
38. Hetzer R, Weng Y, Potapov E et al (2004) First experiences with a novel magnetically suspended axial flow left ventricular assist device. Eur J Cardiothorac Surg 25:964–970
39. LaRose J, Tanez D, Ashenuga M et al (2010) Design concepts and principle of the HeartWare ventricular assist system. ASAIO J 56:285–289
40. Frazier O, Tuzun E, Cohn W et al (2006) Total heart replacement using dual intracorporeal continuous-flow pump in a chronic bovine model: a feasibility study. ASAIO J 52:145–149

# The History of Research on Adult and Paediatric Heart Transplantation

# 31

Johann U. Brink and Yves d'Udekem

*A Bag of Tools*
*Isn't it strange that princes and kings,*
*And clowns that caper in sawdust rings,*
*And common people like you and me,*
*Are builders for eternity?*
*Each is given a bag of tools,*
*A shapeless mass, A book of rules;*
*And each must make—Ere life is flown—*
*A stumbling block or a steppingstone.*

R.L. Sharpe

(A cherished poem echoed at the funeral of Christiaan Barnard when read by his son).

**Abstract**

Heart transplantation has been an unachievable goal since the dawn of humanity. Only by the courage of a few pioneers could this dream become reality. After the pioneering work of Demikhov, the team of Stanford and New York built up the animal experimentation that would enable the first steps in human transplantation. The name Christiaan Barnard will always be remembered for being the first to perform human transplantation: "...as he stared upon

J. U. Brink
Department of Cardiac Surgery, Royal Children's Hospital, Parkville, Australia
e-mail: Jbrink212@gmail.com

Y. d'Udekem (✉)
Department of Pediatrics, Royal Children's Hospital, Murdoch Children's Research Institute, University of Melbourne, Parkville, Australia
e-mail: yves.dudekem@rch.org.au

M. Picichè (ed.), *Dawn and Evolution of Cardiac Procedures*,
DOI: 10.1007/978-88-470-2400-7_31, © Springer-Verlag Italia 2013

a heartless human chest, at that moment, he was struck by reality for the first time of what he was about to perform..." This breakthrough was quickly followed by rapid enthusiasm for this still experimental surgery in the United States. The poor results of this surgery attracted a lot of criticism. It was then considered that heart transplantation had become a "status symbol to the surgical team" rather than a useful adjunct in the fight against heart failure. It was only after further medical advances in the field of immunity that heart transplantation expanded to become what it is today.

The heart is romanticised to be the seat of the soul and the core of emotions. Until the dying moments of the 19th century and for most of history, the heart was considered to be untouchable, an organ too delicate to engage. Over the years, the mysteries of this enchanted organ were unravelled. This research laid the foundation for the impossible: heart transplantation, one of the greatest achievements of the 20th century.

## 31.1 Pioneering Research that Led to First Human Heart Transplantation

Russian pioneer, Vladimir P. Demikhov, one of the most underrated but greatest experimental surgeons of the 20th century, made legendary contributions to transplant medicine. In 1937, he designed the first mechanical cardiac assist device, maintaining circulation of an excised canine heart for 5 h [1]. Working as an assistant in the department of physiology at the M. V. Lomonosov State University in Moscow, he transplanted a heart into the inguinal region of a dog. After unsuccessful attempts, he concluded, "because of its anatomical and physiological features, the heart can only function actively when it is transplanted into the thorax" [2, 3]. After returning from World War II, Demikhov continued his experiments on dogs and in 1946, he performed the world's first successful intrathoracic heterotopic heart transplantation without cardiopulmonary bypass or hypothermia [4]. On 30 June 1946, Demikhov authenticated the technical feasibility of the first successful heterotopic heart–lung transplantation in a dog who survived for almost 10 h [5]. He made the first recorded attempt at orthotopic heart transplantation in 1951. In 1954, he performed the most controversial experimental operation of the 20th century by transplanting a canine head. Making headlines in the Cape Argus newspaper in South Africa, this invigorated Christiaan Barnard, who duplicated the procedure that same afternoon [6].

Based on the principles of cross-circulation coined by Lillehei, Marcus and colleagues introduced their "interim parabiotic perfusion" experimenting with heterotopic heart transplantation in dogs in the early 1950s. The objective of this rather perplexing technique was to sustain perfusion of the donor heart during the transfer by utilising the cardiopulmonary system of a third dog. By 1953, they had applied various modifications of their original technique, performing heterotopic heart and heart–lung transplantations and achieved survival of up to 48 h [7].

In 1953, Wilford Neptune, performed the first complete orthotopic heart–lung transplantation in a dog under deep hypothermic circulatory arrest, relying on speedy surgery [8]. At the time, he cooled the animal down in an ordinary beverage cooler to a rectal temperature of 21–24 °C. The initial results were poor, but with the third attempt the dog survived for 6 h before dying of shock.

Experimental heart transplantation rapidly evolved during the 1960s. Revolutionary contributions were made by pioneers Norman Shumway and Richard Lower at Stanford University Medical Center. In 1959, they published their results on "selective hypothermia of the heart in anoxic cardiac arrest," providing a satisfactory method of myocardial protection with cold Saline at 0–5 °C. Safe reversible cardiac arrest was maintained for up to 1 h [9]. In the same year their results for orthotopic transplantation in dogs became promising. The recipient dog's circulation was maintained with cardiopulmonary bypass under moderate hypothermic conditions (30 °C) while the donor heart was protected by submersion in cold saline (4 °C). Their surgical technique was likely based on the original work of British surgeons, Cass and Brock, leaving both recipient atria intact, thus, minimising ischaemic time. This biatrial cuff method subsequently became known as "Shumway's technique" and is still used in modern times. In 1960, they performed 8 consecutive homotransplantations with 5 animals surviving for 6–21 days. These dogs showed good initial exercise tolerance and normal ECG findings. However, after rapid deterioration, death occurred and histological findings demonstrated myocardial round-cell infiltration, interstitial haemorrhage, oedema and areas of necrosis and Shumway concluded, "observation on these animals suggests that, if the immunologic mechanisms of the host were prevented from destroying the graft, in all likelihood it would continue to function adequately for the normal life span of the animal" [10, 11].

On 23 January 1964, Mississippi surgeon, Dr James Hardy, performed the world's first xenotransplantation. A 68-year-old man was admitted with a gangrenous leg in a shocked state and required resuscitation and a subsequent below-knee amputation. His condition became terminal: "...and it was obvious that if heart transplantation was to be performed it must be done at once." Owing to the lack of human donor availability and the imminent nature of the patient's poor condition, Dr Hardy transplanted the heart of an approximately 45-kg male chimpanzee into the chest of his dying patient [12]. He applied the surgical technique of Lower and Shumway, but unfortunately "the donor heart eventually appeared unable to handle the venous return" and his patient died about 1 h after circulatory support was discontinued. Dr Hardy later admitted that the deranged metabolic state of the recipient was doubtless the major factor of failure of the xenograft and that the biopsy slides revealed absence of hyperacute rejection. This courageous stride might seem like a failure, but was in fact proof that heart transplantation had undoubtedly become technically possible and that recipient and donor selection played a major role.

"From the beginning, we believed that transplantation would prove to be the treatment of choice for infants and children with otherwise lethal cardiac lesions," was the rationale of surgeon Adrian Kantrowitz, at Maimonides Medical Center, Brooklyn, New York. He advocated that a natural heart would have growth potential in a child and that rejection might be less aggressive because of the immaturity of their immune system. Even though debateable, anencephalic infants were identified, morally and ethically, as the most appropriate potential donors. During 1962–1967, heart transplantation was performed in 411 puppies with excellent results. Some puppies survived for up to 213 days without any evidence of rejection. The methodology consisted of a modified Shumway technique and deep hypothermic circulatory arrest. By the beginning of 1966, Kantrowitz had published and presented a vast amount of successful experimental data and had implemented a hospital research committee-approved protocol with his sights on their first human-to-human heart transplantation. His first potential recipient was a cyanotic infant born on 11 May 1966 with pulmonary atresia, a patent ductus arteriosus, an atrial and ventricular septal defect and corrected transposition of the great arteries. On 27 June 1966, an anencephalic infant was delivered in Oregon and was flown to Maimonides the following day as the donor. Three days later his heart stopped beating and the recipient was prepared for the first ever human to human heart transplant in history, but the procedure was abandoned owing to unsuccessful resuscitation of the donor heart [13].

By 1967, the world's leading transplant authority Norman Shumway stated, "we think the way is clear, for a trial of human heart transplantation." This statement was supported by Richard Lower, "we are now quite convinced that cardiac transplant is a perfectly feasible procedure from the technical as well as the physiological standpoint" [14].

## 31.2 The First Transplantations

In 1956, a South African surgeon continued his post-graduate training in cardiac surgery at the University of Minnesota, Minneapolis in the United States under the guidance of Dr. Walton Lillehei. Upon his return to South Africa in 1958, he was appointed cardiac surgeon at the Groote Schuur Hospital as well as Director of Surgical Research at the University of Cape Town. On 3 December 1967, Christiaan Barnard (Fig. 31.1) captivated humanity by performing the first human-to-human heart transplant. Louis Washkansky, a 53-year-old male smoker, was bedridden in Groote Schuur hospital in Cape Town, suffering from diabetes, peripheral vascular disease, severe coronary artery insufficiency and terminal cardiac failure. On 2 December 1967, a young white woman was diagnosed by a neurosurgeon and state pathologist with unrecoverable lethal brain injury after she was hit by a car while crossing the street on the way to the bakery. She was matched as a suitable donor after leukocyte and red cell antigen compatibility screening and both the donor and recipient were taken to adjoining theatres. Published in the *South African*

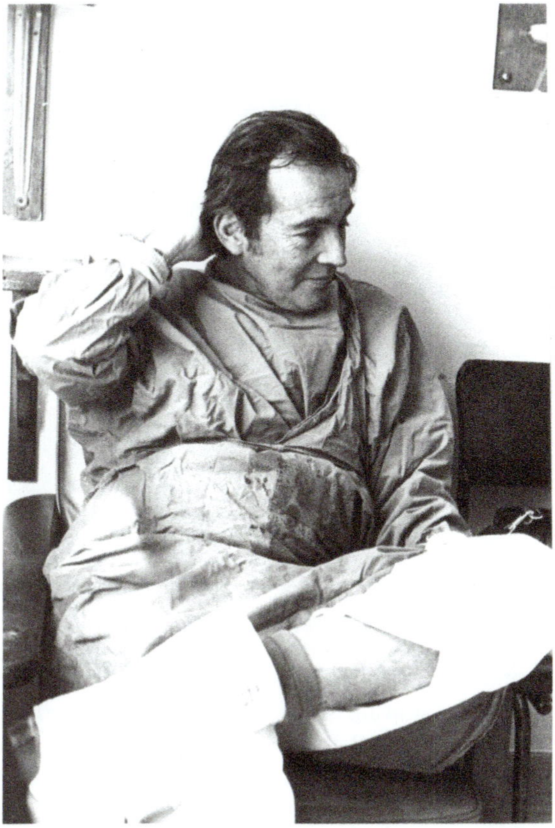

**Fig. 31.1** Prof. Christiaan Barnard relaxing after surgery. Courtesy of the Heart of Cape Town Museum, South Africa

*Medical Journal*, "A human cardiac transplant: an interim report of a successful operation performed at Groote Schuur Hospital, Cape Town", describes the operation [15]. For the first time in Barnard's life, as he stared upon a heartless human chest, at that moment, he was struck by the reality of what he was about to perform (interview on film at the Heart of Cape Town museum). Washkansky made excellent progress for about a fortnight, but his condition deteriorated with pneumonic infiltrates appearing on chest X-ray. The surgical team elected to treat him for lung oedema caused by rejection-related cardiac failure and increased his immunosuppressive therapy. He died on the 18th postoperative day of bilateral pneumonia confirmed at post-mortem [16]. This failure elicited opposing reactions of both the general public and the medical profession, some questioning the ethics and prematurity of organ transplantation as a form of palliation, while others saw this first human transplantation as an enormous achievement. On 2 January 1968, Barnard performed his second orthotopic transplant in 59-year-old Philip Blaiberg, who became the first heart transplant patient to be discharged from hospital and to resume a normal life (Fig. 31.2). He died 19 months later of unanticipated allograft vasculopathy [17], today a well-recognised complication. The success of Blaiberg

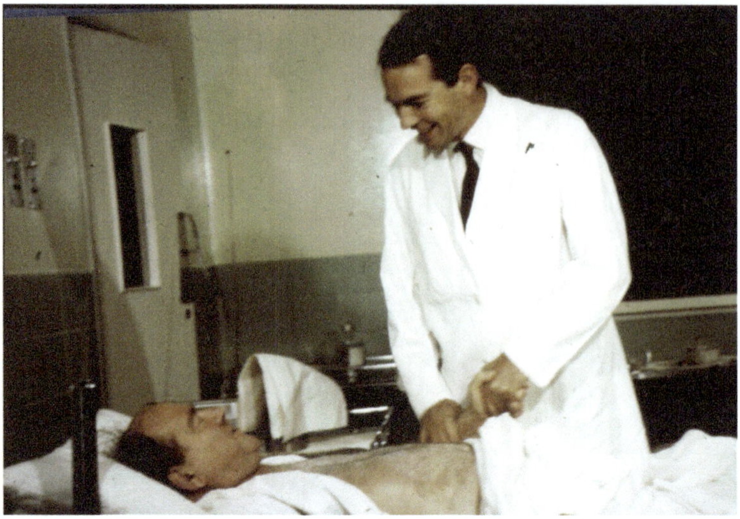

**Fig. 31.2** Prof. Christiaan Barnard greeting Dr Blaiberg, the first heart transplant recipient to be discharged home. Courtesy of the Heart of Cape Town Museum, South Africa

became a sigh of hope that shielded heart transplantation from extinction. Barnard continued to lay the foundation for cardiac transplantation at the Groote Schuur Hospital and of the first 10 transplantations performed, 4 patients lived for more than 1 year and 2 for 13 and 23 years respectively. He made a revolutionary contribution to the development of heterotopic heart transplantation, the concepts of brain death, organ donation and other ethical controversies, organ preservation and hemodynamic and metabolic effects of brain death, and early attempts at xenotransplantation [18].

On the morning of 3 December 1967, the daughter of Adrian Kantrowitz stunned him with the radio broadcast reporting Christiaan Barnard's operation and 3 days later Kantrowitz performed in his Brooklyn hospital in New York, America's first human heart transplant on a 3-week-old infant with Ebstein's anomaly. The infant survived for 6½ h. This procedure was considered to be a failure and Helen Taussig accused Kantrowitz of "clearly trying to be first in the country," and "...playing for the gallery" [13]. One month later, Shumway performed his first human transplant at Stanford [19] and by May 1968, Cooley and his team had performed 10 human heart transplantations [20]. Because of the high initial mortality, heart transplant centres became vulnerable targets and were widely criticised for performing the procedure as a "status symbol to the surgical team." "I don't see why we don't limit transplantation to non fatal organs, or to organs for which we have alternative means of sustaining life in the event of failure, until further improvement in our knowledge," stated Charles Hufnagel [21]. During 1968–1970, the worldwide 2-year survival for cardiac transplantation was only 11 % and had a profoundly negative impact on cardiac transplantation during the 1970s. Only a few major transplant centers continued active research and pushing frontiers [18]. Heart transplantation had to wait for further medical advances to be made in order to reach its full expansion.

## 31.3 Progress in Heart Transplantation

### 31.3.1 ABO and HLA Compatibility

Heart transplantation, technically, had become reality but, now, scientists were faced with the ultimate clinical barrier: the immune system. In 1901, Karl Landsteiner, demonstrated the presence of three different types of iso-agglutinins responsible for clumping of donor red blood cells. In 1909, he classified human blood into groups A, B, AB, and O, and demonstrated the catastrophic reactions of transfusion incompatibility [22]. ABO blood group compatibility became a prerequisite not only for transfusion, but also for transplantation and subsequently restricted donor–recipient matching and extended waiting time on the transplantation list. Because donors were so rare in the pediatric population and it was suspected that younger children may display better tolerance to transplanted organs, the team in Toronto investigated the possibility of ABO-incompatible heart transplantation. In 2001, in a cornerstone publication, West and colleagues demonstrated successful ABO-incompatible heart transplantation in infants. They showed that, before the age of 1 year, serum titers as well as the production of anti-A and anti-B antibodies were low enough to allow ABO-incompatible transplantation [23]. Their analysis also concluded that ABO incompatibility was a risk factor for wait-list death and paved the way for widening the indication for ABO-incompatible transplantation. Today, the United Network for Organ Sharing (policy 3.7.8) recommends a recipient upper age limit of 2 years and pre-transplant isohemagglutinin levels < 1:4.

In 1958, French immunologist and Nobel Prize laureate, Jean Dausset, unravelled the secrets of the immune system by discovering the first human leukocyte antigen, MAC, today known as human major histocompatibility complex HLA-A2 [24, 25], which allowed tissue matching beyond blood types.

### 31.3.2 Cyclosporine and Modern Immunosuppressants

Worldwide interest in heart transplantation was revived in the early 1980s after another immunological milestone, the discovery of cyclosporine A. In 1976, Jean Borel first published on the immunosuppressive effects of cyclosporine A after in vitro and animal experimentation and soon thereafter, the first human clinical trials [26]. This fungal metabolite was isolated from soil fungus from Norway and was the first immunosuppressive agent that targeted lymphocytes selectively with a great degree of potency. Further advancements included the development of tacrolimus, sirolimus, mycophenolate mofetil, monoclonal antibodies, and polyclonal antilymphocyte preparations, which caused a dramatic decrease in graft rejection, bringing heart transplantation to its current level of success.

### 31.3.3 Surgical Technique

Little advancement has been made over the last 40 years since Shumway described the biatrial technique, which is still considered today by some to be the gold standard for orthotopic transplantation because of its simplicity. In 1991, Sievers described the bicaval technique where the donor's left atrium is anastomosed to a recipient cuff containing the four pulmonary veins [27]. The donor's right atrium and superior vena cavae were connected to the inferior and superior vena cavae. The bicaval technique is more time consuming and technically demanding and requires longer bypass time. However, today short-term outcomes support its superiority owing to decreased disruption of atrial geometry, less mitral and tricuspid valve insufficiency, and less sinus node dysfunction with a reduced pacemaker requirement [28, 29].

## 31.4 Heart Transplantation Today

The reality of heart transplantation, as we know it today, was built upon the resilience, the successes and the failures of numerous pioneers. Today, the need for cardiac transplantation by far exceeds the current number performed. Approximately 3,500 heart transplantations are performed annually worldwide [30]. Donor availability is the current "Achilles heel" of cardiac transplantation. The challenges in transplant medicine are superior graft endurance and graft–host immune tolerance. In 1970, cardiac transplantation was more vulnerable than ever before and Christiaan Barnard said:

> To curb transplantation at this stage would be to strangle one of the most promising and exciting fronts of medical endeavour of this century. From the experience gained in the problems of rejection, methods of immunological control will be improved and vital organ replacement will become a routine life-saving procedure. To deny medicine its full thrust in this direction would be irresponsibly short sighted. Indeed, it is difficult not to conclude that withdrawal from this new frontier would be professionally unethical. We have only to continue transplantation on a most active scale [31].

His words seem to resonate through history, and remain valid today.

## References

1. Shumacker HB Jr (1994) A surgeon to remember: notes about Vladimir Demikhov. Ann Thorac Surg 58(4):1196–1198
2. Demikhov VP (1962) Experimental transplantation of vital organs (trans: Basil Haigh). Consultant's Bureau Enterprises, Inc. New York
3. Demikhov VP (1960) Transplantation of vital organs in experiments (in Russian). Medgiz, Moscow
4. Konstantinov IE (1998) A mystery of Vladimir P. Demikhov: the 50th anniversary of the first intrathoracic transplantation. Ann Thorac Surg 65(4):1171–1177
5. Cooper DK (1969) Transplantation of the heart and both lungs. I. Historical review. Thorax 24(4):383–390

6. Westaby S, Bosher C (1997) Landmarks in cardiac surgery. Isis Medical Media Ltd., Oxford
7. Marcus E, Wong SNT, Luisada AA (1953) Technique of interim parabiotic perfusion; 2. Transplantation of the heart in dogs. Arch Surg 66:179
8. Neptune WB, Cookson BA, Bailey CP (1953) Complete homologous heart transplantation. Arch Surg (Chicago) 66:174
9. Shumway NE, Lower RR, Stofer RC (1959) Selective hypothermia of the heart in anoxic cardiac arrest. Surg Gynecol Obstet 109:750–754
10. Lower RR, Shumway NE (1960) Studies on the orthotopic homotransplantation of the canine heart. Surg Forum 11:18–19
11. Lower RR, Stofer RC, Shumway NE (1961) Homovital transplantation of the heart. J Thorac Cardiovasc Surg 41:196–204
12. Hardy JD, Chavez CM, Kurrus FD (1964) Heart transplantation in man. J Am Med Assoc 188:1132–1140
13. Kantrowitz A (1998) America's first human heart transplantation. The concept, the planning, and the furor. ASAIO J 44(4):244–252
14. Cuddihy J (1968) Transplants: modern wonder surgery. Grolier encyclopedia science supplement. CT Grolier, Danbury
15. Barnard CN (1967) The operation. A human cardiac transplant: an interim report of a successful operation performed at Groote Schuur Hospital, Cape Town. S Afr Med J 41(48):1271–1274
16. Barnard CN (1968) What have we learned about heart transplants. J Thorac Cardiovasc Surg 56:457–468
17. Thompson JG (1969) Atheroma in a transplanted heart. Lancet II:1088–1092
18. Brink JG, Hassoulas J (2009) The first human heart transplant and further advances in cardiac transplantation at Groote Schuur Hospital and the University of Cape Town. Cardiovasc J Afr 20(1):30–35, 38
19. Stinson EB, Dong E Jr, Schroeder JS, Harrison DC, Shumway NE (1968) Initial clinical experience with heart transplantation. Am J Cardiol 22:791–803
20. Cooley DA, Hallman GL, Bloodwell RD, Nora JJ, Leachman RD (1968) Human heart transplantation. Experience with twelve cases. Am J Cardiol 22:804–810
21. [no authors listed] (1968) Specialists voice mixed reactions to heart transplantations and its future. J Am Med Assoc 203:39–41
22. Landsteiner K (1961) On agglutination of normal human blood. Transfusion 1:5–8
23. West LJ, Pollock-BarZiv SM, Dipchand AI et al (2001) ABO-incompatible heart transplantation in infants. N Engl J Med 344:793–800
24. Dausset J, Collin M (1958) Research technique for immunologic thrombo-agglutinins; influence of previous heating of platelet suspensions. Rev Fr Etud Clin Biol 3:60–61
25. Dausset J (1984) The birth of MAC. Vox Sang 46:235–237
26. Borel JF (1976) Comparative study of in vitro and in vivo drug effects on cell-mediated cytotoxicity. Immunology 31:631–641
27. Sievers HH, Weyand M, Kraatz EG, Bernhard A (1991) An alternative technique for orthotopic cardiac transplantation, with preservation of the normal anatomy of the right atrium. Thorac Cardiovasc Surg 39(2):70–72
28. Jacob S, Frank S (2009) Is bicaval orthotopic heart transplantation superior to the biatrial technique? Interact Cardiovasc Thorac Surg 9:333–342
29. Davies RR, Russo MJ, Morgan JA, Sorabella RA, Naka Y, Chen JM (2010) Standard versus bicaval techniques for orthotopic heart transplantation: an analysis of the united network for organ sharing database. J Thorac Cardiovasc Surg 140:700–708
30. Stehlik J, Edwards LB, Kucheryavaya AY, Aurora P, Christie JD, Kirk R et al (2010) The registry of the International Society for Heart and Lung Transplantation: twenty-seventh official adult heart transplant report—2010. J Heart Lung Transplant 29(10):1089–1103
31. Barnard CN (1970) Experience with human heart transplantation in "sterilization and preservation of biological tissues by ionizing radiation". International Atomic Agency, Vienna. IAEA-PL-333/10:79–94

# The History of Pediatric Cardiac Surgery After the Advent of Cardiopulmonary Bypass

32

Jean E. Rubay

*The rise of cardiac surgery.*

Dr Owen Wangensteen


**Abstract**

The history of cardiac surgery using cardiopulmonary bypass (CPB) has been closely related to pediatrics since the first achievements were made in this particular field. From this point, the search was orientated towards the best health conditions for children by correction of cardiac defects, as early as possible, and preferably with bi-ventricular repairs under the safest conditions, both at the myocardial and the cerebral level. The congenital field is the largest in cardiac surgery. It was therefore decided to focus on the major steps of anatomical repairs. The next steps in the history of pediatric cardiac surgery will probably open new doors in CPB and miniaturization of assist devices. Myocardial cell developments are fascinating. Future pediatric cardiothoracic teams will face challenging issues like worldwide access to congenital cardiac surgery and an increasing population living with congenital heart disease in adulthood. This is a future chapter for a future edition.


The history of cardiac surgery using cardiopulmonary bypass (CPB) is closely related to pediatrics since the first achievements were made in this particular field.


J. E. Rubay (✉)
Department of Cardiovascular and Thoracic Surgery,
Saint Luc Ucl, Brussels, Belgium
e-mail: jean.rubay@uclouvain.be



M. Picichè (ed.), *Dawn and Evolution of Cardiac Procedures*,
DOI: 10.1007/978-88-470-2400-7_32, © Springer-Verlag Italia 2013

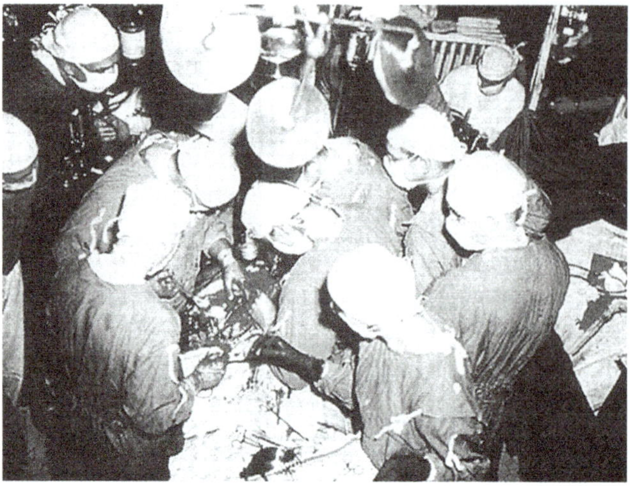

**Fig. 32.1** Dr Lillehei's first cross-circulation performed on 26 March 1954, for repair of a ventricular septal defect. Dr Lillehei is on the patient's right, wearing a headlight. Dr Varco, first assistant. Behind Dr Varco, Dr Gott. On Dr Gott's right: Dr Shumway. On the right of the operative field: the father, who served as biological oxygenator. Reproduced with permission from Elsevier

## 32.1 Dawn

Amazingly, the dawn of open-heart surgery occurred in the early 1950s in the field of pediatrics; soon after successful closure of an atrial septal defect using total-body hypothermia and inflow occlusion at the University of Minnesota on 2 September 1952, by John Lewis, Dr Gibbon [1] performed a monumental achievement on 15 May1953 by closing the same type of defect in Philadelphia, using a screen oxygenator that he had developed.

A general disappointment about open-heart surgery because of the death of the next 4 patients led to the technique almost being abandoned until Dr Lillehei successfully closed a ventricular septal defect on 26 March 1954, again at the University of Minnesota, using cross-circulation (Fig. 32.1).

During the next year, Dr Lillehei operated on 32 children using this type of support, including repairs of ventricular septal defects (VSD), tetralogy of Fallot, and atrioventricular septal defects (AVSD), on beating hearts, without cardiotomy sucker, direct closure of the VSD for most of them, and a remarkably short duration of by-pass [2].

In full agreement with Dr Gott [3], we may consider Walton Lillehei to be as the father of open-heart surgery, not only for his pioneering work in correcting congenital malformations, but also for the tremendous results of his research laboratory, including the Lillehei–DeWall bubble-oxygenator, the first clinical implantation of a pacemaker [4], the first repair of a mitral valve, and the development of many different prosthetic valves.

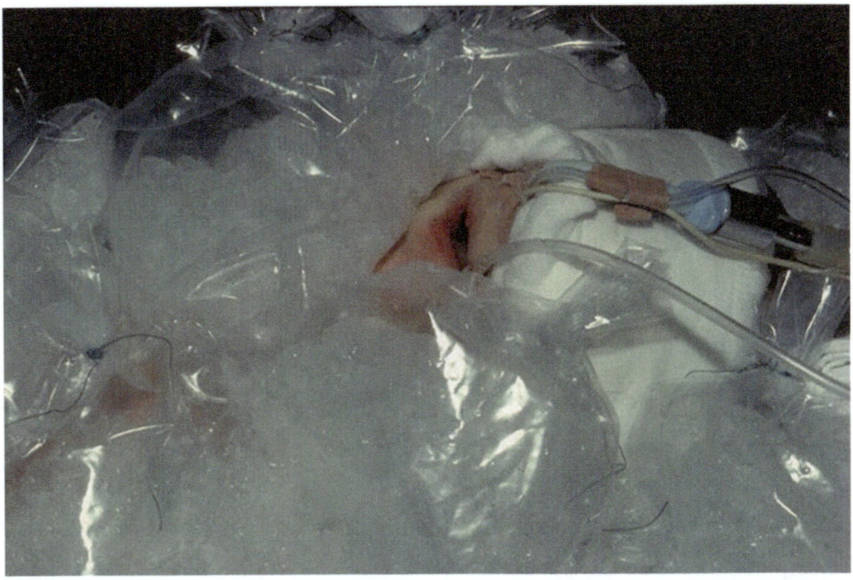

**Fig. 32.2** Two-month-old baby girl with transposition of the great arteries (TGA). Surface cooling. 1977, University Hospital of Louvain, UCL, Belgium

Many of the surgical matters that will be addressed in this review bear Lillehei's stamp, giving the strange feeling that almost nothing new was invented that has not already been described by him or his school.

Parallel to these pioneering works, new insights into myocardial protection and body and brain metabolism were addressed.

## 32.2 From Hypothermia and Deep Hypothermic Circulatory Arrest to Normothermia: from March to the Sun

In 1950, Bigelow [5] introduced the idea that whole body hypothermia might be useful in cardiac surgery. In 1958, Sealy et al. [6] reported successful clinical cases in which hypothermia was used in combination with CPB (Fig. 32.2).

After experimental studies reported by Drew et al. [7] on total circulatory arrest, Dubost et al. [8] in Paris reported the use of profound hypothermia and total circulatory arrest for cardiac surgery.

A combination of surface cooling, which allows a more uniform body temperature and total circulatory arrest up to 60 min at 17° allowed Dillard et al. [9] to repair a total anomalous pulmonary venous connection in 1967 (Fig. 32.3).

Surprisingly, hypothermic CPB, isolated or associated with deep hypothermic circulatory arrest (DHCA) is still widely used in pediatric cardiac surgery [10], despite the numerous demonstrated side effects [11].

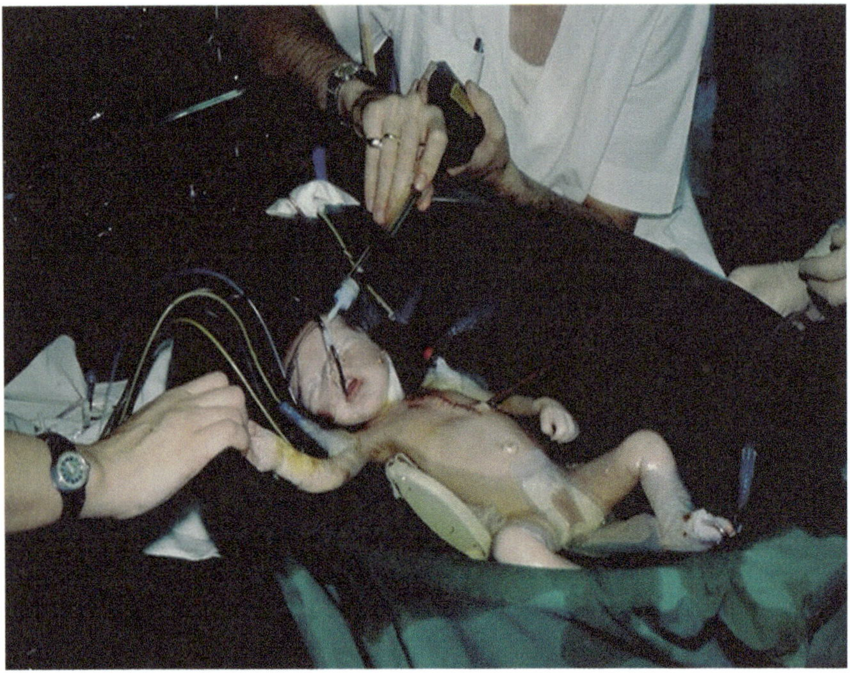

Fig. 32.3 Same patient, after a Senning operation, rewarmed in a basin of warm water

Refinements in technical environment and surgical skills have progressively banished the fear of major bypass accidents, which in turn led to the re-introduction of normothermic CPB.

Several theoretical advantages favor the use of normothermic bypass, including shorter duration of CPB, lower neurological risk, less coagulation disorders, reduced need for hemodilution and simplification of CPB management, regardless of the alpha-stat or pH-stat regulation; other side effects of hypothermia on glucose regulation, on the endocrine system and on the immune system are avoided. The hemoglobin dissociation curve is not further affected by hypothermia and allows better oxygen delivery.

Normothermic CPB was introduced into pediatric cardiac surgery in 1995 by Durandy and Lecompte in Paris [12] and has since been confirmed by large studies on complex repairs [13, 14].

## 32.3 Myocardial Protection: "Some Like it Hot"

In the early years of pediatric cardiac surgery, little mention was made of the possible relationship between fatal or nonfatal low cardiac output postoperatively and the damaging effects of the cardiac operation itself. Myocardial necrosis as a complication of surgery or as a cause of low cardiac output, or temporary depression of myocardial function (stunning) as a result of the operation itself were neglected but deleterious.

In 1974, it was shown that, even after the short and simple repair of an atrial septal defect, all patients had enzymatic evidence of myocardial necrosis [15].

After Melrose [16] advocated elective normothermic cardiac arrest with reduced oxygen consumption, the first deliberate attempts to protect the myocardium were published by Shumway [17] in 1959 and Hufnagel in 1961 [18].

In the mid-1970s, in Europe, Hearse and Braimbridge [19] were exploring the induction of reversible cardiac arrest and soon after Buckberg [20] identified blood as the optimal vehicle for cardioplegic carriage.

Cardioplegic solutions that provide a relaxed, bloodless operating field soon proved attractive to the pediatric cardiac surgeon by facilitating exposure and improving intracardiac repair, especially when this method was demonstrated to be as effective as intermittent cross-clamping [21]. The advantages of warm blood cardioplegia, demonstrated in adults in 1989 [22], was confirmed in congenital heart disease by Durandy from 2001 [13] with the liberal use of intermittent warm blood cardioplegia (IWBC), in combination with normothermia. Our group [23] has demonstrated its effectiveness and safety on various types of cardiac repairs with a randomized trial comparing two randomized cohorts of pediatric patients, with equivalent procedures, the first assigned to moderate hypothermia and cold crystalloid cardioplegia compared with the second group who were operated on under normothermic conditions and IWBC.

Myocardial protection was assessed by various parameters, including myocardial biopsies in order to measure intracellular adenosine triphosphate (ATP). Results demonstrated a clear advantage of the "warm" protocol, with physiological ATP steady state, reflecting the absence of cellular ischemic insult.

## 32.4 The Brain: Terra Incognita

It is generally agreed that the brain has the shortest "safe" circulatory arrest time of any organ or part of the body, both at normal and low temperatures.

Data from near-infrared spectroscopy (INVOS®) and transcranial Doppler monitoring indicate that many maneuvers, unrelated to duration or temperature of CPB, can generate microemboli and cerebral malperfusion, such as cannulae insertion, starting and stopping CPB, clamping, de-airing, and matching flow rates to body temperature. Cerebral physiology and understanding in cardiac surgery has evolved parallel to myocardial protection: first ignored, it was a concern for decades and was anticipated by cooling and DHCA. In the current era common sense makes it obvious that the brain functions better with normal flow and physiological temperature. For decades abundant literature has focused on a haunting question: how far, how deep, and how long do we have to cool to allow the brain to support circulatory arrest? [10]. The answer might be as simple as: do not cool and do not stop the circulation! The ghost of equipment failure leaving little margin of safety is then waived in order to maintain some form of mild hypothermia. We and a few others [13, 14, 23] have followed the history and moved from DHCA in the 1970s, to mild hypothermia in the 1990s and, since the beginning of this millennium, to full normothermic flow, even in neonates and/or patients with complex repairs, demonstrating similar quality of cardiac repair and late neurodevelopmental outcomes.

## 32.5 Transposition of the Great Arteries: the Holy Grail

It is little known that the first attempts of total correction of transposition of the great arteries (TGA) were directed at the arterial level. In 1954, Mustard in Toronto [24] performed an arterial switch operation (ASO) in 7 patients with the transfer of the left coronary artery. The same year, Bailey [25] attempted to switch the great arteries, but without coronary transfer. Soon after, Senning, in Stockholm, tried to correct a TGA/VSD at arterial level [26] by closing the VSD and transferring the pulmonary artery onto the right ventricle.

Idriss at the Children's Hospital in Chicago [27] developed a technique of switching the great arteries including coronary transfer, with an isolated aortic segment containing the ostia. He carried out the procedure in the laboratory followed by 2 patients, a 7-year-old boy on 29 June 1960, who died of left ventricular failure and a 3 month-old girl who died from bleeding.

Failures due to misunderstanding of the physiological pre-requisite left morphological and pulmonary conditions to succeed in anatomical correction, led to the success of the correction at the atrial level, described by Albert [28] in a meeting of the American College of Surgeons in 1954.

The first successful atrial switch was accomplished by Senning in 1957 [26] followed by Mustard [29], who introduced a modification of the original technique by using a pericardial baffle.

Postoperative arrhythmias, systemic ventricular dysfunction, and venous obstructions either at the systemic or the pulmonary level have contributed to the success of the ASO: in 1975, Jatene et al. [30] achieved a major breakthrough by successfully performing the ASO, and was followed by Sir Yacoub [31] and Sir Ross [32].

A major improvement of the technique was proposed by Lecompte [33], who demonstrated that direct reconstruction of the new pulmonary artery was possible when the pulmonary artery bifurcation was transferred to the front of the ascending aorta. The so-called "French Maneuver" eliminated the use of prosthetic conduits and made it very attractive to use as primary repair, even in neonates.

Moreover, the same author [34] proposed a new simplified classification of the complex TGA (transposition, ventricular septal defect, and left outflow tract obstruction) based on the relative position of the great vessels to the ventricular septal defect and the semi-lunar valves.

The "*réparation à l'etage ventriculaire*" (REV) procedure, after resection of the existing infundibular septum, creates a short intraventricular tunnel from the left ventricle toward the aortic valve and, allows, in combination with the French

Maneuver, a complete repair with excellent mid- [35] and long-term results [36] without any prosthetic or homograft tube, being therefore less prone to sternal compression, in contrast to the classical Rastelli operation [37].

More recently, another approach of complex transposition was re-introduced. The Nikaidoh operation [38], described in 1984, was actually a revival of a technique introduced by the same French team in 1980 [39]. This technique is particularly useful in the presence of an inlet or restrictive VSD, or anomalous coronary anatomy interfering with a distal right ventricular outflow tract incision, at the cost of two valves exposed at risk: the aortic, which can be distorted by the translocation maneuver and the pulmonary homograft used for right ventricular outflow tract reconstruction.

## 32.6 Valves: From Steel Work to Art

Valve disease in the pediatric age group defies cardiac surgeons.

When necessary, replacement of the diseased valve in infants and children by prostheses requires consideration of several variables that are unique to this age group, like small annulus, growth, calcium metabolism, and anticoagulation in very active patients. None of the currently available prostheses exhibits the required features of an ideal substitute for valve replacement in children [40].

After liberal use of mechanical valves, despite their high rate of morbidity and mortality in the 1960s, numerous articles appeared in the next decade, which rather enthusiastically proclaimed the tissue valves to be the best choice for use in children [41]. It rapidly became obvious that these valves should not be used in children, owing to accelerated degeneration [42]. Initial encouraging results with fresh [43] and subsequently cryopreserved aortic homografts [44] led to the same disappointment and contributed to the renewed interest in the Ross procedure [45] with excellent hemodynamic results [46].

Despite improvements in prosthetic valve technology and implantation techniques, repairs are better alternatives and the basic principle is to preserve the native valvular tissue. Good immediate hemodynamics and persistent long-term results are mandatory when reconstructing a functional valve in children. Left [2] and right [47] atrio-ventricular valves have been soon amenable for repair. Mitral valve repair in children with congenital malformations was precisely outlined according to pathology by Carpentier in 1976 [48].

Aortic valve repair is more recent in the pediatric armamentarium. Introduced into adults in the early 1990s [49] for aortic incompetence and aneurysm, this technique is particularly suitable in the setting of Marfan syndrome, giving a clear advantage over aortic replacement in terms of valve-related complications [50].

Since the initial report by Senning [51] on the use of fascia lata to reconstruct the aortic valve, several surgical techniques have used the glutharaldehyde-treated [52] or untreated [53] autologous pericardium cusp extension technique with reasonable mid-term results.

Tricuspid valve reconstruction in Ebstein's anomaly using the initial technique described by Lillehei [47] benefited from new insights by Carpentier [54] before achieving excellent results in the modern era [55].

## 32.7 Transplantation

On 3rd of December 1967, word of the first successful human transplantation astonished the world [56]. Although the patient survived only 18 days, no operation in history had ever generated such publicity. Just 3 days after this first transplantation, New York surgeon, Adrian Kantrowitz, carried out a transplant in a 2-week-old neonate. But it was actually another of Lillelei's trainees who had perfected heart transplantation in Stanford, over years of research, namely, Shumway [57]. He was ready to move from the laboratory into the operating room, but was delayed in doing so by a major impediment: in the USA, the clinical definition of death was still based on a heart that no longer beats. This was not the case in South Africa for Christian Barnard. Shumway had to wait until 6 January 1968 and became the world's most experienced heart-transplant surgeon, with more than a thousand operations by the time of his retirement.

After the first event, cardiac transplantation was begun in many centers around the world, but few patients were more than short-term survivors and by the early 1970s, it had largely disappeared from clinical practice.

The experience of "Baby Fae" in Linda [58] astonished the scientific community and opened the door to cardiac replacement therapy for a wide variety of congenital and acquired cardiac conditions in pediatrics.

The introduction of immunosuppression in the early 1980s led to the revival of transplantation as an acceptable therapeutic modality.

## 32.8 What Else ?

The next steps in the history of pediatric cardiac surgery will probably open new doors in CPB and the miniaturization of assist devices. Developments in myocardial cells are fascinating. Future pediatric cardiothoracic teams will face challenging issues like worldwide access to congenital cardiac surgery and an increasing population living with congenital heart disease in adulthood. This is a future chapter for a future edition.

## References

1. Gibbon JH (1954) Application of a mechanical heart-lung apparatus to cardiac surgery. Minn Med 37:171–180
2. Lillehei CW, Cohen M, Warden HE, Varco RL (1955) The direct-vision intracardiac correction of congenital anomalies by controlled cross circulation: results in thirty-two

patients with ventricular septal defects, tetralogy of Fallot, and atrioventricularis communis defects. Surgery 38:11–29
3. Gott VL (2005) Lillehei, Lewis, and Wangensteen: the right mix for giant achievements in cardiac surgery. Ann Thorac Surg 79:S2210–S2213
4. Lillehei CW, Gott VL, Hodges PC Jr, Long DM, Bakken EE (1960) Transistor pacemaker for treatment of complete atrioventricular dissociation. J Am Med Assoc 30(172):2006–2010
5. Bigelow WG, Lindsay WK, Greenwood WF (1950) Hypothermia—its possible role in cardiac surgery: an investigation of factors governing survival in dogs at low body temperatures. Ann Surg 132:849–866
6. Sealy WC, Brown IW, Young WG (1958) A report on the use of both extracorporeal circulation and hypothermia for open heart surgery. Ann Surg 147:603–613
7. Drew CE, Keen G, Benazon DB (1959) Profound hypothermia. Lancet 1:745–750
8. Piwnica A, Weiss M, Lenfant C, Dubost C (1960) Circulatory arrest with deep hypothermia induced with a pump oxygenator system and a heat exchanger. J Cardiovasc Surg 1:74–80
9. Dillard DH, Mohri H, Hessel EA, Anderson HN, Nelson RJ, Crawford EW, Morgan BC, Winterscheid LC, Merendino KA (1967) Correction of total anomalous pulmonary venous drainage in infancy utilizing deep hypothermia with total circulatory arrest. Circulation 35(I):105–110
10. Hanley F (2005) Religion, politics....deep hypothermic circulatory arrest. J Thorac Cardiovasc Surg 130:1236–1241
11. Lichtenstein SV, Ashe KA, El Dalati H, Cusimano RJ, Panos A, Slutsky AS (1991) Warm heart surgery. J Thorac Cardiovasc Surg 101:269–274
12. Durandy Y, Hulin S, Lecompte Y (2002) Normothermic cardiopulmonary bypass in pediatric surgery. J Thorac Cardiovasc Surg 123:194
13. Durandy Y, Hulin S (2007) Intermittent warm blood cardioplegia in the surgical treatment of congenital heart disease: clinical experience with 1400 cases. J Thorac Cardiovasc Surg 133:241–246
14. Pouard P, Mauriat P, Ek F, Haydar A, Gioanni S, Laquay N, Vaccaroni L, Vouhé PR (2006) Normothermic cardiopulmonary bypass and myocardial cardioplegic protection for neonatal arterial switch operation. Eur J Cardiothorac Surg 30:695–699
15. Neutze JM, Drakely MJ, Barratt-Boyes BG, Hubbert K (1974) Serum enzymes after cardiac surgery using cardiopulmonary bypass. Am Heart J 88:425–442
16. Melrose DG, Dieger DB, Bentall HH, Baker JBE (1955) Elective cardiac arrest: preliminary communication. Lancet 2:21–22
17. Shumway NE, Lower RE, Stofer RC (1959) Selective hypothermia of the heart in anoxic cardiac arrest. Surg Gynecol Obstet 109:750–754
18. Hufnagel CA, Conrad PW, Schanno J, Pifarre R (1961) Profound cardiac hypothermia. Ann Surg 153:790–796
19. Hearse DJ, Stewart DA, Braimbridge MV (1976) Cellular protection during myocardial ischemia: the development and characterization of a procedure for the induction of reversible ischemic arrest. Circulation 54:193–202
20. Buckberg GD (1979) A proposed "solution" to the cardioplegic controversy. J Thorac Cardiovasc Surg 77:803–815
21. Bull C, Cooper J, Stark J (1984) Cardioplegic protection of the child's heart. J Thorac Cardiovasc Surg 88:287–293
22. Lichtenstein SV, El Dalati H, Panos A, Slutsky AS (1989) Long cross-clamp time with warm heart surgery. Lancet 1:1443
23. Poncelet AJ, Van Steenberghe M, Moniotte S, Detaille T, Beauloye C, Bertrand L, Nassogne MC, Rubay JE (2011) Cardiac and neurological assessment of normothermia/warm blood cardioplegia versus hypothermia/cold crystalloid cardioplegia in pediatric cardiac surgery: insights from a prospective randomized trial. Eur J Cardiothorac Surg 40(6):1384–1390
24. Mustard WT, Chute AL, Keith JD, Sirek A, Rowe R, Vlad PA (1954) Surgical approach to transposition of the great vessels with extracorporeal circuit. Surgery 36:31–51

25. Bailey CP, Cookson BA, Downing DF, Neptune WB (1954) Cardiac surgery under hypothermia. J Thorac Surg 27:73–91
26. Senning A (1959) Surgical correction of transposition of the great vessels. Surgery 45:966–980
27. Idriss FS, Goldstein IR, Grana L, French D, Potts WJ (1961) A new technique for complete correction of transposition of the great vessels. An experimental study with a preliminary clinical report. Circulation 24:5–11
28. Albert HM (1954) Surgical correction of transposition of the great vessels. Surg Forum 5:74–77
29. Mustard WT, Keith JD, Trusler GA, Fowler R, Kidd L (1964) The surgical management of transposition of the great vessels. J Thorac Cardiovasc Surg 48:953–958
30. Jatene AD, Fontes VF, Paulista PP, Souza LC, Neger F, Galantier M, Sousa JE (1976) Anatomic correction of transposition of the great vessels. J Thorac Cardiovasc Surg 72:364–370
31. Yacoub MH, Radley-Smith R, Hilton CJ (1976) Anatomical correction of complete transposition of the great arteries and ventricular septal defect in infancy. Br Med J 1:1112–1114
32. Ross D, Rickards A, Somerville J (1976) Transposition of the great arteries: logical anatomical arterial correction. Br Med J 1:1109–1111
33. Lecompte Y, Zannini L, Hazan E, Jarreau MM, Tran Viet Tu, Neveux JY (1981) Anatomic correction of transposition of the great arteries. New technique without use of a prosthetic conduit. J Thorac Cardiovasc Surg 82:629–631
34. Sakata R, Lecompte Y, Batisse A, Borromée L, Durandy Y (1986) Anatomic repair of ventriculoarterial connection associated with ventricular septal defect. Criteria of surgical decision. J Thorac Cardiovasc Surg 95:90–95
35. Rubay JE, Lecompte Y, Batisse A, Durandy Y, Dibie A, Lemoine G, Vouhé P (1988) Anatomic repair of anomalies of ventriculo-arterial connection (REV). Results of a new technique in cases associated with pulmonary outflow tract obstruction. Eur J Cardiothorac Surg 2:305–311
36. Lecompte Y (2008) Rastelli repair for transposition of the great arteries: still the best choice? J Thorac Cardiovasc Surg 1:192–193
37. Rastelli GC, Wallace RB, Ongley PA (1969) Complete repair of transposition of the great arteries with pulmonary stenosis. A review and report of a case corrected by using a new surgical technique. Circulation 39:83–95
38. Nikaidoh H (1984) Aortic translocation and biventricular outflow tract reconstruction. A new surgical repair for transposition of the great arteries associated with ventricular septal defect and pulmonary stenosis. J Thorac Cardiovasc Surg 88:365–372
39. Bex JP, Lecompte Y, Baillot F, Hazan E (1980) Anatomical correction of transposition of the great arteries. Ann Thorac Surg 29:86–88
40. Roberts WC (1976) Choosing a substitute cardiac valve: type, size, surgeon. Am Heart Cardiol 38:633–644
41. Sade RMN, Ballenger JF, Hohn AR, Arants JE, Riopel DA, Taylor AB (1979) Cardiac valve replacement in children: a comparison of tissue with mechanical prosthesis. J Thorac Cardiovasc Surg 78:123–127
42. Geha AS, Laks H Jr (1979) Late failure of porcine valve heterografts in children. J Thorac Cardiovasc Surg 78:351–361
43. DN Ross (1962) Homograft replacement of aortic valve. Lancet 2:487
44. O'Brien MF, Stafford G, Gardner M, Pohlner P, McGiffin DC (1987) A comparison of aortic valve replacement with viable cryopreserved and fresh allograft valves, with a note on chromosomal studies. J Thorac Cardiovasc Surg 94:812–823
45. Ross DN (1969) Replacement of aortic and mitral valves with a pulmonary autograft. Lancet 2:956–958
46. Rubay JE, Shango P, Clement S, Ovaert C, Matta A, Vliers A, Sluysmans Th (1997) Ross procedure in congenital patients: results and left ventricular function. Eur J Cardiothorac Surg 11:92–99

47. Hunter SW, Lillehei CW (1958) Ebstein's malformation of the tricuspid valve with suggestions of a new form of surgical therapy. Dis Chest 33:297–304
48. Carpentier A, Branchini B, Cour JC, Asfaou E, Villani M, Deloche A, Relland J, D'Allaines C, Blondeau P, Piwnica A, Parenzan L, Brom G (1976) Congenital malformation of the mitral valve in children. Pathology and surgical treatment. J Thorac Cardiovasc Surg 72:854–866
49. David TE, Feintel CM (1992) An aortic valve-sparing operation for patients with aortic incompetence and aneurysm of the ascending aorta. J Thorac Cardiovasc Surg 103:617–622
50. De Oliveira NC, David TE, Ivanov J, Armstrong S, Eriksson MJ, Rakowski H, Webb G (2003) Results of surgery for aortic root aneurysm in patients with Marfan syndrome. J Thorac Cardiovasc Surg 125:789–796
51. Senning A (1967) Fascia lata replacement of aortic valves. J Thorac Cardiovasc Surg 54:465–470
52. Odim J, Laks H, Allada V, Child J, Wilson S, Gjertson D (2005) Results of aortic valve-sparing and restoration with autologous pericardial leaflet extensions in congenital heart disease. Ann Thorac Surg 80:647–654
53. Kalangos A, Beghetti M, Baldovinos A, Vala D, Bichel T, Mermillod B, Murith N, Oberhansli I, Friedli B, Faidutti B (1999) Aortic valve repair by cusp extension with the use of fresh autologous pericardium in children with rheumatic aortic insufficiency. J Thorac Cardiovasc Surg 118:225–236
54. Carpentier A, Chauvaud S, Mace L, Relland J, Mihaileanu S, Marino JP, Abry B, Guibourt PJ (1988) A new reconstructive operation for Ebstein's anomaly of the tricuspid valve. Thorac Cardiovasc Surg 96:92–101
55. Da Silva PJ, Baumgratz JF, da Fonseca L, Meiken Franchi S, Lopes LM, Tavares MP, Soares AM, Moreira LP, Barbero-Marcial M (2007) The cone reconstruction of the tricuspid valve in Ebstein's anomaly. The operation: early and midterm results. J Thorac Cardiovasc Surg 133:215–223
56. Barnard CN (1967) The Operation. A human cardiac transplant: an interim report of a successful operation performed at Groote Schuur hospital, Cape Town. S Afr Med J 41:1271–1274
57. Lower RR, Dong E, Shumway NE (1965) Long-term survival of cardiac homografts. Surgery 58:110–119
58. Bailey LL, Nehlsen-Cannarella SL, Doroshow RW, Jacobson GJ, Martin RD, Allard MW, Hyde MR, Dang Bui RH, Petry EL (1986) Cardiac allotransplantation in newborns as therapy for hypoplastic left heart syndrome. N Engl J Med 315:949–963

# Minimally Invasive and Robotic Cardiac Surgery

# 33

Loris Salvador

*If a man will begin with certainties, he shall end in doubts, but if he will content to begin with doubts, he shall end in certainties.*
Francis Bacon

**Abstract**

In this chapter the discussion will be confined to the ministernotomy approach, the thoracoscopic video-assisted or video-guided surgery (port access), and robot-assisted surgery. The growing evidence of interest and the increasing number of published articles are reflecting the attention that cardiac surgeons pay to this subject. Port access and robotic surgery are stimulating techniques that require a new attitude for surgeons: different incision (minithoracotomy and ports), different view (screens and monitors and 3D vision), different surgeon location (sitting a few meters from the patient on the robotic platform).

Minimally invasive cardiac surgery is a surgical approach that reflects a philosophy, a commitment to improve surgical techniques or integrate the latest technologies providing evident benefits such as reduction of pain, smaller incisions, short hospitalization, and reduction of surgical risks and complications. In the definition of minimally invasive should be included any operation performed that reduces the impact of the conventional full sternotomy surgery and the use of extracorporeal circulation. Surgery carried out through any limited access, such as ministernotomy, or any operation conducted off pump should be included in this classification.

In this chapter the discussion will be confined to the ministernotomy approach, the thoracoscopic video-assisted or video-guided surgery (port access), and robot-

L. Salvador (✉)
Cardiac Surgery Unit, Department of Cardiovascular Science,
San Bortolo Hospital, Vicenza, Italy
e-mail: medloris@yahoo.it

M. Picichè (ed.), *Dawn and Evolution of Cardiac Procedures*,
DOI: 10.1007/978-88-470-2400-7_33, © Springer-Verlag Italia 2013

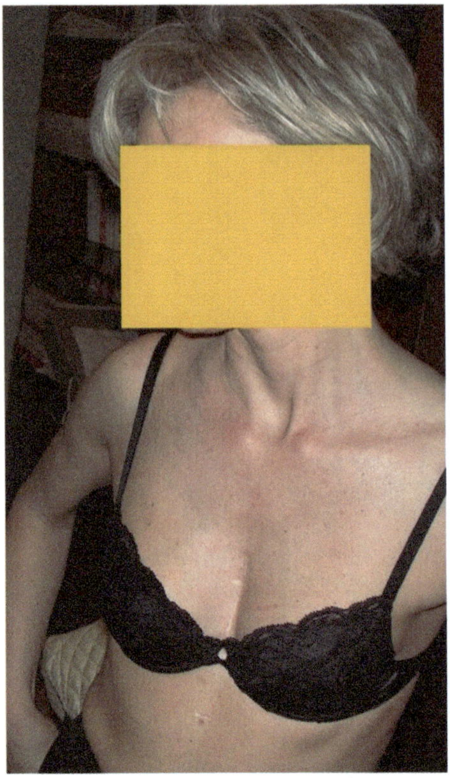

**Fig. 33.1** Mitral Valve surgery via ministernotomy: good cosmetic result 1 year after operation

assisted surgery. The growing evidence of interest and the increasing number of published articles are reflecting the attention that cardiac surgeons pay to this subject. Port access and robotic surgery are stimulating techniques that require a new attitude for surgeons: different incision (minithoracotomy and ports), different view (screens and monitors and 3D vision), different surgeon location (sitting a few meters from the patient on the robotic platform).

Over the years, minimally invasive cardiac surgery has evolved and impressive advances have been made to improve success and safety. Clinical evidence of additional benefits has emerged after more than 15 years of multiple publications and reports, and minimally invasive surgery is becoming a standard practice for many surgeons [1]. Despite the reluctance of a significant part of the cardiac surgical community, minimally invasive surgery is expected to have a major impact on the management of patients with valvular heart disease over the next few years [2]

## 33.1 History

Cardiac surgery has probably been the last surgical specialty to adopt minimally invasive video-thoracoscopic techniques. Tributes should be acknowledged to pioneers who have had little to do with cardiac surgery. Raoul Palmer, an American surgeon working in France, performed in the early 1950s the first diagnostic laparoscopy [3]. Kurt Semm, a German gynecologist, performed the first laparoscopic appendectomy in May 30, 1980 [4]. Erich Muhe of Böblingen, Germany, carried out the first laparoscopic cholecystectomy on 12 September 1985 [5].

The technique of video-assisted thoracic surgery (VATS) pulmonary lobectomy was first reported in the early 1990s simultaneously by several authors [6, 7].

First use of a video-thoracoscopic system in cardiac surgery was reported in 1993 by Burke and Chang [8] in congenital heart surgery. In adult cardiac surgery, the first publications were submitted by Furuse et al. [9] in 1995 on aortic valve repair and Kaneko et al. [10] on mitral valve replacement, both via full sternotomy.

At that time, videoscopy [11] was adopted to improve the visualization and magnification of anatomically inaccessible structures and the definition of "minimally invasive cardiac surgery" was finally proposed.

In 1996, a team from the University of Stanford performed the first mitral valve replacement [12] using an aortic balloon, and this was the beginning of the Endoclamp age. In the same year, Carpentier [13] successfully performed the first video-assisted procedure, and in 1998 [14] performed the first successful open heart surgery (Atrial septal defect correction) using the Da Vinci Robotic System (Intuitive Surgical Inc., Mountain View, CA, USA).

In the middle of the 1990s, Cosgrove [15, 16] and Cohn et al. [17], started using routinely mini-sternotomy for their valve operations, either with a parasternal incision or hemisternotomy. Main advantages of this approach, over the mini-thoracotomy, are superior anatomical exposure in the case of aortic valve surgery and a more familiar setting for the surgeon that allows easy extension to a full sternotomy if there are complications during the procedure.

However, the evolution of cardiac minimally invasive surgery was not possible without the improvement of other various aspects of cardiac surgery: perfusion, as new cannulas were developed and vacuum-assisted extracorporeal circulation was introduced; the use of $CO^2$ to reduce the risk of air embolism; the intraoperative transesophageal echocardiography, essential in confirming the right position of the cannulas, analyzing the cardiac structures, verifying the results.

## 33.2 Rationale and Learning Curve

Minimally invasive surgery is considered safe and efficient when it is obtainable at no adjunctive risk and is giving the same quality of treatment in comparison to conventional sternotomy surgery. The key benefits are described in Table 33.1.

Some authors recommend this approach in specific groups of patients, as in those over 70 years of age [18], or in the presence of obesity [19]. Surprisingly, McCreath [20] at Duke University found a better renal outcome in patients operated on with minimally invasive surgery compared with open chest surgery. In personal experience COPD patients comprise another group that can benefit from this surgery, as well those patients who require a mitral operation after previous complicated cardiac surgery.

**Table 33.1** Advantages of minimally invasive surgery

| Advantages |
|---|
| Shorter hospitalization |
| Faster healing and faster recovery to normal life |
| Reduction in tissue damage |
| Reduction of pain |
| Reduction in blood transfusion |
| Reduction in risk of infection |
| Smaller incisions, better cosmetic result, and superior psychological acceptance |
| Reduction in risk at second operation |
| Lower global cost |

Selection of patients is mandatory at the beginning of a minimally invasive program and the surgeon must be completely trained in cardiac conventional surgery. After acquiring appropriate experience, virtually all patients with valve pathologies can be operated on with this technique. In port access cases, adequate training and proctoring are essential because surgeons approaching this technique must be aware that it cannot be performed confidently after just a few cases; simulation, tutoring, team involvement are the keys to reaching the high standard of surgery and the consequent safety that patients expect from such an operation. Centers with an adequate volume of mitral cases can successfully and safely substitute or integrate a minimally invasive program alongside their conventional surgery and into their training programs with a standardized plan. An adequate number of minimally invasive surgeries can be arbitrarily quantified as 40–50 cases per year, about 1 case per week, in order to keep well trained all professionals involved in this program and to achieve a good standard of care.

Four steps are recommended according to the Carpentier–Loulmet Classification of Degrees of Surgical Invasiveness (Table 33.2).

Indications and contraindications for this technique are described in Table 33.3

## 33.3 Techniques

There is no best technique, or best approach; several technical options are available and every surgeon can find his own way to perform operations in minimally invasive settings. The most popular operative models are described below.

**Table 33.2** The Carpentier–Loulmet Classification of Degrees of Surgical Invasiveness

| Classification | Invasiveness |
|---|---|
| Level I | Incision of 10–12 cm |
| | Direct vision |
| Level II | Incision of 4–6 cm |
| | Video-assisted |
| Level III | Incision of 1–2 cm (port) |
| | Video-directed |
| Level IV | Port incision with robotic instruments |
| | Video-directed |

**Table 33.3** Indications and contraindications for minimally invasive surgery

| Indications | Contraindications |
|---|---|
| Mitral valve repair or replacement | Multiple concomitant procedures. |
| Atrial septal defect closure | Heavy right pleural adhesions |
| Myxomas and other benign neoplasm removal | |
| Tricuspid valve surgery | |
| Aortic valve surgery | |
| Atrial fibrillation treatment | |

## 33.3.1 Port Access Approach

### 33.3.1.1 Patient Preparation

Single or double lumen intubation, central line inserted, body and face up, right chest elevated 30–45°; external defibrillation pads. Usually one radial artery line is monitored, but both radial arteries are monitored if Endoclamp, IntraClude or EndoDirect (Edwards Lifesciences, Irvine, CA, USA) systems are used.

### 33.3.1.2 Arterial perfusion

Ascending Aorta cannulation: Endodirect ® or¯StrightShot||® Cannula (Edwards Lifes.,Irvine,CA; USA) are good solutions. Peripheral cannulation: one Femoral Artery is used, both if the caliber is too small. Other option: Subclavian Artery. In femoral cannulation, standard cannulas are usually adopted while Endoreturn® cannula (Edwards Lifesciences, Irvine,CA,USA) is utilized if Endoclamp or IntraClude is expected to apply.

#### 33.3.1.3 Venous Drainage

A single cannula inserted in the femoral vein reaching the superior vena cava (negative pressure of 40 mmHg is recommended) is adequate for the majority of cases. Double drainage: 14–17 F cannula inserted via the jugular internal vein and 22–25 F cannula inserted via the femoral vein into the inferior vena cava (optional negative pressure) are the alternatives, but are recommended if a right atrium opening has to be performed.

#### 33.3.1.4 Port Access Incisions

One main incision: 4–6 cm in length on the 3rd or 4rd intercostal space in a submammary position or between the anterior and mid-axillary lines. Muscles are divided and soft tissue or regular costal retractor is inserted into the intercostal space. Two satellite 5-mm ports are necessary, one with a side connection for $CO_2$ delivery. These ports are used to introduce into the right pleural cavity the vent cannula and the 0° or 30° camera.

#### 33.3.1.5 Pericardium

The pericardium is opened about 2–3 cm anterior to the phrenic nerve and retracted.

#### 33.3.1.6 Ventricular Unloading

Regular vent cannula for ventricular decompression is used, EndoVent ® pulmonary catheter (Edwards Lifesciences) introduced through the right internal jugular vein or the left subclavian vein can be an alternative.

#### 33.3.1.7 Cardioplegia

Antegrade delivery can be obtained by standard or longer cardioplegic cannula inserted into the ascending aorta secured with a purse string or delivered via the Endoclamp, IntraClude or Endodirect systems. Retrograde delivery can be obtained using a specifically designed cannula (Endoplege®) inserted under transesophageal echo control via the jugular vein or directly through the port access incision.

#### 33.3.1.8 Aortic occlusion

Direct external aortic occlusion is achieved by transthoracic aortic cross-clamps with the Chitwood Clamp (Scanlan International, Minneapolis, MN, USA), or Portaclamp® FLEX (Cardio Life Research, Louvain La Neuve, Belgium). These are introduced through an additional chest port, while the Cygnet Clamp (Vitalitec Surgical, Domalain, France), a malleable external clamp, is introduced through the same minithoracotomy incision. Intra-aortic occlusion is conversely obtained by the Endoclamp® IntraClude and EndoDirect®; these systems are designed to occlude the ascending aorta, inflating a balloon inside the aortic lumen with a predetermined volume of saline.

In selected patients with poor ventricles or heavy adhesions from a previous operation, the procedure can be carried out with a beating or fibrillating heart without aortic cross-clamping.

Body temperature is maintained in moderate hypothermia; this is helpful since the heart is in a closed environment and faster rewarming of the myocardium has been detected [21].

### 33.3.2 Ministernotomy Approach

#### 33.3.2.1 Patient Preparation

The same as in conventional surgery, but external defibrillation pads are mandatory since it is impossible to use internal pads.

#### 33.3.2.2 Arterial and Venous Perfusion

Either central or peripheral cannulation is possible; if direct right atrium drainage is preferred, a small caliber cannula and negative pressure can be useful in order to reduce encumbrance and to have more space for surgical maneuvers.

#### 33.3.2.3 Incision

Several approaches have been adopted following surgeon preference: in aortic valve surgery a skin incision of 5–7 cm is made in the upper third of the sternum, and the bone is divided following a reverse "C" [22], "I" [23], "J" [24, 25], "S" [26], reverse "T" [27], "Z" [28] shape. A right parasternal incision is also proposed [15, 25, 29]. Mammary arteries are usually spared in most of these approaches. A small retractor is inserted and usually the aorta and right atrium are visualized. In the case of mitral valve surgery the incision is usually made in the lower segment of the sternum, resulting in good cosmetic result (Fig. 33.1). Peripheral cannulation is preferred in order to avoid obstacles during the procedure. Interatrial septal incision is favored entering the left atrium.

Ventricle unloading, aorta cross-clamping, cardioplegia delivery, and surgical techniques for valve correction are the same as for the full sternotomy approach.

## 33.4 Clinical Evidence

### 33.4.1 Port Access

Suri et al. [30], at the Mayo Clinic, investigated the outcomes of mitral valve repair performed through a minithoracotomy approach in 350 patients versus 365 operated through full sternotomy between 1999 and 2006. After a propensity score analysis they conclude that despite longer cross-clamp and cardiopulmonary bypass time, early outcomes were similar, demonstrating the "non-inferiority" of the port access technique in comparison with the open approach in their Institution. In addition to shorter postoperative ventilator support, no other significant differences were identified in the two groups comparing length of stay, reoperation, blood transfusion. No analysis was performed regarding stroke and early mortality because there were too few events. Some results of these authors are in contrast with others [31–33] with respect to blood transfusion, length of stay, and reoperation. The review by Richardson [22] that searched for the best evidence of the superiority of port access mitral valve repair versus sternotomy, concluded that in several cohort studies minimally invasive mitral valve repair is reported to result in a shorter ICU and hospital stay, reduced postoperative bleeding and pain, and a shorter time before resuming normal activities. This is at the expense of longer bypass and operative times.

No difference in long-term outcomes can be detected for mitral valves that are repaired with a minimally invasive approach and those operated in the conventional manner, according to findings reported by Galloway [34] in a decade of minimally invasive surgery and 1,601 patients included in the study. The same good results were registered by the group of Mohr [35] in Leipzig, which evaluated 1,230 patients operated on from 1999 to 2007.

The conversion rate, was 3.8% in the Port Access Registry [36] published in 2000.

Neurological events are one of the major issues that opponents of this technique argue in order to emphasize a supposedly higher risk in patients operated on with minimally invasive surgery. This argument has been definitively clarified. In the systematic review published by Modi [37] ten studies reported no difference in the incidence of stroke, while two showed a reduced incidence with a minimally invasive approach. A higher rate of neurological events, however, was reported at the initial experiences, when $CO_2$ was not adopted. The use of $CO_2$ played a significant role in improving these results since it is evident to all surgeons performing this type of surgery that the small entity of microbubbles at the TEE ECHO after aorta declamping is the opposite of a major presence of air entrapped in the cardiac chambers after conventional surgery.

Lower rates of wound infection are also reported [36], while incidence of postoperative atrial fibrillation remains the same as in conventional surgery.

The risk of aortic dissection is now greatly reduced [37] by the use of external aortic clamp, central cannulation, and increased attention to cannula insertion maneuvers in peripheral arteries.

Interesting results were finally demonstrated in patients with previous sternotomy operated with port access according to the articles of Ricci et al. [38], Mihos et al. [39], and Arcidi et al. [40], they electively recommend this approach in this subset of patients.

Quality of life and other psychological aspects are under study in our Center and reports in the literature confirm a better psychological outcome, which can be related to the outstanding cosmetic result.

### 33.4.2 Ministernotomy

Several authors demonstrated that ministernotomy access results in a shorter length of stay, less incisional pain, shorter duration of ventilation, less blood loss, less blood transfusion, earlier recovery, and minor costs compared with a full sternotomy [17, 25]. Others did not find the same differences except for a cosmetic benefit [41]. However, avoiding full sternotomy seems to have real benefits in Centers where this technique is adopted routinely, with mortality, safety, and efficacy at least similar to those of conventional surgery. Deep sternal infection is reported with a very low incidence with this technique. In patients with severe COPD, the stability of the undivided sternum allows a shorter ventilation time and a reduced risk of pneumonia [25]. After an adequate learning curve cardiopulmonary by-pass time is not significantly different from surgery carried out with a full sternotomy, and almost all valve pathologies can be treated with this approach.

## 33.5 Robotic Cardiac Surgery

Although robotic surgery is performed with sophisticated devices, the operation is not completely automated since the handling of the platform is still managed by the surgeon. The history of this recent technology started during the late 1980s, when the Defense Advanced Research Project Administration (DARPA) made by researchers of SRI International (Menlo Park, CA, USA), cultivated the idea of developing a system able to operate on injured soldiers in the battlefield, under the control of a surgeon placed in a remote location [42]. It was imagined that the robotic manipulator arms would be mounted in a mobile vehicle for Medical Forward Advanced Surgical Treatment (MEDFAST) while the surgical workstation with the operative surgeon would be placed in the Mobile Advanced Surgical Hospital (MASH). In 1995 this project expanded into a new company called Intuitive Surgical, (Mountain View, CA, USA), which afterward introduced into a clinical setting the Da Vinci Robotic surgical platform. In 1997, the first robotic surgical procedure on a patient was performed in Brussels, Belgium, by Jacques Himpens, MD, and Guy Cardiere, MD [43].

Other projects were independently developed during those years: RoboDoc for hip replacement surgery, the German ARTEMIS (Advanced Robot and Telemanipulator System for Minimally Invasive Surgery), which was initially developed for telemanipulation of nuclear waste. In 1985 a robot, the PUMA 560, was used to place a needle for a brain biopsy using CT guidance. Other devices based on the primary design derived from the IBM Puma Arm were developed, but lack of funds stopped most of these programs.

In 1993, Alberto Rovetta [44] was able to successfully perform a liver biopsy on a pig liver with the surgeon's station being at the NASA Jet Propulsion Lab (JPL) in Pasadena, CA, USA, and the manipulators and pig liver in his laboratory in Milan, Italy.

Yulun Wang, [45] founded Computer Motion (Goleta, CA, USA) in 1989 and developed the Automated Endoscopic System for Optimal Positioning (AESOP), a voice activated arm supporting an endoscope, part of a NASA project to allow surgeons on earth to treat medical emergencies on the Shuttle and on the international space station. AESOP was the first step of a more sophisticated program:

Zeus, a three-armed robot controlled by a surgical workstation, and Socrates, a Robotic Telecollaboration System that allows a surgeon at a remote location to connect to an operating room. In September 2001 the Zeus system was used for the first trans-Atlantic robotic surgery (called Operation Lindbergh) between New York and Strasbourg, France by Jacques Marescaux and Michele Gagner [46]. A laparoscopic cholecystectomy was performed.

The rationale of this project was exciting: to give expert support and assistance to surgeons in remote areas.

The first to use a robot in cardiac surgery, the Aesop 3,000 device, was Mohr in 1997 [47]. Vision was 2D and long instruments were used to carry out the surgery. The first successful mitral valve repair using the Da Vinci System, was reported by Carpentier and Loulmet in 1998. In the same year Mohr performed the first coronary artery bypass using the Da Vinci System, and the following year Reichenspurner reported the first successful clinical use of ZEUS for coronary artery bypass [48].

In 2003, after years of litigation cases for patent infringement, Intuitive Surgical and Computer Motion merged into one company. The computer motion devices were then discontinued and the Da Vinci System is the only robotic surgery platform currently available.

With the Da Vinci System, a four-armed robot with 3D vision, it is likewise possible to perform operations at a distance, but some obstacles remain to be overcome, such as latency, the time delay between the doctor's action and the robotic arm's response, since input data are transmitted via internet broadband or satellite broadcasting. At present, the surgeon is working in the same operative room; in this way, robotic arms can react promptly to the hand movements.

Micro-electro-mechanical systems (MEMS) and nanotechnology are already areas of interest and several robots are under construction; nevertheless, it will be necessary to continue the research for decades before these projects can be applied for clinical use.

## 33.6 Controversies on Robotic Surgery

The Da Vinci System is used primarily for mitral valve surgery and totally endoscopic coronary artery by-pass (TECAB). Robotics has been established in surgical practice in many cardiac surgery programs. According to surgeons who use the Da Vinci System in their practice [49], the robotic platform is an improvement of the endoscopic instrumentation that with only four degrees of freedom reduces the dexterity, and the loss of depth perception by using two-dimensional video monitors further increases operative difficulty. Robotic surgery, however, is a new technology and efficacy has not yet been well established. Most studies are carried out to demonstrate feasibility [50, 51], but no large, long-term follow-up studies are available to confirm or deny its effectiveness.

Several surgeons, with extensive experience of video-directed minimally invasive surgery, claim that the same results in terms of cosmetics and invasiveness are also reached using the port access technique. The 3D superior visualization of the operative field, the six degrees of movement of the Da Vinci System are not sufficient elements to balance against the lack of haptic (tactile) sensation and the cost of the robotic technology.

Nevertheless, the robotic platform is promising and able to overcome some human defects, such as tremor. There is an absence of tremors with telemanipulation because tremor cancellation algorithms are able to filter the surgeon's hand movements. The 3D image gives the surgeon the illusion of being directly in the surgical field and the instruments seem to be moved naturally by the intuitive hand controllers.

## 33.7 Conclusion

Minimally invasive surgery is an appealing technique, but is not for all surgeons. Although the ministernotomy approach is adopted today by an increasing number of cardiac surgeons, the port access technique is far less widespread, sometimes because of a low mitral valve caseload. According to Bolling et al. [52], based on the STS database, the median number of mitral valve operations for a cardiac surgeon in USA is five per year. Based on this assumption, it seems unreasonable to start a mitral minimally invasive surgery program in all cardiac surgery units if an adequate case volume is not available. To reduce invasiveness and morbidity associated with the traditional surgical techniques, minimally invasive approaches are an attractive option, but must be performed in the right environment to achieve the expected results.

Robotics is also an encouraging option, but despite good results being published, there are still some relevant drawbacks, such as time, cost, efficiency, and compatibility with current hospital systems.

## References

1. Casselman FP, Van Slycke S, Wellens F, De Geest R, Degrieck I, Van Praet F, Vermeulen Y, Vanermen H (2003) Mitral valve surgery can now routinely be performed endoscopically. Circulation 108(Suppl 1):II48–II54
2. Rosengart TK, Feldman T, Borger MA, Vassiliades TA, Gillinov AM, Hoercher KJ, Vahanian A, Bonow RO, O'Neill W (2008) Percutaneous and minimally invasive valve procedures. A scientific statement from the american heart association council on cardiovascular surgery and anesthesia, council on clinical cardiology, functional genomics and translational biology interdisciplinary working group, and quality of care and outcomes research interdisciplinary working group. Circulation 117:1750–1767
3. Litynski GS (1997) Raoul palmer, world war II, and transabdominal coelioscopy. Laparoscopy extends into gynecology. JSLS 1(3):289–292

4. Morgenstern L (2005) Against the tide: kurt karl stephan semm (1927–2003). Surg Innov 12(1):5–6
5. Reynolds Walker Jr (2001) The first laparoscopic cholecystectomy. JSLS 5(1):89–94
6. Kirby TJ, Rice TW (1993) Thoracoscopic lobectomy. Ann Thorac Surg 56:784–786
7. Lewis RJ (1993) The role of video-assisted thoracic surgery for cancer of the lung: wedge resection to lobectomy by simultaneous stapling. Ann Thorac Surg 56:762–768
8. Burke RP, Chang AC (1993) Video-assisted thoracoscopic division of a vascular ring in an infant. J Card Surg 8:537–540
9. Furuse A, Kohno T, Ohtsuka T (1995) Intraoperative visualization of the aortic valve from the left ventricle. J Thorac Cardiovasc Surg 109:395
10. Kaneko Y, Kohno T, Ohtsuka T, Ohbuchi T, Furuse A, Konishi T (1996) Video-assisted observation in mitral valve surgery. J Thorac Cardiovasc Surg 111:279–280
11. Peters WS (1993) Minimally invasive cardiac surgery by cardioscopy. Aust J Cardiac Thorac Surg 2:152–154
12. Pompili MF, Yakub A, Siegel LC, Stevens JH, Awang Y, Burdon TA (1996) Port-access mitral valve replacement: initial clinical experience. Circulation 94(Suppl 1):533
13. Carpentier A, Loulmet D, Carpentier A, Le Bret E, Haugades B, Dassier P, Guibourt P (1996) Open heart operation under videosurgery and minithoracotomy: first case (mitral valvuloplasty) operated with success. C R Acad Sci III 319:219–223
14. Carpentier A, Loulmet D, Aupècle B et al (1998) Computer assisted open heart surgery. First case operated on with success. C R Acad Sci III 321:437–442
15. Cosgrove DM, Sabik JF (1996) Minimally invasive approach for aortic operations. Ann Thorac Surg 62:596–597
16. Navia JL, Cosgrove DM (1996) Minimally invasive mitral valve operations. Ann Thorac Surg 62:1542–1544
17. Cohn LH, Adams DH, Couper GS, Bichell DP, Rosborough DM, Sears SP, Aranki SF (1997) Minimally invasive cardiac valve surgery improves patient satisfaction while reducing costs of cardiac valve replacement and repair. Ann Surg 4:421–428
18. Holzhey DM, Shi W, Borger MA, Seeburger J, Garbade J, Pfannmüller B, Mohr FW (2011) Minimally invasive versus sternotomy approach for mitral valve surgery in patients greater than 70 years old: a propensity-matched comparison. Ann Thorac Surg 91(2):401–405
19. Santana O, Reyna J, Grana R, Buendia M, Lamas GA, Lamelas J (2011) Outcomes of minimally invasive valve surgery versus standard sternotomy in obese patients undergoing isolated valve surgery. Ann Thorac Surg 91(2):406–410
20. McCreath BJ, Swaminathan M, Booth JV, Phillips-Bute B, Chew STH, Glower DD, Stafford-Smith M (2009) Mitral valve surgery and acute renal injury: port access versus median sternotomy. Ann Thorac Surg 75:812–819
21. Loulmet D, Carpentier A, Cho PW, Berrebi A, d'Attellis N, Austin CB, Couëtil JP, Lajos P (1998) Less invasive techniques for mitral valve surgery. J Thorac Cardiovasc Surg 115:772–779
22. Aris A (1999) Reversed 'C' ministernotomy for aortic valve replacement. Ann Thorac Surg 67:1806–1807
23. Chang YS, Lin PJ, Chang CH, Chu JJ, Tan PP (1999) 'I' ministernotomy for aortic valve replacement. Ann Thorac Surg 68:40–45
24. Svensson LG (1997) Minimal-access 'J' or 'j' sternotomy for valvular, aortic, and coronary operations or reoperations. Ann Thorac Surg 64:1501–1503
25. Tabata M, Umakanthan R, Cohn LH, Bolman RM 3rd, Shekar PS, Chen FY, Couper GS, Aranki SF (2008) Early and late outcomes of 1000 minimally invasive aortic valve operations. Eur J Cardiothorac Surg 33(4):537–541
26. Autschbach R, Walther T, Falk V, Diegeler A, Metz S, Mohr FW (1998) S-shaped in comparison to L-shaped partial sternotomy for less invasive aortic valve replacement. Eur J Cardiothorac Surg 14(Suppl 1):S117–S121 453

27. Gundry SR, Shattuck OH, Razzouk AJ, del Rio MJ, Sardari FF, Bailey LL (1998) Facile minimally invasive cardiac surgery via ministernotomy. Ann Thorac Surg 65(4):1100–1104
28. Nair RU, Sharpe DA (1998) Minimally invasive reversed Z sternotomy for aortic valve replacement. Ann Thorac Surg 65:1165–1166
29. Kasegawa H, Shimokawa T, Matsushita Y, Kamata S, Ida T, Kawase M (1998) Right-sided partial sternotomy for minimally invasive valve operation: 'open door method'. Ann Thorac Surg 65:569–570
30. Suri RM, Schaff HV, Meyer SR, Hargrove WC III (2009) Thoracoscopic versus open mitral valve repair: a propensity score analysis of early outcomes. Ann Thorac Surg 88:1185–1190
31. Raanani E, Spiegelstein D, Sternik L, Preisman S, Moshkovitz Y, Smolinsky AK, Shinfeld A (2010) Quality of mitral valve repair: median sternotomy versus port-access approach. J Thorac Cardiovasc Surg 140(1):86–90
32. Iribarne A, Russo MJ, Easterwood R, Hong KN, Yang J, Cheema FH, Smith CR, Argenziano M (2010) Minimally invasive versus sternotomy approach for mitral valve surgery: a propensity analysis. Ann Thorac Surg 90(5):1471–1478
33. Richardson L, Richardson M, Hunter S (2008) Is a port-access mitral valve repair superior to the sternotomy approach in accelerating postoperative recovery? Interact Cardiovasc Thorac Surg 7(4):678–683
34. Galloway AC, Schwartz CF, Ribakove GH, Crooke GA, Gogoladze G, Ursomanno P, Mirabella M, Culliford AT, Grossi EA (2009) A decade of minimally invasive mitral repair: long-term outcomes. Ann Thorac Surg 88(4):1180–1184
35. Seeburger J, Borger MA, Doll N, Walther T, Passage J, Falk V, Mohr FW (2009) Comparison of outcomes of minimally invasive mitral valve surgery for posterior, anterior and bileaflet prolapse. Eur J Cardiothorac Surg 36:532–553
36. Glower DD, Siegel LC, Frischmeyer KJ, Galloway AC, Ribakove GH, Grossi EA, Robinson NB, Ryan WH, Colvin SB (2000) Predictors of outcome in a multicenter port-access valve registry. Ann Thorac Surg 70(3):1054–1059
37. Modi P, Hassan A, Chitwood WR Jr (2009) Minimally invasive mitral valve surgery: a systematic review and meta-analysis. Eur J Cardiothorac Surg 34(5):943–952
38. Ricci D, Pellegrini C, Aiello M, Alloni A, Cattadori B, D'Armini AM, Rinaldi M, Viganò M (2010) Port-access surgery as elective approach for mitral valve operation in re-do procedures. Eur J Cardiothorac Surg 37(4):920–925
39. Mihos CG, Santana O, Lamas GA, Lamelas J (2011) Outcomes of right minithoracotomy mitral valve surgery in patients with previous sternotomy. Ann Thorac Surg 91(6):1824–1827
40. Arcidi JM Jr, Rodriguez E, Elbeery JR, Nifong LW, Efird JT, Chitwood WR Jr (2011) Fifteen-year experience with minimally invasive approach for reoperations involving the mitral valve. J Thorac Cardiovasc Surg
41. Szwerc MF, Benckart DH, Wiechmann RJ, Savage EB, Szydlowski GW, Magovern GJ Jr, Magovern JA (1999) Partial versus full sternotomy for aortic valve replacement. Ann Thorac Surg 68:2209–2214
42. Rebello KJ (2004) Applications of MEMES in surgery. Proc IEEE 92:43–55
43. Himpens J, Leman G, Cardiere GB (1998) Telesurgical laparoscopic cholecystectomy. Surg Endosc 12:1091
44. Rovetta A, Sala R, Cosmi F, Wen X, Sabbadini D, Milanesi S, Toqno A, Angelini L, Bejczy AK (1993) Telerobotics surgery in a transatlantic experiment: application in laparoscopy. In: Kim WS (ed) Telemanipulator technology and space telerobotics. Proceedings of SPIE, vol 2057. pp 337–344
45. Wang Y, Sackier J (1994) Robotically enhanced surgery: from concept to development. Surg Endosc 8:63–66
46. Marescaux J, Leroy J, Gagner M, Rubino F, Mutter D, Vix M, Butner ES, Smith KM (2001) Transatlantic robot-assisted telesurgery. Nature 413:379–380
47. Falk V, Walther T, Autschbach R et al (1998) Robot-assisted minimallyinvasive solo mitral valve operation. J Thorac Cardiovasc Surg 115:470–471

48. Reichenspurner H, Damiano RJ, Mack M, Boehm DH, Gulbins H, Detter C et al (1999) Use ofthe voice-controlled and computer-assisted surgical system ZEUS for endoscopic coronaryartery bypass grafting. J Thorac Cardiovasc Surg 118(1):11–16
49. Modi P, Rodriguez E, Chitwood WR Jr (2009) Robot-assisted cardiac surgery. Interact Cardiovasc Thorac Surg 9:500–505
50. Chitwood WR, Rodriguez E, Chu MWA, Hassan A, Ferguson TB, Vos PW, Nifong LW (2008) Robotic mitral valve repairs in 300 patients: a single center experience. J Thorac Cardiovasc Surg 136:436–441
51. Argenziano M, Katz M, Bonatti J, Srivastava S, Murphy D, Poirier R, Loulmet D, Siwek L, Kreaden U, Ligon D (2006) TECAB trial investigators. Results of the prospective multicenter trial of robotically assisted totally endoscopic coronary artery bypass grafting. Ann Thorac Surg 81(5):1666–1674
52. Bolling SF, Li S, O'Brien SM, Brennan JM, Prager RL, Gammie JS (2010) Predictors of mitral valve repair: clinical and surgeon factors. Ann Thorac Surg 90(6):1904–1911

# The History of Research on Percutaneous, Transapical, and Sutureless Aortic Valve Replacement

34

Thierry Aymard and Thierry Carrel

*Knowing is not enough; we must apply. Willing is not enough; we must do.*

Johann Wolfgang von Goethe


**Abstract**

A large number of scientific inventions evolved from research in different fields of interest. Only a few people with a visionary mind are able to see the future practical implications that transform a good idea into revolutionary process. For over 30 years the surgical replacement of a diseased aortic valve represented the golden standard of curative treatment for severe symptomatic aortic valve stenosis and significant regurgitation. Only recently has the operative risk declined crucially and the functional results are excellent. Long-term survival is very satisfactory, even for patients >80 years of age and has become close to that of non-operated patients of the same age. Despite these excellent results, surgery was found to be practiced preferentially in patients in good condition, whereas a substantial proportion of patients were not referred to surgery because the perioperative risk was estimated to be high owing to advanced age or significant comorbidities [1]. These patients would need an alternative technique to replace the diseased valve in order to re-establish normal valvular function. Recently, the development of two new techniques has changed the approach of patients considered to be at high risk of being refused conventional intervention: the insertion of a sutureless prosthesis and thus reducing substantially the surgery time and the transcatheter technique known as transcatheter aortic valve implantation (TAVI) allowing a tremendous decrease in the invasiveness of surgery. This new concept could profit from the already well-established method of cardiac catheterization.



An erratum to this chapter is available at doi:10.1007/978-88-470-2400-7_35.



T. Aymard (✉) · T. Carrel
Clinic for Cardiovascular Surgery, Inselspital Berne, Berne University Hospital and University of Berne, Freiburgstrasse, 3010 Berne, Switzerland
e-mail: thierry.aymard@insel.ch



M. Picichè (ed.), *Dawn and Evolution of Cardiac Procedures*,
DOI: 10.1007/978-88-470-2400-7_34, © Springer-Verlag Italia 2013

## 34.1 The Transcatheter Aortic Valve Implantation

### 34.1.1 First Step: To Reopen a Human Heart Valve

On 13 July 1912 the French surgeon, Theodore Tuffier, carried out the first clinical attempt to dilate a stenotic aortic valve through a transaortic approach using his finger [2]. Unfortunately, excessive mortality made it impossible to continue clinical research in this field. In 1922, in St Louis, Missouri, Evart Graham and Duff Allen decided that intervention for diseased valves required direct vision and they invented a cardioscope that could come into direct contact with the valves [3]. The instrument was introduced through the left ventricular apex or the subclavian artery and a knife was carried alongside to cut the stenosed valve. These two surgeons can be considered the inventors of the transcatheter technique, being the first to approach this pathology through a peripheral vessel. As early as 1923 Graham was the first surgeon to successfully perform a pneumonectomy, opening a new horizon in thoracic surgery [4]. Harvey Cushing [5], surgeon-in-chief at the newly opened Peter Bent Brigham Hospital, followed by Elliott Cutler, worked on a mitral valvulotomy procedure through the left ventricle apex in the laboratory. The first patient underwent successful operation in May 1923, using a keratotomy knife [6]. In 1925 Dr Souttar, an English surgeon, performed a mitral valvulotomy using his finger [7]. Charles Bailey in 1949 published his clinical experience in 60 mongrel dogs: *The Surgical Treatment of Mitral Stenosis* [8]. Owing to the high mortality of his patients, he became "famous" as the "butcher of Hahnemann Hospital." On 10 June 1948, he scheduled two new cases. The first patient died. The second operation in another hospital started promptly before the bad outcome was known and before the administration was able to cancel the procedure. The surgery was completed and 1 week later Bailey presented the triumphant case to the American College of Chest Physicians [9].

### 34.1.2 Development of Aortic Valve Prostheses

In the early 1950s, two surgeons, Charles Hufnagel [10] in Washington DC and Campbell [11] in Oklahoma, independently developed and implanted artificial valves in the descending aorta of dogs. The valves consisted of a mobile ball within a chamber made of a single piece of methacrylate with fixation rings of nylon on both ends. The valve was inserted through a left thoracotomy after mobilization of the descending aorta. After presenting this first model of a mechanical prosthesis at the American College of Surgeons meeting in 1949, Hufnagel applied this concept for the treatment of aortic insufficiency in September 1952. His experience was published in *Surgery* in 1954 [12] in a study of 23 patients. The hospital mortality reached 20%, but 24 years later few patients were still alive with satisfactory results. Hufnagel's caged ball valve used multiple-point fixation rings to secure the apparatus to the aorta and can be considered today to be the precursor of the actual sutureless valve. Besides the high mortality rate and the cumbersome insertion patients complained about the noise of the bouncing metal ball, which was soon replaced by a silicone-covered ball. Dr Dwight Harken performed the first operation using a caged ball valve in 1960 in a subcoronary position [13]. In the same year Starr and Edwards [14] replaced the mitral valve using a self-designed caged ball valve. By 1967, 2,000 Starr–Edward valves had been implanted and the use of their prosthesis represented the established standard.

### 34.1.3 Development of Cardiac Catheterization and Implantation of Devices

Ancient Egyptians in 3000 BC as well as the Greek Hippocrates from Kos in 400 BC, using metallic pipes, tried to push water or air into a cadaver's vasculature. Harvey in 1651 catheterized the inferior vena cava. During the next three centuries physiologists introduced needles into the vasculature for intracardiac measurements. In 1953 Sven-Ivar Seldinger described the technique of inserting a catheter over a needle puncture [15]. Finally, in 1956, Cournand, Forssmann, and Richards received the Nobel Price for their contribution on cardiac catheterization [16]. In 1970, in Zurich, Switzerland, Andreas Grüntzig invented the concept of balloon angioplasty. In May 1977, he performed the first coronary angioplasty [17] and Ulrich Sigwart et al. in 1987 implanted the first stent in a human coronary artery [18]. In 1985 Alain Cribier performed the first adult balloon aortic valvuloplasty [19] in Rouen, France. The technique was never very successful in terms of clinical use because it suffered from the comparison with the excellent results obtained by conventional open-chest aortic valve replacement. Only a few patients being rejected for surgery could profit from this evolving technique.

### 34.1.4 Temporary Implantable Prosthetic Heart Valves in Animal Models

In 1965, Hywel Davies from Guy's Hospital in London described a catheter-mounted valve for temporary relief of aortic insufficiency and tried it in dogs [20]. The item consisted of a cone shaped unicusp valve like a parachute with wires and was attached to the tip of a 5 F catheter. The catheter reached the descending aorta through the femoral artery. The proximal part of the catheter was fixed to the skin of the leg. The valve collapsed during systole and opened during diastole. The catheter was part of the system and the device was indicated only for temporary use as a bridge to surgery, but not for definitive implantation. Dr Davies now lives in Sion, Switzerland and devotes most of his time to writing. In 1959, he gave the first comprehensive description of chest deformities that accompany large ventricular septal defects and are known as the "Thorax of Davies" [21]. In 1971 Moulopoulos [22] and Phillips [23] designed three different temporary catheter-mounted aortic valves that they inserted into the ascending aorta in dogs. One valve had an umbrella design and the other two showed balloon systems. The balloons were fixed at the end of a polyethylene catheter and inflated during diastole in order to prevent the diastolic backflow. The catheter was proximally connected to a pump that synchronized inflation and deflation according to diastole and systole. In 1977, Boretos and Poirier described a catheter-mounted valve, shaped as a cone with a broad circular basis pointing in the direction of the left ventricle and with flexible valves of the cone extending downstream [24]. In 1992, Matsubara presented a balloon catheter with check valves: a latex balloon was mounted on the end of the catheter and inflated to occlude the aorta. Two proximal and two distal holes allowed blood to pass through the balloon during systole and two latex valves were attached to the proximal apertures to avoid regurgitation during diastole [25]. The endovascular anchoring was not proposed and the technique was limited to temporary use. Despite the technical development none of these inventions went into clinical use and none of them were applicable for permanent use.

### 34.1.5 The New Idea: A Percutaneous Catheter-Mounted Valve

In the year 1988 the Danish registrar Andersen was captivated by the lecture over of a new technique of balloon dilation within coronary vessels [26]. Fascinated by the new concept Andersen soon came up with a revolutionary idea: the non-invasive insertion of a valve without open surgery and performed on a beating heart. Using the valves of porcine hearts bought at the local butcher, Andersen constructed the initial device consisting of the stent valve, the sheets, and the catheters. He excised the aortic valve free and placed it on a latticed, metal tube (two 0.55-mm surgical stainless steel wires normally used to close the sternum after sternotomy, folded into 15 loops, 8 mm high each), which he squeezed around a balloon. A bulky 41 F delivery device helped to insert the valve. The ascending or the descending aorta was the only access. The proof of concept (with a nonsterilized or treated valve) was documented in pigs and in vitro models. He introduced the balloon into the heart and inflated it so that the stent and the valve expanded and became wedged against the cardiac wall. At that time in the late 1980s, the Institute of Clinical Medicine consisted only of a small room, whereas today it is one of the major research institutes at the University of Aarhus. The University had to confess that when they had finished operating on the patients upstairs, the surgeons sometimes moved the pigs directly into the operating room. On 1 May 1989 they succeeded: the first pig to survive with a new heart valve in the descending aorta. In November of the same year, the first subcoronary implantation was performed. Dr Andersen had reached his goal and was convinced that he would have a publication accepted by one of the major cardiovascular journals. But neither the periodicals nor the companies that produced heart valves were interested. Finally the article was published in the *European Heart Journal* [27]. Andersen and colleagues sold the patent to a small American company, Percutaneous Valve Technologies (PVT), Fort Lee, NJ, USA, for USD 10,000. Despite this lack of enthusiasm, Andersen continued his clinical research. Although nobody believed him, he was regularly invited to speak about his invention around the world. Eventually one day in 1992, an English doctor inserted a heart valve in a patient using the Andersen Patent. The valved stent technique was ready for a broader clinical application. PVT worked in collaboration with 3F

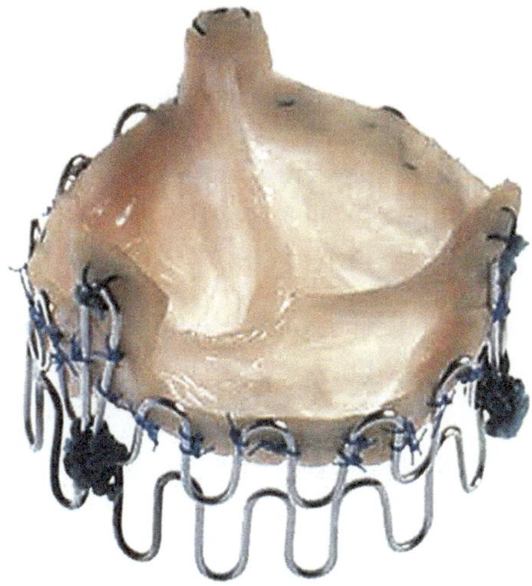

**Fig. 34.1** The Cribier–Edwards prosthetic heart valve

Therapeutic to develop the technology and sold it out to Edwards Lifesciences in 2004, which has a third of the world market for heart valve surgery, for about USD 125 million [28]. The company had only one asset—the Andersen Patent. Andersen did not regret having sold the patent in such a nonlucrative manner: "The only thing that I regret is that I did not contribute to developing the idea until it could be used in humans." Edwards soon came up with a prosthetic heart valve product, the Cribier–Edwards (Fig. 34.1) followed by the Sapien–Edwards in collaboration with Alain Cribier from Rouen in France who was the first to implant the device in 2002 [29]. Andersen was the first to patent a device, but was not the only one; the radiologist Dusan Pavcnik from Prague, Czech Republic, demonstrated the feasibility of transcatheter implantation of a caged ball valve in an infracoronary position in dogs [30]. A caged self-expanding stent was positioned in the native valve and the expandable balloon ball was placed within the cage and expanded with air, contrast medium, or a polymerizing silicon substrate. The early valve function was excellent, but after some hours the ball escaped. In 1996, Nader Moazami in St Louis described the technique with a bovine trileaflet pericardial bioprosthesis mounted in a collapsible stent [31]. Despite academic interest from around the world, the new technology did not gain much attention for another few years. The interest from the industry was minimal. Bonhoeffer and Boudjemline in 2000 reported the first implantation of a valved stent in a pulmonary position in lambs [32] in Paris, France. The device consisted of a biological bovine jugular vein conduit sutured into a platinum–iridium alloy stent. The first human valved stent was reported in October 2000 in a degenerated conduit between the right ventricle and the pulmonary artery [33]. The same group also investigated aortic devices in the descending aorta [34, 35]. In 2002, Georg Lutter, a cardiac surgeon working in Freiburg, Germany, successfully deployed a porcine valved nitinol 21-mm stent in a porcine aorta. Alain Cribier, the pioneer of aortic balloon valvuloplasty, achieved the next step. He successfully implanted the first in-human aortic valved stent on 16 April 2002, as a lifesaving last-resort option [27]. The patient survived for 17 weeks and died of noncardiac causes. In 2005, The Core Valve Company proposed the concept of a biological valve mounted on a self-expanding nitinol-based stent [36]. The access, through the subclavian artery, provided a different route in the case of peripheral vessel disease. Encouraged by these positive and promising achievements, numerous groups worldwide started to become involved in transcatheter valve therapies, research, and engineering. After having been inserted only for compassionate indications, transcatheter prostheses are now available on the European market and are implanted preferentially but not exclusively in patients at high risk of conventional surgery.

### 34.1.6 Transapical Access

The transapical access was absolutely not considered during initialization of transcatheter valves, even if Graham in 1922 had already introduced a cardioscope with a knife in the apex of the left ventricle in order to open an aortic valve [3]. In February 2004 the transapical access was presented for the first time at the International Society of Endovascular Specialists by a young Swiss surgeon, Christoph Hubert [37]. His experimental results in 12 pigs were excellent, with eight successfully placed devices and good hemodynamic results observed with intracardiac ultrasound [38]. Although the transfemoral arterial procedure has proven to be successful, a substantial number of patients are not suitable for this approach because of the small size of the iliacofemoral arteries, tortuosity or severe atheromatous or calcific lesions in the aorto-iliac bifurcation. The group of Webb in Vancouver, Canada developed the initial animal porcine model using direct catheter implantation through the left ventricular apex [39]. This approach was thought to have numerous advantages in a certain group of patients. They reported the first case using the transarterial delivery system to implant an aortic valve via the apex of the left ventricle [40, 41]. Since 2005, many groups all over the world have started a program of TAVI [42, 43]. In common with all transcatheter techniques is the fact that the diseased valve is not excised and further evolution remains unpredictable [44, 45].

## 34.2 The Sutureless Aortic Valve Replacement

### 34.2.1 The Precursors

In September 1952 Charles Hufnagel, director of the surgical research laboratory of Georgetown University Medical Center, inserted a sutureless artificial valve into the aorta of a 30-year-old woman. The concept of sutureless valves was designed again in the early 1960s, in order to facilitate implantation and shorten ischemic and perfusion times. In the 1960s it took at least 45 min to suture the valve in place without efficient myocardial protection. Facing a 90% mortality rate in his patients, Magovern, Chief of Cardiothoracic Surgery at the University of Pittsburgh Medical Center, was about ready to quit doing these operations. To face this time-saving problem he decided to conceive a sutureless valve. Thinking about the design, he entered a machine shop in Aspinwall, and met an eager employee, Mr Harry Cromie, a machinist engineer who worked ambitiously in his garage on his own machine interventions and who was about to create the Surgitool Company [46]. Through this lucky coincidence the two men started a partnership and developed a ball valve that incorporated a unique sutureless fixation. The valve was inserted by rotating an implantation tool to engage the multiple vertical pins in the aortic annulus (Fig. 34.2). It took only about 3 or 4 min to put the sutureless valve in place. This change in insertion time represented tremendous progress in changing a 90% mortality rate to a 90% survival rate. Cromie obtained the patent on the valve, and eventually worked for Baxter Healthcare of Deerfield, IL, USA, which purchased the rights of the invention, bought the Surgitool Company and is still one of the leaders in medical technologies. The valve was described by Magovern in 1963 and remained in use by Magovern's group until 1991 [47]. In 1989, Magovern reported on his 25-year experience in 728 patients between 1962 and 1988; ball variance occurred in 14 patients (2%), and necessitated 12 reoperations with two deaths. Just as with the Starr–Edwards valves, ball variance was virtually eliminated in the mid-1960s with the postmold heat cure process. In 1964, a silicone rubber cuff was attached to the upper plate and the poppet was impregnated with barium sulfate to convey radiolucency. Despite the concept being abandoned because of numerous complications, such as paravalvular leaks and valve-related thromboembolic events, some implants were very successful. In 2007 an Israeli surgeon found a Magovern–Cromie valve during a redo-cardiac surgery. The surgeon was surprised to discover a metal "ball and cage" valve that was not held in place by stitches, but by several tiny U-shaped hooks. The valve had worked flawlessly for 42 years, and was still functioning [48]. Production of the Magovern–Cromie ball valves ceased in 1980, although Magovern continued to implant this valve for several more years [47].

### 34.2.2 The Modern Era

Owing to the rapid development of transcatheter valve technologies, there is renewed interest in sutureless aortic valve implantation, mostly realized by mounting a biological aortic valve into a metal stent and compressing it into a catheter sleeve [49, 50]. To date, there are more than 40 patents for sutureless valve technologies and three different types of sutureless prostheses have been actually implanted. The 3f® Enable (Fig. 34.3) aortic bioprosthesis model 6000 from ATS, now Medtronic, received CE market approval in 2010. It was the first sutureless prototype to be tested [51] based upon the already known stentless 3f® Aortic Bioprosthesis Model 1000 mounted in a nitinol stent that unfolds at normal temperature. Nitinol is a metal alloy of nickel and titanium with two unique

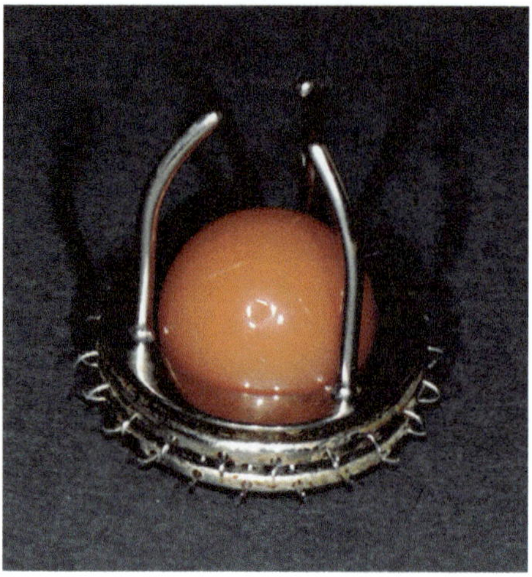

**Fig. 34.2** Magovern–Cromie ball valve

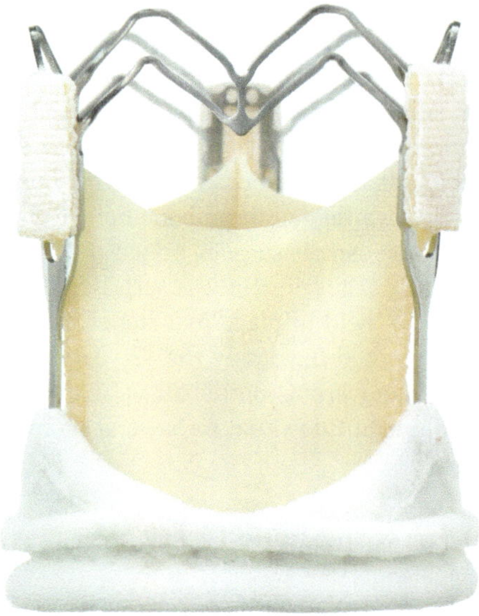

**Fig. 34.3** The 3f® Enable aortic bioprosthesis model

properties, shape memory and superelasticity capable of recoverable deformation (approximately 8–10 times that of steel), regaining its initial shape when stress is removed (a deformation-driven superelastic effect). The valve is assembled from three equal sections of glutaraldehyde-fixed equine pericardial tissue. Results of the in vitro and in vivo studies compare favorably with commercially available stentless and stented valves and the experience with this valve is based on more than 10,000 patients over the last 10 years. Sorin proposed the Perceval, similar in concept to the Enable. Like the Sorin Solo stentless bioprosthesis from bovine pericardium [52], which is CE approved, the Perceval is mounted in a nitinol stent with double ring geometry. The concept was applied in numerous European departments and received the CE market approval in February 2011 [53]. Finally, Edwards, the third cardiac valve company, taking advantage of their expertise in the field of transcatheter technologies and stent mounted bioprosthesis, started a pilot clinical investigation (Triton) for their own sutureless aortic valve, named Intuity. The device consists of a balloon-expandable frame with subvalvular fixation of a stainless steel stent.

Within the past 50 years remarkable progress has been achieved in the development of heart prostheses. Within only 5 years a new concept of less invasive and more applicable transcatheter valves (TAVI) and sutureless techniques emerged and thus made it possible to enlarge the operable group of patients. These technologies have matured and will compete with the conventional therapeutic approaches in the future.

## References

1. Iung B et al (2003) A prospective survey of patients with valvular heart disease in Europe: the Euro heart survey on valvular heart disease. Eur Heart J 24(13):1231–1243
2. Tuffier T (1913) Etat actuel de la chirurgie intrathoracique. Trans Int Congr Med (London 1914), 7; Surgery 1914;2:249
3. Allen DS, Graham EA (1922) Intracardiac surgery—a new method: preliminary report. J Am Med Assoc 79(13):1028–1030
4. Graham EA (1949) The first total pneumonectomy. Tex Cancer Bull 2:2–4
5. Cushing H, Branch JRB (1908) Experimental and clinical notes on chronic valvular lesions in the dog and their possible relation to a future surgery of the cardiac valves. J Med Res 17:471
6. Cohn LH (2007) Cardiac surgery in the adult. McGraw-Hill Professional, New York
7. Souttar HS (1925) Surgical treatment of mitral stenosis. Br Med J 2:603
8. Bailey CP (1949) The surgical treatment of mitral stenosis. Dis Chest 15:377
9. Naef AP (1990) The story of thoracic surgery. Hogrefe & Huber, New York, p 94
10. Hufnagel CA (1951) Aortic plastic valvular prostheses. Bull Georgetown Med Cent 4:128
11. Campbell JM (1958) Artificial aortic valve. J Thorac Cardiovasc Surg 19:312
12. Hufnagel CA, Harvey WP, Rabil PJ et al (1954) Surgical correction of aortic insufficiency. Surgery 35:673
13. Harken DE, Soroff HS, Taylor WJ et al (1960) Partial and complete prostheses in aortic insufficiency. J Thorac Cardiovasc Surg 40:744
14. Starr A, Edwards ML (1961) Mitral replacement: clinical experience with a ball-valve prosthesis. Ann Surg 154:726
15. Seldinger SI (1953) Catheter replacement of the needle in percutaneous arteriography: a new technique. Acta Radiol 39:368–376
16. The Nobel Prize in Physiology or Medicine (1956) www.Nobelprize.org. Accessed 14 July 2011
17. Grüntzig AR, Myler RK, Hanna ES et al (1977) Coronary transluminal angioplasty. Circulation 84:55–56
18. Sigwart U, Puel J, Mirkovitch V et al (1987) Intravascular stents to prevent occlusion and restenosis after transluminal angioplasty. N Eng J Med 316:701–706
19. Cribier A, Savin T, Saudi N et al (1986) Percutaneous transluminal valvuloplasty of acquired aortic stenosis in elderly patients: an alternative to valve replacement? Lancet 1(8472):63–67
20. Davies H (1965) Catheter-mounted valve for temporary relief of aortic insufficiency. Lancet 1:250
21. Davies H (1959) Chest deformities in congenital heart disease. Brit J Dis Chest 53:151–155

22. Moulopoulos SD, Anthopoulos L, Stamatelopoulos S et al (1971) Catheter mounted aortic valves. Ann Thorac Surg 11:423–430
23. Phillips SJ, Ciborski M, Freed PS et al (1976) A temporary catheter-tip aortic valve: hemodynamic effects on experimental acute aortic insufficiency. Ann Thorac Surg 21:134–137
24. Boretos JW, Poirier RA (1977) Aortic heart valve catheter. US Patent 1977 4,056,854
25. Matsubara T, Yamazoe M, Tamura Y et al (1992) Balloon catheter with check valves for experimental relief of acute aortic regurgitation. Am Heart J 124:1002–1008
26. International Congress on Endovascular Interventions (2004) Arizona Heart Institute Foundation, Arizona, 8–12 Feb 2004
27. Andersen HR, Knudsen LL, Hasenkam JM (1992) Transluminal implantation of artificial heart valves. Description of a new expandable aortic valve and initial results with implantation by catheter technique in closed chest pigs. Eur Heart J 13:704–708
28. Edwards Lifesciences: Edwards Lifesciences to acquire Percutaneous Valve Technologies, Inc. for $125 Million. http://www.edwards.com/newsroom/Pages/nr20031215.aspx
29. Cribier A, Eltchaninoff H, Bash A et al (2002) Percutaneous transcatheter implantation of an aortic valve prosthesis for calcific aortic stenosis: first human case description. Circulation 106:3006–3008
30. Pavcnik D, Wright KC, Wallace S (1992) Development and initial experimental evaluation of a prosthetic aortic valve for transcatheter placement: work in progress. Radiology 183:151–154
31. Moazami N, Bessler M, Argenziano M, Choudhri AF, Cabreriza SE, Allendorf JD, Rose EA, Oz MC (1996) Transluminal aortic valveaortic valve placement. A feasibility study with a newly designed collapsible aortic valve. ASAIO J 42(5):M381–M385
32. Bonhoeffer P, Boudjemline Y, Saliba Z et al (2000) Transcatheter implantation of a bovine valve in pulmonary position: a lamb study. Circulation 102:813–816
33. Bonhoeffer P, Boudjemline Y, Saliba Z et al (2000) Percutaneous replacement of pulmonary valve in a right-ventricular to pulmonary-artery prosthetic conduit with valve dysfunction. Lancet 356:1403–1405
34. Boudjemline Y, Bonhoeffer P (2002) Percutaneous implantation of a valve in the descending aorta in lambs. Eur Heart J 23:1045–1049
35. Boudjemline Y, Bonhoeffer P (2002) Steps towards percutaneous aortic valve replacement. Circulation 105:775–778
36. Grube E, Laborde JC, Zinkmann B et al (2005) First report on a human percutaneous transluminal implantation of a self-expanding valve prosthesis for interventional treatment of aortic valve stenosis. Cathet Cardiovasc Interv 66:465–469
37. Huber C, Nasratullah M, Augstburger M, von Segesser LK (2004) New tools for new goals: ultrasound navigation through the heart for off-pump aortic valved stent implantation. International Congress XVII on Endovascular Interventions. Arizona Heart Institute Foundation, Arizona, 8–12 February 2004
38. Huber C, Cohn LH, von Segesser LK (2005) Direct-access valve replacement—a novel approach for off pump valve implantation using valved stents. J Am Coll Cardiol 46(2):366–370
39. Webb JG, Munt B, Makkar R, Naqvi T, Dang N (2004) A percutaneous stent-mounted valve for treatment of aortic or pulmonary valve disease. Catheter Cardiovasc Interv 63:89–93
40. Ye J, Cheung A, Lichtenstein SV, Carere RG, Thompson CR, Pasupati S, Webb JG (2006) Transapical aortic valve implantation in man. J Thorac Cardiovasc Surg 131:1194–1196
41. Lichtenstein SV (2006) Closed heart surgery: back to the future. J Thorac Cardiovasc Surg 131:941–943
42. Walther T, Kasimir MT, Doss M, Schuler G, Simon P, Schächinger V, Mohr FW, Wimmer-Greinecker G (2010) One-year interim follow-up results of the TRAVERCE trial: the initial feasibility study for trans-apical aortic-valve implantation. Eur J Cardiothorac Surg 39:532–537
43. Lichtenstein SV, Cheung A, Ye J et al (2006) Transapical transcatheter aortic valve implantation in humans. Initial clinical experience. Circulation 114:591–596
44. Hanzel GS, O'Neill WW (2006) Complications of percutaneous aortic valve replacement: experience with the Cribier–Edwards percutaneous heart valve. Eurointervention Suppl 1:A3–A8

45. Piazza N, van Gameren M, Jüni P, Wenaweser P, Carrel T, Onuma Y et al (2009) A comparison of patients characteristics and 30 days mortality outcome after transcatheter aortic valve implantation and surgical aortic valve replacement for the treatment of aortic stenosis: a two-centre study. Eurointervention 5:580–588
46. DeWall RA, Qasim N, Carr L (2000) Evolution of mechanical heart valves. Ann Thorac Surg 69:1612–1621
47. Magovern GJ, Liebler GA, Park SB, Burkholder JA, Sakert T, Simpson A (1989) Twenty-five-year review of the Magovern–Cromie sutureless aortic valve. Ann Thorac Surg 48:S33–S34
48. Zlotnick AY, Shiran A, Lewis BS, Aravot D (2008) A perfectly functioning Magovern-Cromie sutureless prosthetic aortic valve 42 years after implantation. Circulation 117:e1–e2
49. Webb JG, Pasupati S, Humphries K, Thompson C, Altwegg L, Moss R et al (2007) Percutaneous transarterial aortic valve replacement in selected high-risk patients with aortic stenosis. Circulation 116:755–763
50. Walther T, Simon P, Dewey T, Wimmer-Greinecker G, Falf V, Kasimir MT et al (2007) Transapical minimal invasive aortic valve implantation. Circulation 116 [Suppl I]:I-240–I-245
51. Aymard T, Kadner A, Walpoth N, Göber V, Englberger L, Stalder M, Eckstein F, Zobrist C, Carrel T (2010) Clinical experience with the second-generation 3f Enable sutureless aortic valve prosthesis. J Thorac Cardiovasc Surg 140(2):313–316
52. Aymard T, Eckstein F, Englberger L, Stalder M, Kadner A, Carrel T (2010) The Sorin Freedom SOLO stentless aortic valve: technique of implantation and operative results in 109 patients. J Thorac Cardiovasc Surg 139(3):775–777
53. Shrestha M, Folliguet T, Meuris B, Dibie A, Bara C, Herregods MC, Khaladj N, Hagl C, Flameng W, Laborde F, Haverich A (2009) Sutureless Perceval S aortic valve replacement: a multicenter, prospective pilot trial. J Heart Valve Dis 18(6):698–702

# Erratum to: The History of Research on Percutaneous, Transapical, and Sutureless Aortic Valve Replacement

35

Thierry Aymard and Thierry Carrel

## Erratum to: The History of Research on Percutaneous, Transapical, and Sutureless Aortic Valve Replacement, DOI: 10.1007/978-88-470-2400-7_34

| Pages | Item or line | Corrections |
|---|---|---|
| 343 | Chapter 34 | Replace old caption of 34.1 with the new caption "**a** The Cribier-Edwards bioprosthesis from Edwards, **b** the Edwards Sapien Transcatheter Heart Valve from Edwards, **c** the CoreValve System bioprosthesis from Medtronic". |
| 346 | Chapter 34 | Replace old caption of 34.2 with the new caption "**a** The Magovern-Cromie sutureless prosthetic aortic valve, **b** the 3f® Enable aortic bioprosthesis model 6000 from ATS (Medtronic), **c** the Perceval S bioprosthesis from Sorin". |

The online version of the original chapters can be found at doi:10.1007/978-88-470-2400-7_34.

T. Aymard (✉) · T. Carrel
Clinic for Cardiovascular Surgery, Inselspital Berne, Berne University Hospital and University of Berne, Freiburgstrasse, 3010 Berne, Switzerland
e-mail: thierry.aymard@insel.ch

M. Picichè (ed.), *Dawn and Evolution of Cardiac Procedures*,
DOI: 10.1007/978-88-470-2400-7_35, © Springer-Verlag Italia 2013

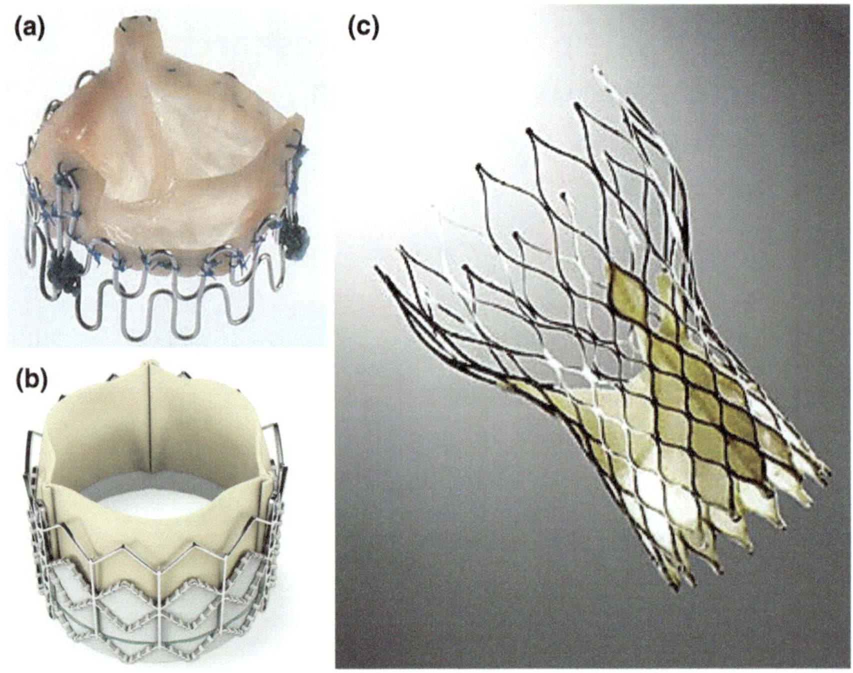


**Fig. 34.1** **a** The Cribier-Edwards bioprosthesis from Edwards, **b** the Edwards Sapien Transcatheter Heart Valve from Edwards, **c** the CoreValve System bioprosthesis from Medtronic

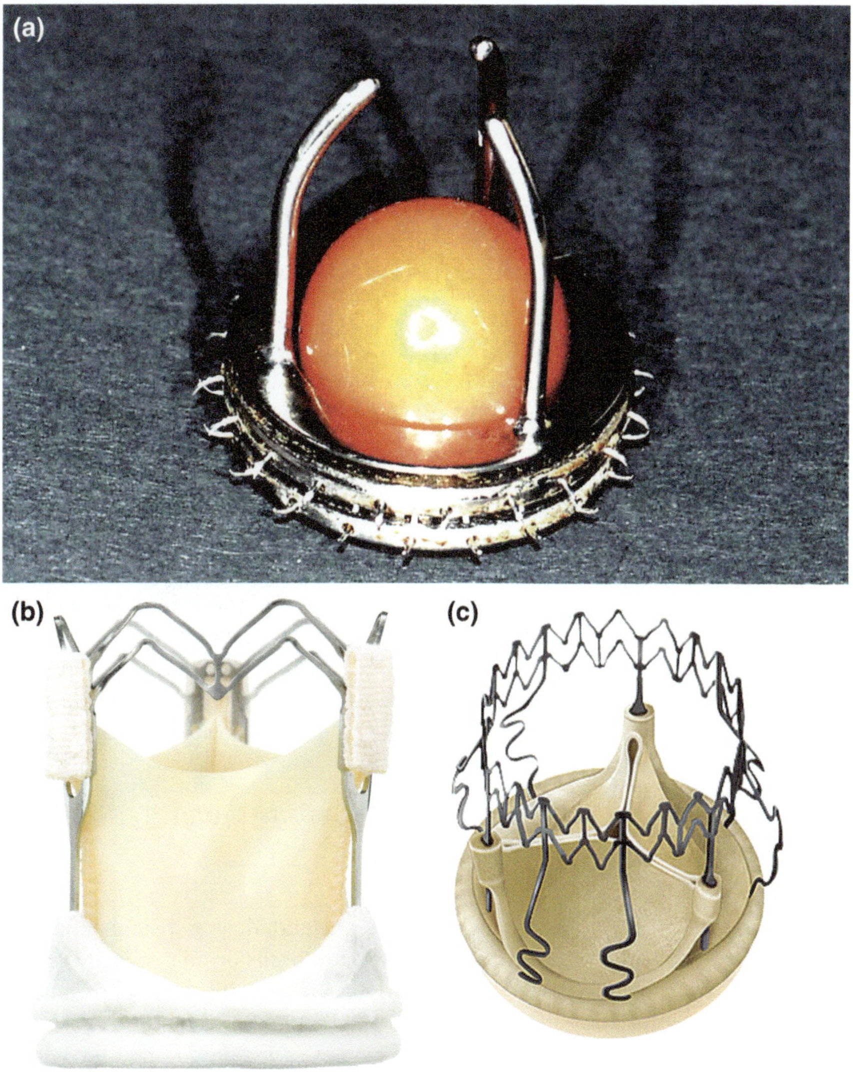

**Fig. 34.2** **a** The Magovern-Cromie sutureless prosthetic aortic valve, **b** the 3f® Enable aortic bioprosthesis model 6000 from ATS (Medtronic), **c** the Perceval S bioprosthesis from Sorin

# Index



M. Picichè (ed.), *Dawn and Evolution of Cardiac Procedures*,
DOI: 10.1007/978-88-470-2400-7, 

Batch number: 10166241

Printed by Printforce, the Netherlands